ORAL DEVELOPMENT AND HISTOLOGY
Second Edition

Editor

James K. Avery, D.D.S., Ph.D.

Professor Emeritus, Dentistry, Anatomy, and Cell Biology
University of Michigan
School of Dentistry and Medical School
Ann Arbor, Michigan

Associate Editor
Pauline F. Steele, B.S., R.D.H., B.S.(Educ.), M.A.
Professor Emeritus and Director of Dental Hygiene
School of Dentistry
University of Michigan
Ann Arbor, Michigan

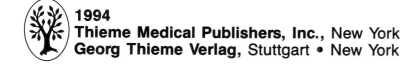
1994
Thieme Medical Publishers, Inc., New York
Georg Thieme Verlag, Stuttgart • New York

Thieme Medical Publishers, Inc.
318 Park Avenue South
New York, New York 10016

Oral Development and Histology, Second Edition
James K. Avery

Library of Congress Cataloging-in-Publication Data

Oral development and histology / editor, James K. Avery. — 2nd ed.
  p.   cm.
  Includes bibliographical references and index.
  ISBN 0-86577-553-2 (Thieme Medical Publishers).—ISBN
3-13-100192-5 (Georg Thieme Verlag)
  1. Mouth—Anatomy. 2. Teeth—Anatomy. 3. Mouth—Histology,
4. Teeth—Histology. 5. Embryology, Human. I. Avery, James K.
  [DNLM: 1. Stomatognathic System. WU 101 063 1994]
RK280.0683 1994
611'.31—dc20
DNLM/DLC   94-30332
for Library of Congress   CIP

Important note: Medicine is an ever-changing science. Research and clinical experience are continually broadening our knowledge, in particular our knowledge of proper treatment and drug therapy. Insofar as this book mentions any dosage or application, readers may rest assured that the authors, editors, and publishers have made every effort to ensure that such references are strictly in accordance with the state of knowledge at the time of production of the book. Nevertheless, every user is requested to carefully examine the manufacturers' leaflets accompanying each drug to check on his own responsibility whether the dosage schedules recommended therein or the contraindications stated by the manufacturers differ from the statements made in the present book. Such examination is particularly important with drugs that are either rarely used or have been newly released on the market.

Some of the product names, patents, and registered designs referred to in this book are in fact registered trademarks or proprietary names even though specific reference to this fact is not always made in the text. Therefore, the appearance of a name without designation as proprietary is not to be construed as a representation by the publisher that it is in the public domain.

Printed in the United States of America.

5 4 3 2 1

TMP ISBN 0-86577-553-2
GTV ISBN 3-13-100192-5

Preface

Dentistry is continually changing as both the basic and clinical sciences modify with advances in knowledge. The dental profession is constantly being updated with progress through research, and therefore attains changing perspectives as new developments and innovations occur. This thereby provides increased knowledge and improved techniques for performing new tasks.

The role of this book is to enhance the student's capability to assimilate needed biological concepts and to increase his or her ability to understand new technologies. This approach is provided in each chapter's discussion. Each chapter also includes the following features: Objectives, Clinical Applications, Summary, and Self-Evaluation Review. Some overlap occurs between chapters, although each one is constructed as a self-contained unit. This deliberate approach gives the instructor the benefit of flexibility in designing an individualized curriculum and augments student learning with a side-by-side format of text and visual aids.

This book is a compilation of discussions on numerous dental subjects contributed by recognized authorities who are knowledgeable about specific areas within the dental curriculum. Their knowledge has been gained through many years of research within their specific subjects. This second edition has had the advantage of revision by being updated and refined, which provides both student and instructor these benefits.

James K. Avery, Editor

Acknowledgments

Oral Development and Histology was initiated as a group effort by the instructors of this course at the University of Michigan School of Dentistry. Initially Dr. Donald Strachan inspired the development of a series of slide tapes as a basis of presenting this course. The tapes soon evolved into a class manual developed with the capable assistance of the staff of the Educational Resources Department. A number of dental students contributed to these manuals, especially in the early editions. We are grateful to Dr. Norman Wilhelmson and Dr. James McNamara, who carried out the studies on tooth movement; Drs. John Gregg and David Johnsen, who contributed to our knowledge of tooth eruption; and Dr. Carla Evans, who researched facial growth. Drs. Jim Jackson, Thomas Simpson, and Arthur Tomaro assisted with studies on the effects of vitamins and hormones, oxytalan fibers, and taste and olfaction, respectively.

The medical illustrations in this book were initially drawn by very capable dental students—Dr. Jeff Clark, who did those in the earlier chapters, and Alayne Spencer Evans, who did the majority of those throughout the book. In this second edition Mrs. Patricia Whittler and Chris Jung contributed other illustrations. There were several excellent dental student photographers who contributed to the first edition: Steve Olsen, Gary Bilik, and Thomas Simmons. Also, Mr. John Virey and Mr. Warren Wheeler provided excellent micrographs for the book. We are also grateful to Drs. Charles Cox and Soo D. Lee for many of the electron micrographs in this text, and Mr. John Baker for the histologic tissue preparation. The authors are grateful to those who typed manuscripts: Mrs. Wadsworth, now deceased, and Mrs. Lewicki, Mrs. Lopatin, and Mrs. Gerlach.

We are deeply indebted to Dr. Sol Bernick, of the University of Southern California, now deceased, who made a number of trips to Ann Arbor to demonstrate his famous thick section celloidin technique. He produced a number of the micrographs in this book. We are also grateful to Dr. Nagat ElNesr of the University of Alexandria, Egypt, who did a sabbatical year with us and contributed to a number of chapters. Dr. Charles F. Cox of our histology department, now at the University of Alabama, was a person we relied on to get various jobs done whether large or small and who made it possible to meet various deadlines. He has inspired numerous dental students and faculty alike and contributed greatly to the first edition. We also thank Dr. Daniel Chiego, Jr., a fellow colleague whose suggestions have immeasurably improved the neuroscience sections in the book.

In this second edition authors were selected because of their expertise in their specialties concerning the structure and function of oral tissues. Each has made a major contribution to this textbook in the preparation of materials aimed at enhancing student understanding of the various subjects. In this edition we are grateful to have the assistance of a very patient and meticulous editor, Professor Pauline Steele, who has made a great effort to improve the presentation of the material and eliminate errors that were missed in the first edition. Finally, I am grateful again to my wife Dody, who has been understanding of my desire to complete this second edition. Thanks to all.

J.K.A.

Contributors

James K. Avery, D.D.S., Ph.D.
Professor Emeritus, Dentistry
School of Dentistry
University of Michigan
Ann Arbor, Michigan

Sol Bernick, Ph.D. (Deceased)
Professor of Anatomy
Department of Anatomy
University of Southern California
Los Angeles, California

Daniel J. Chiego, Jr., M.S., Ph.D.
Associate Professor
Department of Cariology, Restorative Sciences and
  Endodontics, and Biologic and Materials Sciences
School of Dentistry
University of Michigan
Ann Arbor, Michigan

**Marion J. Edge, D.M.D., F.A.C.D., F.I.C.D.,
A.C.O.P., A.O.**
Assistant Professor
Department of Prosthodontics
School of Dentistry
University of Michigan
Ann Arbor, Michigan

Nagat M. ElNesr, B.D.S., Ph.D.
Professor, Department of Oral Biology
Faculty of Dentistry
Alexandria University
Alexandria, Egypt

Carla A. Evans, D.D.S., D.M.Sc.
Associate Professor and Head
Department of Orthodontics
University of Illinois
Chicago, Illinois

David C. Johnsen, D.D.S., M.S.
Professor and Head
Department of Pediatric Dentistry
School of Dentistry
Case Western Reserve University
Cleveland, Ohio

Robert M. Klein, Ph.D.
Professor
Department of Anatomy and Cell Biology
School of Medicine
University of Kansas
Kansas City, Kansas

Robert B. O'Neal, D.M.D., M.S.
Assistant Professor
Department of Periodontics
School of Dentistry
University of Michigan
Ann Arbor, Michigan

Nicholas P. Piesco, Ph.D.
Assistant Professor
Division of Oral Biology
Department of Anatomy/Histology
School of Dental Medicine
University of Pittsburgh
Pittsburgh, Pennsylvania

Francisco Rivera-Hidalgó, B.S., D.M.D., M.S.
Associate Professor of Periodontics
Baylor College of Dentistry
Dallas, Texas

James W. Simmelink, Ph.D.
Director of Research
Associate Professor of Restorative Dentistry
School of Dentistry
Case Western Reserve University
Cleveland, Ohio

Donald S. Strachan, D.D.S., Ph.D.
Professor of Dentistry
School of Dentistry
Associate Professor of Anatomy and Cell Biology
Medical School
University of Michigan
Ann Arbor, Michigan

Dennis F. Turner, D.D.S., M.B.A.
Associate Professor and Assistant Dean
School of Dentistry
University of Michigan
Ann Arbor, Michigan

Contents

SECTION I

Development and Maturation of the Craniofacial Area

SECTION II

Development of the Teeth and Supporting Structures

Structure of the Periodontium and the Temporomandibular Joint

Structure of the Teeth

Structure of the Soft Tissues

SECTION I

Development and Maturation of the Craniofacial Region

CHAPTERS 1–4

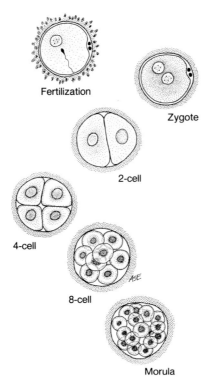

Figure 1–3. Cleavage stages.

- Fertilization
- Zygote
- 2-cell
- 4-cell
- 8-cell
- Morula

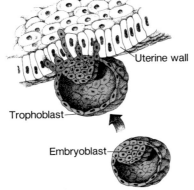

Figure 1–4. Implantation.

- Uterine wall
- Trophoblast
- Embryoblast

uterus, it is a many-celled mass called a "morula" (Fig. 1–3). As the cell mass divides, it enlarges and gains a fluid-filled inner cavity termed the blastocele. The blastocele separates the cells into two parts: an outer cell layer, the trophoblast; and an inner cell mass, the embryoblast. This is called the "blastocyst stage" (Fig. 1–4) and occurs at 4.5 days after conception and shortly before implantation.

On the 6th day, implantation takes place. The trophoblast at the embryonic pole attaches to the sticky endometrial surface on the posterior wall of the body of the uterus (Fig. 1–2). The wall has developed increased vascularity to receive the cell mass. The surface cells of the trophoblast produce enzymes that digest the uterine endometrial cells, which allows a deeper penetration of the cell mass (Fig. 1–4).

Periods of Prenatal Development

Implantation and enlargement of the blastocyst, which contains the embryonic tissues, occur rapidly and are termed the "proliferative period." This period persists for the first 2 weeks. During this time, fertilization, implantation, and formation of the embryonic disc takes place. After the second week, this mass of cells begins to take the form of an embryo, so the period of 2 to 8 weeks is appropriately termed the "embryonic period." During this period, the different types of tissues develop, organizing to form organ systems located in various areas of the embryo. The heart forms and begins to beat. The face and oral structures develop. At 8 weeks, the embryo takes on a more human appearance and passes into the fetal period, which extends until birth (Fig. 1–5). The increase in body weight and size reflects the beginning of various organs and systems.

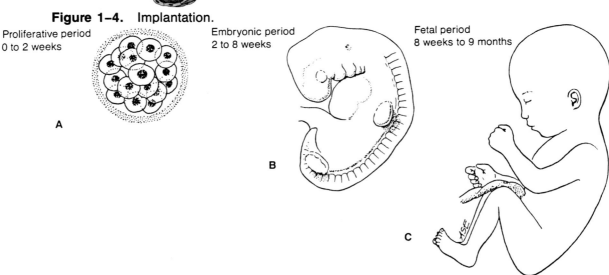

Proliferative period
0 to 2 weeks

Embryonic period
2 to 8 weeks

Fetal period
8 weeks to 9 months

A

B

C

Figure 1–5. The developing human passes through three periods: (A). The proliferative two-week period, when cell division is prevalent. (B). The embryonic period, which extends from the second to the eighth weeks. (C). The fetal period from the eighth week to birth.

In the second week, cells of the inner cell mass of the growing blastocyst differentiate into two cell types (Fig. 1–6): columnar-shaped ectodermal cells and cuboidal-shaped endodermal cells adjacent to the blastocele. The amniotic cavity appears between the ectodermal cells and the overlying trophoblast (Fig. 1–6). Later in the developmental process the amnion expands, filling the entire extraembryonic coelom and eventually extending from the umbilical cord to the inner wall of the placenta, to which it adheres. Thus, in its final form, the amnion is a free membrane enclosing a fluid-filled space around the embryo. Again, cells grow from the trophoblast and the embryonic disc, to form a primitive yolk sac (Fig. 1–7). During the second week, the blastocyst becomes embedded in the endometrium, and fibrin plugs the endometrial implantation site. The placenta will develop from the highly vascularized tissue surrounding the enlarging blastocyst.

On day 15, a groove called the "primitive streak" appears on the surface in the midline of the dorsal aspect of the ectoderm of the embryonic disc. By day 16, a primitive knot of cells (Hensen's node) appears at the cephalic end of the primitive streak. This knot gives rise to the cells that form the notochordal process (Fig. 1–8), which grows cranially in the midline to define the primitive axis of the embryo. Cells from the primitive streak and notochordal process migrate laterally between the ectodermal and endodermal layers of the embryonic shield. These cells form the third germ layer, which is called the "mesodermal layer" (Fig. 1–9). By the end of the third week, the mesoderm migrates in a lateral direction between the ectoderm and the endoderm, except at the anterior prochordal plate and posterior cloacal membrane. The anterior plate forms the future oropharyngeal membrane (Fig. 1–10). Finally, mesodermal cells of the embryonic disc migrate peripherally to join the extraembryonic mesoderm on the amnion and yolk sac. Anteriorly, mesodermal cells pass on either side of the prochordal plate to meet each other in front of this area (Fig. 1–9).

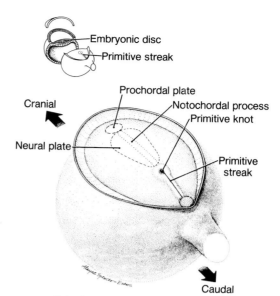

Figure 1–8. Primitive knot and streak on embryonic disc.

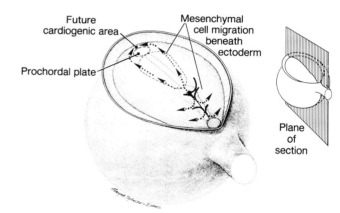

Figure 1–9. Formation of mesoderm.

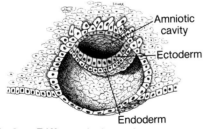

Figure 1–6. Differentiation of ectoderm and endoderm.

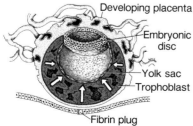

Figure 1–7. Formation of embryonic disc.

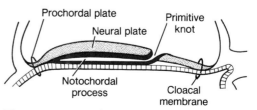

Figure 1–10. Sagittal view of notochord.

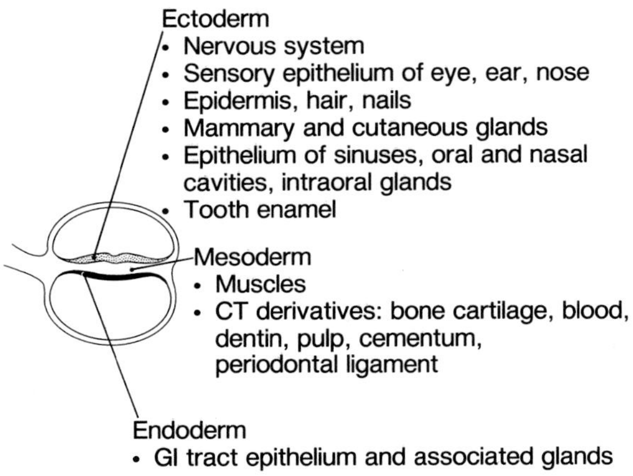

Ectoderm
- Nervous system
- Sensory epithelium of eye, ear, nose
- Epidermis, hair, nails
- Mammary and cutaneous glands
- Epithelium of sinuses, oral and nasal cavities, intraoral glands
- Tooth enamel

Mesoderm
- Muscles
- CT derivatives: bone cartilage, blood, dentin, pulp, cementum, periodontal ligament

Endoderm
- GI tract epithelium and associated glands

Figure 1–11. Derivatives of germ layers.

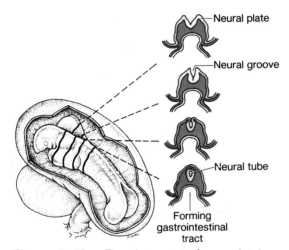

Figure 1–12. Development of neural tube.

Neural plate

Neural groove

Neural tube

Forming gastrointestinal tract

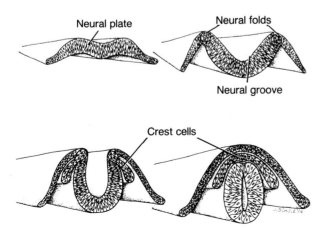

Neural plate

Neural folds

Neural groove

Crest cells

Figure 1–13. Development of neural crest.

Ectodermal cells will give rise to the nervous system, the epidermis and its appendages (hair, nails, and sebaceous and sweat glands), the epithelium lining the oral cavity, nasal cavities and sinuses, a part of the intraoral glands, and the enamel of the teeth. Endodermal cells will form the epithelial lining of the gastrointestinal tract and all associated organs. The mesoderm will give rise to the muscles and all the structures derived from connective tissues—for instance, bone, cartilage, blood, dentin, pulp, cementum, and the periodontal ligament (Fig. 1–11).

The embryonic disc will soon become altered by bends and folds necessary for the further development of the human body.

Development of Nervous System

On day 18, the developing notochord and adjacent mesenchyme affect (induce) the overlying ectoderm to form the neural plate (Figs. 1–12 and 1–13). Induction is the net influence exerted by cells or their products on adjacent cells or tissues. It usually occurs for a limited time during early development and results in a thickening of the ectoderm dorsal to the notochord (Fig. 1–8). The neural plate then bends along its central axis to form a groove, and the raised margins along both sides of this groove form neural folds. The neural folds gradually approach each other in the midline, where they fuse (Fig. 1–12). Fusion of these folds to form the neural tube begins in the central body region and proceeds in cephalic and caudal directions. The folds remain temporarily open at the cranial and caudal ends forming the anterior and posterior neuropores (Fig. 1–12). The neuropores close during the fourth week, and the central nervous system is established. At the time of neural tube closure, a unique population of cells known as the "neural crest cells" separate from the crest of the folds (Fig. 1–13). These cells undergo extensive migration beneath the surface ectoderm, especially in the head and neck region (Fig. 1–14) and give rise to a variety of different cells that form components of many tissues, such as the sensory ganglia, sympathetic neurons, Schwann cells, pigment cells, meninges, and cartilage of the branchial arches. They contribute to the formation of the embryonic connective tissue of the facial region, which includes connective tissue dental

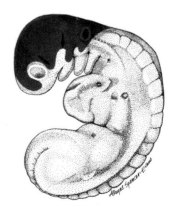

Figure 1–14. Neural crest migration.

structures (dentin, pulp, and cementum). Although the neural crest cells are ectodermal in origin, they exhibit some properties of mesenchyme. As a result, the tissue they form is called "ectomesenchyme." Growth and differentiation of the neural tube are greatest anteriorly. By the fourth week, the fused neural folds have formed three primary brain vesicles: forebrain, midbrain, and hindbrain. Secondary vesicles rapidly develop from these primary vesicles. Figure 1–15 is a diagram of these vesicles and their adult derivatives.

A lateral view of the developing brain and cranial nerves at the third, fourth, fifth, and seventh prenatal weeks is seen in Figure 1–16. The brain enlarges and bends, whereas the cranial nerves develop downward from the floor of the brain and are included in the developing tissues of the face, neck, and lower body.

Development of Gastrointestinal System

The closing neural tube and the developing gastrointestinal tube lie adjacent to each other. In the area between these two developing tubes, the somites form sheets of muscle from the mesoderm (Fig. 1–17).

As the gastrointestinal tract lengthens, a number of structures develop as outpouchings. Craniocaudally, the first structures to appear are the thyroid glands, lungs, liver, pancreas, and urinary bladder (allantois) (Fig. 1–18A). The thyroid

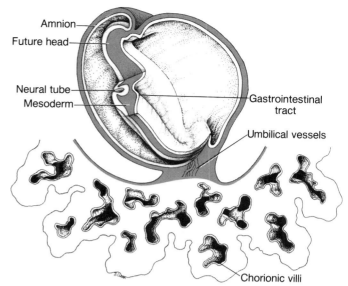
Figure 1–17. Development of GI tract.

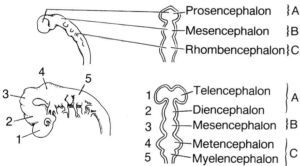
Figure 1–15. Development of brain vesicles.

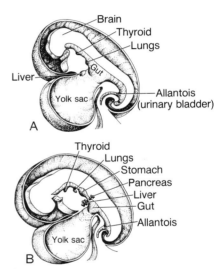
Figure 1–18. Derivatives of GI tract at (A) 4.5 and (B) 5 weeks.

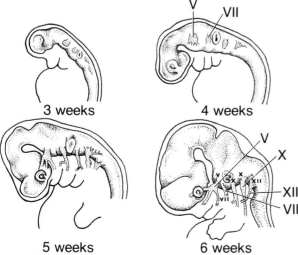
Figure 1–16. Development of cranial nerves.

Clinical Application

Ovulation is a monthly cyclic event controlled by the endocrine secretions of estrogen and progesterone. The ova matures and is expelled from the ovary, and if fertilized, it will implant and be nourished in the uterine wall seven days after fertilization. The "pill" functions to maintain an increased level of progesterone and a decreased level of estrogen that will prevent follicle maturation (of the ovum) or ovulation. Without the ovum pregnancy will not occur.

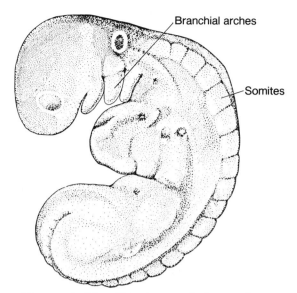

Figure 1–19. Development of muscles.

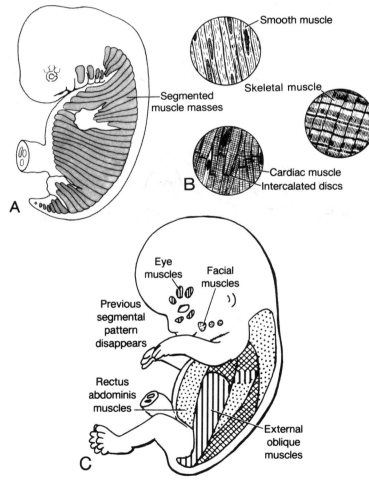

Figure 1–20. (A). Development of skeletal muscle. (B). Muscle types. (C). Differentiation of skeletal muscle.

glands begin to develop in the fourth prenatal week. The bilateral lung buds enlarge and differentiate but do not inflate and function until birth. The stomach develops as a localized enlargement of the anterior gut (Fig. 1–18B). The liver grows rapidly during prenatal life, and by 6 weeks it functions in red blood cell development and in conversion and storage of nutritional elements. The pancreas and its product, insulin, develop early. Insulin secretion, which functions initially as a growth hormone and later in carbohydrate metabolism, begins by 20 weeks. The midgut undergoes rotation and expands into the umbilical cord in the sixth week. By the 10th week, the body has increased sufficiently in size to allow return of the gut to the abdominal cavity. The midgut forms the rest of the duodenum, the entire small intestine, and the ascending and transverse colon of the large intestine. The hindgut forms the descending colon and the terminal parts of the alimentary canal. The urinary bladder develops in conjunction with the genitourinary system.

Development of Muscular System

The muscular system is composed of specialized cells (arising from mesoderm) in which the property of contractility has been highly developed. On the basis of microscopic structure and function, three types of muscles are recognized: (1) skeletal muscle, attached to and responsible for movement of the body framework; (2) smooth muscles, found characteristically in the walls of the hollow viscera, ducts, and blood vessels; and (3) cardiac muscles, found only in the heart.

Skeletal Muscle

At the end of 3 weeks postconception, the body appears to have five to seven paired somites lateral to the neural tube. Somites are segmentations of mesodermal tissue that will form the axial skeleton and muscle masses. By the 35th day, 44 pairs will have formed; 4 will be occipital; 8, cervical; 12, thoracic; 5, lumbar, 5, sacral; and 8 to 10, coccygeal (Fig. 1–19A). The first occipital and five to seven coccygeal somites will later disappear. The somites contribute to the vertebral column, the dermis of the skin, the muscles of the trunk and limbs, and some of the muscles of the orofacial region (Fig. 1–19B). By 10 weeks, muscle cells (myoblasts) have begun migration and specialization into elongated multinucleated muscle fibers (Fig. 1–20A and 1–20B). These fibers divide into groups: epimers, which supply the dorsal surface of the limb; and hypomers, which supply the ventral parts of the limbs. They also split into superficial and deep layers of muscle. In early development, the muscles follow the segmental pattern from the somites, but by the eighth week this pattern disappears (Fig. 1–20C).

Smooth Muscle

At a very early stage of development, wandering mesenchymal cells concentrate around the epithelial linings of such structures as the gut tube, the urogenital ducts, and the large vascular channels. These mesenchymal cells arrange themselves in zones from which involuntary muscles are destined to develop and then lengthen in the direction in which their contractile power will be exerted. These developing smooth muscle (Fig. 1–20B) and cardiac cells (Fig. 1–20B) are both controlled by the autonomic nervous system.

Cardiac Muscle

In the early stages of differentiation, cardiac muscle cells are packed closely together around the developing heart tube and exhibit no definite plan or arrangement (Fig. 1–21). As the developing tissue is pulled into spiral bands about the chamber of the heart, the strands become more regular in arrangement until they appear as groups of fibers running in a generally parallel fashion. The last characteristic feature to appear in the development of cardiac muscle is the intercalated discs (Fig. 1–20B). Electron microscopic studies have shown these transverse markings to be highly modified cell boundaries. Myofibrils on either side of the disc are attached in such a manner that their contractile power can function through the interaction of many cells.

Development of Heart and Blood–Vascular System

The developing embryo is attached to the placenta by a connective tissue stalk that will elongate to become the umbilical cord. Blood vessels have formed in this stalk, which will carry oxygen and nutrition to the embryo (Fig. 1–22). The blood is supplied to the developing embryo by both the vitelline and the umbilical circulatory system. During the first 3 weeks of development, the embryo receives nourishment from the yolk sac through the vitelline system. Yolk sac–derived nutrition is much more prevalent in lower animals than in humans. The umbilical circulation develops rapidly in the third week and conducts oxygenated blood from the uterine placenta to the embryonic heart. At the end of the first month, the embryonic heart begins to beat. Oxygen is then transported from the maternal capillaries of the placenta across a membrane separating the two systems, to the fetal blood cells developed from the embryonic yolk sac. Both systems are seen in Figure 1–22. Nutrition-bearing vitelline vessels from the yolk sac enter the heart, and a single umbilical vein carrying oxygenated blood enters the embryo and then the heart. Observe the vessels (shaded area) that carry the oxygen and nutrients to the body. After this blood circulates throughout the body, the umbilical and vitelline arteries carry the then-deoxygenated blood back to the yolk sac and placenta (Fig. 1–22). At birth, when the lungs replace the placenta in this system, the arteries will conduct the oxygenated blood from the fetal lungs.

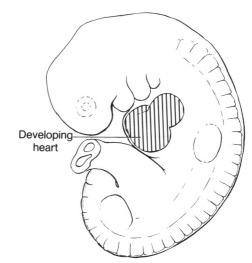

Figure 1–21. Cardiac muscle.

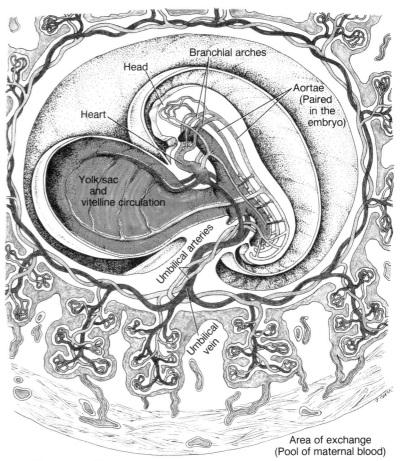

Figure 1–22. Development of blood–vascular system.

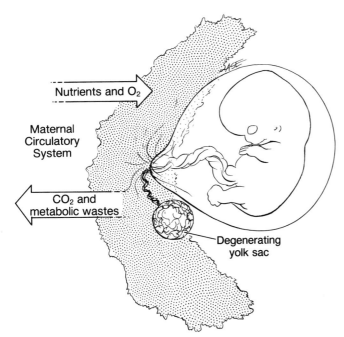

Figure 1–23. Placenta and exchange.

The placenta functions as a nutritional link between mother and fetus (Fig. 1–23). Absorption of nutritional elements and oxygen from the maternal blood occurs in the placenta. Conversely, the elimination of embryonic metabolic wastes such as carbon dioxide is also accomplished in the placenta. Thus, exchange of oxygen and carbon dioxide occurs in the placenta, even though there is no direct flow of blood between mother and fetus. The fetus produces its own blood cells.

Heart

The embryonic heart initially develops from a single vessel created by the fusion of two lateral endothelial heart tubes. In a series of steps (Fig. 1–24) this vessel then enlarges, bends on itself, and differentiates. The septum divides it into right and left chambers. Septa and valves develop that separate the atria from the ventricles. In the embryonic heart, the blood collects in the right atrium, where most of it passes directly to the left atrium via the foramen ovale. It then passes

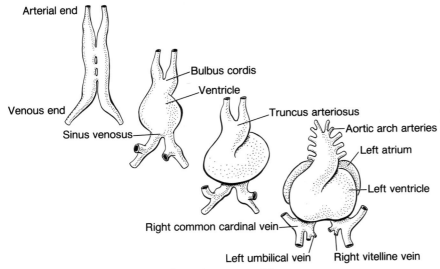

Arterial end

Bulbus cordis

Ventricle

Venous end

Truncus arteriosus

Sinus venosus

Aortic arch arteries

Left atrium

Left ventricle

Right common cardinal vein

Left umbilical vein   Right vitelline vein

Figure 1–24. Development of heart.

Clinical Application

One dramatic change at birth is the transformation from the closed system of the heart to an open one. Before birth this is accomplished by using blood flow from the placenta and conducting it to and through the heart, and then circulating it to the rest of the body. At birth the heart then forces the blood into the lungs, where it is oxygenated. Then, the blood is returned to the heart and pumped to the rest of the body.

to the left ventricle and is carried to the body by the aorta (Fig. 1–25A). Very little blood passes from the right atrium to the right ventricle, where the pulmonary artery carries it to the developing lungs. At this point, blood can also bypass the lung through the ductus arteriosus. The heart is large in the prenatal embryo, as it pumps approximately eight times more blood than does the postnatal heart because of the large placental field. Both oxygenated and nonoxygenated blood are brought to the right atrium. Thus, this mixture is pumped to the rest of the body and then to the placenta by the umbilical arteries.

At birth, several changes occur in this system (Fig. 1–25B). When the infant takes the first breath, the lungs inflate and a small slip of muscle slides over the foramen ovale. This closure forces all of the blood entering the right atrium to pass to the right ventricle and into the pulmonary artery to the lungs. A short time after birth, the ductus arteriosus begins to close, which prevents blood from passing directly from the pulmonary artery to the aorta. From the lungs, the oxygenated blood passes to the left atrium, to the left ventricle, and then to the dorsal aorta. (These changes at birth are vital to assure that a "blue baby" does not develop.) As a result, in the postnatal life all blood is oxygenated before its circulation to the rest of the body.

Skeletal Development

The skeletal and articular systems develop from mesodermal somites, which divide and differentiate into sclerotomes and dermomyotomes. The sclerotomes will form cartilage, bones, and ligaments (Fig. 1–26). Bone develops by two types of connective tissue formation, either intramembranous or endochondral (see Fig. 1–28).

Cartilage

The first skeleton to develop in the embryo is composed of cartilage and has a segmented pattern, as does muscle. Cartilage appears in the embryo's arms, legs, hands, and feet, as well as in the axial skeleton and the base of the skull and face (Fig. 1–27). These cartilages first arise from mesenchyme during the fifth embryonic week and later are gradually transformed into bone by a process termed "endochondral bone development." By the 20th week of prenatal life, bone has replaced much of the early formed cartilage skeleton. Cartilage is then limited to a few locations, such as the nasal septum, alar cartilages, trachea, and external ear, and that covering the ends of long bones.

Bone

Bone may develop as a replacement of cartilage (endochondral) or by transformation of connective tissue independent of cartilage, which is called intramembranous bone. Regardless of the manner in which bones form, however, the resulting bony skeleton will consist of compact or dense bones

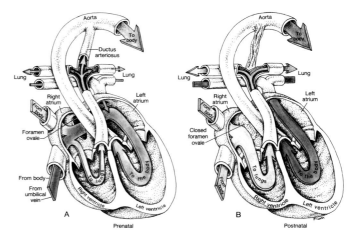

Figure 1–25. (A). Prenatal heart. Both oxygenated and nonoxygenated blood collected in right atrium to right ventricle and mixed blood pumped to the body. (B). Postnatal heart. At birth, foramen ovale (between atria) closes, forcing blood to the right ventricle, then to the lungs, and returns oxygenated to left atria, then to left ventricle and is pumped to the body.

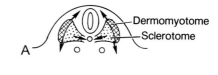

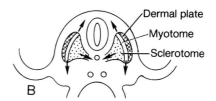

Figure 1–26. Differentiation of bone, cartilage, ligaments, and muscle.

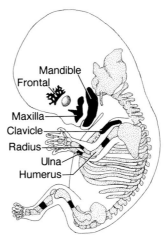

Figure 1–27. Development of cartilage and bone. ■, bone; ▨, cartilage.

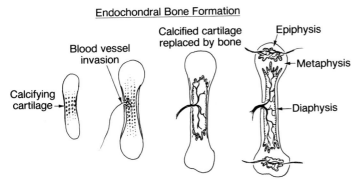

Membranous Bone Formation

Newly formed bone

Osteoblasts

Endochondral Bone Formation

Blood vessel invasion

Calcified cartilage replaced by bone

Epiphysis

Metaphysis

Calcifying cartilage

Diaphysis

Figure 1–28. Types of bone formation.

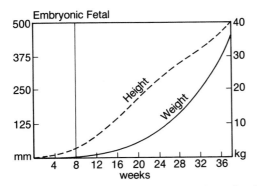

Embryonic Fetal

Height

Weight

Figure 1–29. Increase in weight and length of body.

and cancellous or "spongy" bones. The external portions of bone are usually compact in nature; the internal portions are cancellous (Fig. 1–28). The developing skull consists of both membrane and cartilage components.

Morphologic Change during Prenatal Development

Embryos increase in size by cell multiplication, growth of individual cells, and increase in intercellular substance. From ovum stage to birth, the human increases in length from 140 μm to more than 50 cm, and increase in weight from a few milligrams to more than 3000 g in approximately 266 days (Fig. 1–29). Thus, from fertilization until birth, the embryo increases in size a million times. The embryonic period is one of rapid growth and differentiation of cells, tissues, organs, and organ systems. All major features are established during this time. If the rate of growth during the first 8 weeks were to continue, the human would stand taller than our tallest skyscrapers. Growth may be interstitial–that is, an increase in bulk within a tissue or organ–or appositional–that is, enlargement resulting from surface deposition of tissue. Interstitial growth is characteristic of soft tissues, whereas appositional growth is characteristic of mineralized tissue (bone and hard dental tissues). Differential growth of the various areas is essential to produce the changes in size and shape that cause differences in the size of body parts. After 8 to 10 weeks, the embryo has a relatively human appearance; hence, it is termed a "fetus." The fetal period extends from the eighth prenatal week until birth and is a period of slower growth. The head is proportionately large in early

Clinical Application

All cells have a limited lifetime. The life span of a white blood cell is only a few hours to a few days. On the other hand, red blood cells live approximately 120 days and are then destroyed by macrophages. Surface-covering cells, such as the skin, hair, or nails, renew as they are lost. Cells of the respiratory, urinary, and GI tracts may regenerate throughout life. Other cells in the body do not normally renew after maturity unless they have been injured, such as cells of the liver, kidneys, and thyroid glands; then, they may regenerate to some extent.

development; it represents one-half of the total body at 3 months and reduces to one third of the total body at 5 months and one fourth at birth (Fig. 1–30).

During the first 2 prenatal months the heart develops, blood begins to circulate, the body elongates, and the human face develops (Fig. 1–31). At the end of the third month the upper limbs reach a length relative to the rest of the body. By the end of the fourth month ossification centers have made their appearance in most of the bones, and individual differences become apparent. At the end of the fifth month the fetus is about half the length of the full-term fetus. Its weight is about 500 g, only one sixth of its birth weight. By the end of the sixth month, the face is infantlike, although the skin is wrinkled because of its rapid growth. By the end of the seventh month, however, the fetus has developed subcutaneous fat, eliminating the skin wrinkles. At this time, the eyelids are no longer fused. During this time, body movement patterns become progressively more noticeable. Movement of the lower jaw begins as early as the 10th week, but minor movements are not felt by the mother. Gradually, arm and leg flexing begins as joints mature, and these movements may be quite noticeable. During the eighth and ninth months, hair and fingernails increase in length, and the body becomes plumper. In the last prenatal months, a rapid increase in weight occurs until the fetus reaches 7 lb, the average weight of an infant at birth.

Birth

Parturition or labor begins with muscular contractions when the fetus has attained the proper position deep in the pelvis. The amniotic fluid is squeezed into the thin part of the chorion that overlies the uterine cervix. This acts as the preliminary dilator of the cervical canal. As contractions become more powerful and frequent, the investing membranes of this region rupture, and the infant is freed from the fetal envelope; amniotic fluid starts to flow from the mother, which lubricates the birth canal (Fig. 1–32). Because the process of birth usually lasts several hours, it is important that the placenta remain attached to the uterus. If the fetus were prematurely cut off from its maternal associations, it could not survive the prolonged interruption of its oxygen supply.

Continued contractions of smooth muscle in the uterus, aided by contractions of abdominal skeletal muscles, literally squeeze the fetus into the slowly dilating cervical canal. When dilation is sufficient, the fetus is pushed out of the uterus. This is the first phase of labor. The second phase of labor is much briefer than the first. The fetus, after passing through the cervical canal, moves promptly through the vagina and "presents" itself. The vulval orifice dilates rapidly, and when the head passes this outlet, the rest of the body emerges quickly. With delivery and the tying and cutting of the umbilical cord, maternal connections are ended, and for the first time, the newborn subsists independently of another individual.

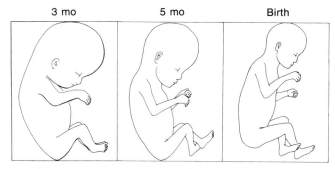

Figure 1–30. Changes in body proportion.

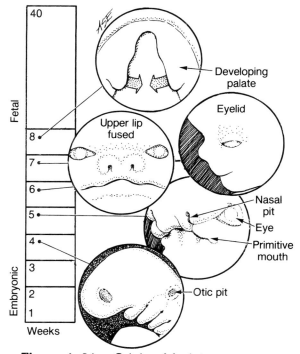

Figure 1–31. Origin of facial process.

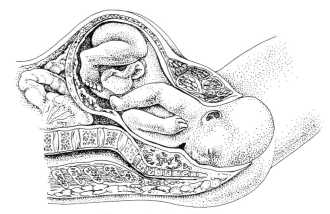

Figure 1–32. Birth.

Approximately 15 to 20 min after the fetus is delivered, the uterus begins another series of contractions, which serve to loosen and expel the placenta and amniotic remnant. This entire mass is referred to as the "afterbirth." This abrupt shedding of tissue from the uterus involves some hemorrhage, but the continued contractions minimize blood loss by compressing the ruptured vessels, which thereby facilitates coagulation. Following parturition, there is a period of repair of the uterine lining that is similar to the one that occurs after menstruation.

The process of birth usually occurs about 9 to 9.5 months after conception. A complete environmental transformation takes place at that time. The infant is catapulted from a dark, quiet environment, in which it has been submerged in fluid at a body temperature of 98 °F, into a lighted, noisy environment, 20 °F colder, in which it must support itself by breathing air through its own lungs and live independently. Thus, at birth the infant must survive a number of physiological changes, such as the inspiration of air and major changes in the circulatory pattern, which can be observed in Fig. 1–25A and B).

Abnormal Development

The causes of congenital malformations may be hereditary and/or environmental (genetic and epigenetic). The majority of congenital defects are the result of interaction between hereditary and environmental factors occurring at a specific time of development.

Beyond prenatal examinations and parental counseling, not much can be done to reduce hereditary hazards in humans. Recent experiments are being directed toward altering the effects of abnormal genetic endowment through changes in the environment, such as the administration of supplementary vitamins.

Our increased knowledge of noxious environmental agents (teratogens) and of the time of their maximal effects on fetal development is of great importance in the understanding and prevention of such malformations. The developing human is least susceptible to teratogens during the proliferation period (first 2 or 3 weeks). At that time, any injury may be compensated for by the remaining cells that have not yet become committed or differentiated. The embryonic period (end of the second or third week to the end of the eighth week) is the most critical time period because it is the period of differentiation of organs and systems. At this time, teratogenic agents may be highly effective and result in numerous malformations. During the fetal period (end of the eighth week until birth), susceptibility to teratogens rapidly declines and may cause only minor defects (Fig. 1–33).

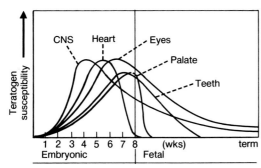

Figure 1–33. Decrease in susceptibility to teratogens with prenatal age.

Hereditary Causes of Congenital Malformations

Hereditary causes of congenital malformations can be attributed to either chromosomal or genetic abnormalities.

Chromosomal Abnormalities

Many congenital defects are now known to be the result of an abnormal number of chromosomes. The abnormality in number is expressed as either a decrease or an increase in the normal number of chromosomes (46 in humans). A decrease in one chromosome, monosomy (45 chromosomes), is usually lethal. An increase in one or more chromosomes is teratogenic and results in congenital malformations. The extra chromosome may be an autosome or a sex chromosome. If an extra chromosome member is present, a condition known as trisomy develops. The best-known example is trisomy 21 or Down's syndrome, also called "mongolism" (Fig. 1–34 and 1–35). In this condition, three members of chromosome 21 are present in the somatic cells of the affected individual, which results in the cells containing 47 chromosomes each. The malformation is characterized by mental retardation, upward slanting palpebral fissures, a flat nasal bridge, and a fissured protruding tongue (macroglossia).

Genetic Abnormalities

Genes are segments of the DNA chain for stored information that can perpetuate from one generation to another. Abnormal development may be the result of expression of defective genes, which may be dominant or recessive. A dominant gene expresses itself whether it is present on one member of the pair of homologous chromosomes (heterozygous) or on both members (homozygous). A recessive gene expresses itself only when it is present on both members of the homologous pair of chromosomes (Fig. 1–36). The following abnormalities are examples of autosomal dominant genes: acrocephalosyndactyly (see Fig. 1–37), achondroplasia,

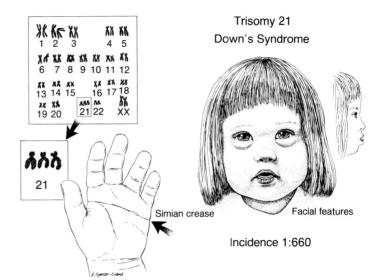

Figure 1–35. Chromosome abnormalities.

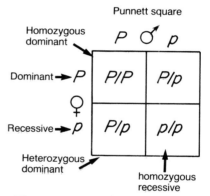

Figure 1–36. Gene expression.

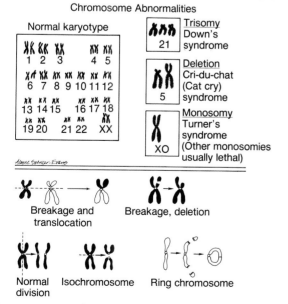

Figure 1–34. Comparison of three types of chromosome abnormalities.

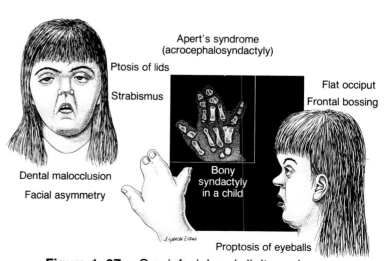

Figure 1–37. Craniofacial and digit syndrome.

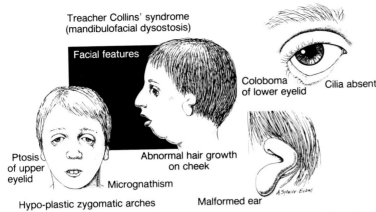

Figure 1-38. Lack of neural crest cell migration resulting in multiple facial abnormalities.

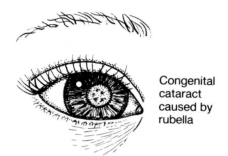

Figure 1-39. Congenital cataract caused by rubella.

Clinical Application

The period from 3 to 8 weeks is one of greatest sensitivity to the action of teratogens. After 8 weeks there is a decreasing sensitivity to the effects of environmental factors. The tissues are no longer undergoing as many differentiative factors as in the early weeks. The risk of malformation is thus greatest during embryogenesis.

cleidocranial dysostosis, mandibulofacial dysostosis, and dentinogenesis imperfecta. Achondroplasia is a condition of defective development of bones ossified in cartilage (particularly the long bones). On the other hand, cleidocranial dysostosis is a condition of defective development of bone ossified in membrane (cranial vault, face, and clavicle). Some of the defects, therefore, are facial and dental malformations. Mandibulofacial dysostosis, also called Treacher Collins' syndrome, results from a defective gene that seems to cause disturbance in the migration and distribution of the neural crest cells. This is expressed as an underdeveloped face (Fig. 1-38). Dentinogenesis imperfecta, a hereditary condition, results in defective dentin formation.

Environmental Causes of Congenital Malformations

Environmental causes of congenital malformations may be classified as infectious agents; radiation; drugs; hormones; nutritional disorders; and teratogenic habits, such as smoking and the imbibition of alcohol- or caffeine-containing products.

Infectious Agents

Viral infections mainly affecting the mother during early pregnancy can cause congenital malformations in the offspring. A well-known example is rubella virus, which causes German measles. When a pregnant woman is infected with rubella, many developmental defects in the child, including cleft palate, malformed teeth, central nervous system anomalies, and congenital cataracts, may result (Fig. 1-39).

Radiation

The direct teratogenic effects of X-ray on the embryo results in specific congenital malformations including cleft palate. The indirect effect of irradiation causes gene mutation (alteration) in the germ cells. This leads to the occurrence of congenital malformations in succeeding generations. To alleviate the dangerous effect of radiation, all personnel dealing with X-ray should use the proper protective measures for both themselves and their patients. They should also protect all women of reproductive age as though these women were pregnant.

Drugs

Although few specific drugs used during pregnancy have been implicated as teratogens, drugs should be avoided during early pregnancy. Remember the tragic effect of thalidomide, a drug once considered to be a safe hypnotic and antinauseant. It caused partial or total absence of the limbs (Fig. 1–40). Aminopterin is another dangerous drug used to induce abortion during pregnancy. It can cause congenital malformations, including cleft lip and palate, when it fails to terminate pregnancy. Tetracycline taken during the second and third trimesters of pregnancy causes permanent brownish discoloration and hypoplasia of the enamel of the deciduous teeth. The permanent teeth will not be affected. So far, little is known about the teratogenicity of interacting drugs.

Hormones

The action of hormones as teratogens is not definitely known in humans. Cortisone, however, has been shown to cause cleft lip and plate in some experimental animals.

Nutritional Disorders

Nutritional disorders have been reported in the case histories of humans. These reports are few, and most relate to the effects of nutritional disorders on developing teeth. Vitamin deficiencies and hypervitaminosis A, C, and D have been reported as teratogenic in animals. Hypervitaminosis A is also implicated in some forms of malformations in humans.

Teratogenic Habits (Smoking, Alcohol, and Caffeine)

Infants of heavy-smoking mothers were shown to have a higher incidence of cleft lip and palate. Alcohol abuse during pregnancy may also produce congenital defects such as mental retardation, growth deficiency, and maxillary hypoplasia. Even excessive caffeine consumption has recently been implicated in some developmental defects.

In general, to reduce teratogenic hazards, all women of reproductive age should avoid drugs and all questionable habits at the time of the first missed menstrual period and for at least 12 weeks thereafter. This will protect the developing human embyro during the time when it is most susceptible to teratogens.

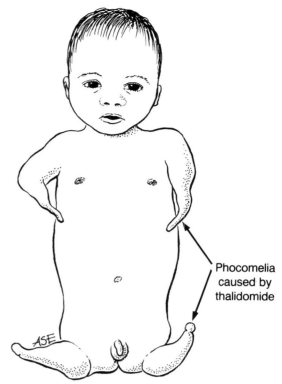

Phocomelia caused by thalidomide

Figure 1–40. Effects of thalidomide.

Summary

The contact of sperm with the egg results in fertilization and production of the fertilized egg or zygote, which rapidly divides as it moves toward the uterus to undergo implantation. As the resulting trophoblast enlarges an embryoblast develops within it. This disk is at first composed of two germ layers, the ectoderm derived from the amnion and the endoderm from the yolk sac. As this disk flattens a third layer, the mesoderm, develops. A longitudinal axis appears as the notochord develops, and a neural tube appears adjacent and above it. This tube soon enlarges to form the bilateral cerebral and cerebellar hemispheres. The gastrointestinal (GI) tract elongates and forms an enlargement for the stomach, specialization for the large and small intestines, and outpouchings for the developing lungs, pancreas, gall bladder, and urinary bladder. Meanwhile, masses appear segmented along the neural tube, termed "somites," which form the muscles and supporting skeletal tissue of the limbs and body wall. By the end of the embryonic period at 8 weeks, all major organ systems, such as the vascular, lymphatic, urinary, digestive, and reproductive, have differentiated into specific structures, and external features are apparent. As the fetal period begins at 9 weeks and extends until birth, there is a general increase in body size and specialization takes place. At birth, there are a number of very rapid changes, such as a shift from the placental intake of oxygen to air breathing as the lungs inflate, and the changes from life at body temperature to room temperature and from life of immersion in a fluid environment. The embryonic period is especially vulnerable to environmental stresses, with an increase in resistance as the fetal period advances.

Self-Evaluation Review

1. Describe how an embryoblast is formed.
2. Define the terms ovulation, fertilization, and implantation.
3. What do somites contribute to embryo development?
4. Describe the two vascular systems of the embryo and the contribution of each.
5. From what does the gastrointestinal tract develop and what organs arise from this tract?
6. What are the three types of muscle and their similarities and differences?
7. Describe the prenatal and postnatal heart and the important changes that the heart undergoes at birth.
8. What are the derivatives of the three germ layers and the neural crest cells?
9. Bone develops by what two methods?
10. What changes in environment does the human experience at the time of birth?

Acknowledgments

Dr. Alphonse R. Burdi provided Figures 1–35, 1–37, and 1–38.

Suggested Readings

Avery JK. Development and structure of cells and tissues. In: Steck PF, ed. *Essentials of Oral Histology and Development*. St. Louis, Mo: Mosby Year Book Inc.; 1992:1–16.

England M. *Color Atlas of Life before Birth*. Chicago, Ill.: Year Book Medical Publishers; 1983.

Moore KL. *Essentials of Human Embryology*. Toronto: BC Decker Inc.; 1988.

Moore KL. *The Developing Human*. 2nd ed. Philadelphia, Pa: WB Saunders; 1977.

Nishimura H., Okamoto N. *Sequential Atlas of Human Congenital Malformations*. Baltimore, Md: University Park Press; 1976.

Poswillo D. The pathogenesis of the first and second branchial arch syndrome. *Oral Surg*. 1973;35:302–328.

Sadler T, ed. *Langmans Medical Embryology*. 5th ed. Baltimore, Md: Williams and Wilkins; 1985.

Sperber GH. *Craniofacial Embryology*. 4th ed. London: Butterworth; 1989.

Tortora GJ. *Principals of Human Anatomy*. 5th ed. New York, NY: Harper and Row, 1989.

2

Development of the Branchial Arches, Face, and Palate

James K. Avery

Introduction

Initiation of the oral cavity occurs in the late third prenatal week as a pit or invagination of the tissues underlying the forebrain. This pit will develop into the future oral cavity, and the tissues surrounding it will form the face. The branchial arches appear as bars of tissue extending horizontally on both sides of the oral pit located on the sides of the neck. As the branchial arches contribute to the face externally, they form the tissues surrounding the oropharynx internally. The initial facial tissues develop as swellings from the first branchial arch forming the future lower jaw, cheeks, and tissues overlying the forebrain region, above which forms the forehead. These swellings appear initially as tissue enlargements delineated by grooves. The union of these tissue masses occurs by merging (or filling in by growth of tissues between these masses). Also, contact between separate masses occurs by the process of fusion (and then elimination of any intervening epithelium [Fig. 2–1]). There are four primary facial masses: frontal mass above the oral pit, two maxillary masses lateral to this pit, and the mandibular mass or first branchial arch beneath it. Another process important to facial development is the appearance and growth of facial placodes. These thickenings of the surface ectoderm, which initially appear, give rise to such adult structures as the lens of the eyes; the auditory, or organs of hearing; and the nasal placodes, or organ of smell. Many other placodes later appear throughout the oropharynx to form the pituitary in the roof of the oral pit, the tooth organs, the salivary glands in the oral cavity, the thyroid and parathyroids, and the thymus in the oropharynx. Our focus is on the 2nd month of prenatal life, involving tissues of the oral cavity and the tissues surrounding it.

Objectives

After reading this chapter, you should be able to describe the formative process of the primitive oral cavity, appearance of the branchial arches (and the overgrowth of the tissue that then eliminates their appearance), and development and

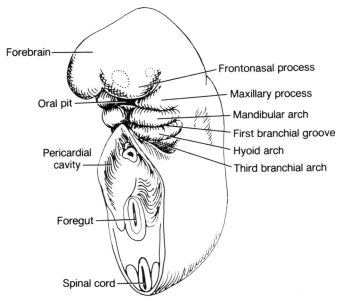

Forebrain

Frontonasal process

Maxillary process

Oral pit

Mandibular arch

First branchial groove

Hyoid arch

Pericardial cavity

Third branchial arch

Foregut

Spinal cord

Figure 2–1. Development of face, 4 weeks.

function of the pharyngeal pouches. You should also be able to describe the normal development of the face, the formation of the palate, and the process of its elevation. You should also be able to discuss how the process of branchial clefts, thyroglossal ducts, cysts, and malformations of the face and palate occur.

Development of Primitive Oral Cavity (Oronasal Cavity)

The primitive oral pit, or stomodeum, is an invagination of surface epithelium lying between the cranial forebrain and the adjacent ventrally developing heart (Fig. 2–1). This invagination appears as a result of the forebrain's anterior growth and enlargement of the developing heart. The oral cavity becomes positioned under the forebrain (Figs. 2–2, 2–3, and 2–4).

During the 3rd prenatal week, at the deep end of the stomodeum, the oral ectoderm is in close contact with the foregut endoderm (Fig. 2–1). This is termed the "oropharyngeal membrane," as it separates the stomodeum from the foregut or pharynx. The oropharyngeal membrane disintegrates to establish continuity between the two cavities (see Figs. 2–5 and 2–6) in the fourth week.

As the oral cavity enlarges, two important endocrine glands develop. From the oral cavity roof, an ectodermal lined pouch, Rathke's pouch, grows dorsally into the floor of the brain and gives rise to the middle and posterior lobes of the anterior pituitary. In the floor of the oral cavity a second epithelial pouch develops and grows downward into the anterior neck, giving rise to the thyroid gland. This gland will later exert control over body metabolism. Both of these important endocrine glands develop from oral tissue.

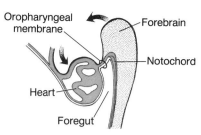

Figure 2–2. Anterior growth of brain vesicles, 2.5 weeks.

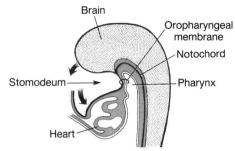

Figure 2–3. Further growth of the brain anteriorly, 3 weeks.

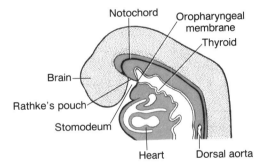

Figure 2–4. Development of stomodeum, 3.5 weeks.

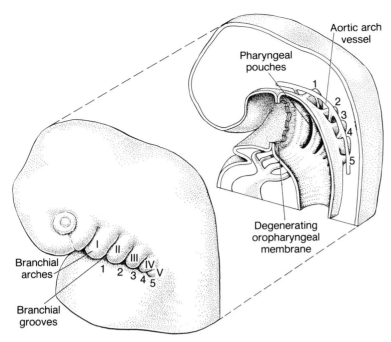

Figure 2–5. Sagittal view of branchial region at 4 weeks. Observe the blood vessels that arise from the heart below and pass through each branchial arch.

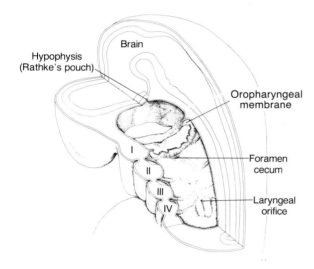

Figure 2–6. Posterior lateral view of pharyngeal-oral cavity loss of oropharyngeal membrane.

Branchial Arches

The tissues bordering the oral pit inferiorly and laterally develop into five or six pairs of bars that form the lower parts of the face and neck. These bars are termed "branchial arches."

The first four branchial arches (numbered I to IV craniocaudally) are well developed in humans. Only the first and second arches extend to the midline, and each arch is progressively smaller (from the first to the last). The mandibular branchial arch is the first branchial arch to develop (Figs. 2–5 and 2–6). The hyoid is the second arch to develop (Fig. 2–7).

The third, fourth, and fifth arches also consist of paired bars of epithelial-covered mesoderm, which are divided in the midline by the developing heart (Fig. 2–4). Each arch is positioned horizontally in the neck and is separated from adjacent ones by shallow branchial grooves externally and by deep pharyngeal pouches internally (Figs. 2–5 and 2–6). The outer surface of the branchial arches and grooves is covered by ectoderm; the inner (pharyngeal) surface is lined by endoderm, except for the first, and possibly the second, arch.

Within branchial arches are neural crest cells beneath the epithelium that surround a core of mesodermal cells in each arch. In each arch, there will be a gradual differentiation of muscles, nerves, cartilages, and blood vessels.

Figures 2–5 and 2–6 are illustrations of the external and pharyngeal views of the branchial arch system. The branchial arches are denoted by Roman numerals I to V; the branchial grooves and the corresponding pharyngeal pouches are designated by Arabic numerals 1 to 5.

The first branchial groove deepens to form the external auditory meatus, or ear canal. The ectodermal membrane in the depth of the groove persists and, together with mesoderm and endoderm from the adjacent first pharyngeal pouch, forms the tympanic membrane (Fig. 2–6). The external

Clinical Application

The lack of normal growth changes in the branchial arches may cause defects to appear in the lateral aspects of the neck. These defects may develop into cysts, causing swellings or fistulas that drain mucous secretions.

features of the second, third, and fourth branchial grooves become obliterated by the caudal overgrowth of the second branchial arch; this overgrowth then provides the smooth contour of the neck (Figs. 2–7 and 2–8).

Endodermal epithelium covering the pharyngeal pouches differentiates into a variety of important organs. From the first pouch, the middle ear and the eustachian tube develop. Palatine tonsils originate from the second pouch. The inferior parathyroid gland and thymus arise from the third pouch. From the fourth pouch, the superior parathyroid gland develops; and the fifth pouch forms the ultimobranchial body (Figs. 2–8B and 2–9).

The thymus gland is relatively large at birth and continues to grow only until puberty. Thereafter, it gradually atrophies and completely disappears later in life. The ultimobranchial body fuses with the thyroid and contributes parafollicular cells to this gland. The parathyroid glands function throughout life in calcium regulation; the tonsils function in lymphocyte development and immunologic factors.

Thyroid Gland

In the fourth week, the thyroid gland appears as a depression and epithelial thickening in the floor of the pharynx (Fig. 2–7). This appears at a point between the body and the base of the tongue. This point becomes an invagination (blind duct) termed the "foramen cecum," from which the thyroid primordium develops and descends in the neck as a bilobed diverticulum, to reach its final destination in front of the trachea in the seventh week (Fig. 2–9). During this migration, the gland remains connected to the floor of the oral cavity by an epithelial cord or duct, the thyroglossal duct, which later becomes a solid core of cells. The foramen cecum, which is a concavity, remains at its site of origin. The thyroid gland begins to function at the end of the third month, when colloid-containing follicles appear.

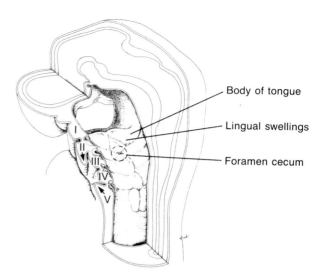

Figure 2–7.   Branchial arches I to V.

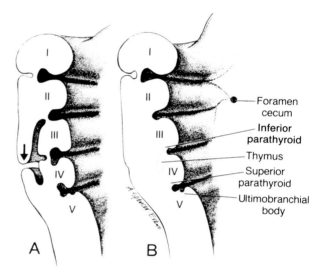

Figure 2–8.   (A). Overgrowth of the second branchial arch to the fifth arch on the external surface. (B). Development of the pharyngeal pouches and their derivatives in the pharynx.

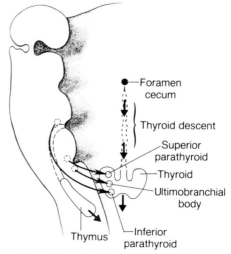

Figure 2–9.   Site of endocrine glands in pharyngeal pouches in oropharynx.

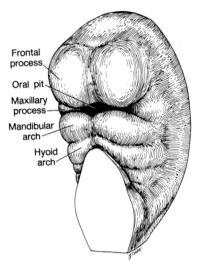

Figure 2–10. Development of face, 4 weeks.

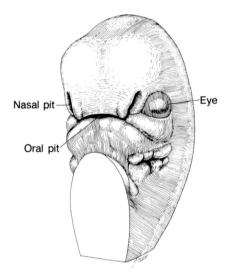

Figure 2–11. Development of face, 5 weeks.

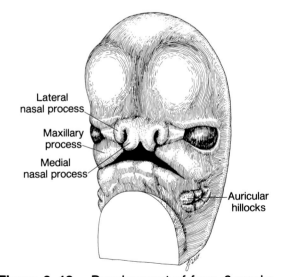

Figure 2–12. Development of face, 6 weeks.

Facial Development

The face develops during the fifth to seventh week of intrauterine life from four primordia that surround a central depression, the primitive oral pit. These primordia are the frontal process, which is a single cranially located process; the two bilaterally located maxillary processes; and the mandibular process, with each of the latter derived from the first branchial arch (Fig. 2–10). The mandibular process appears initially as a partially divided bilateral structure, but soon merges at the median line and eliminates the groove. This process or arch will give rise to the mandible, the lower part of the face, and the body of the tongue. The mandibular branchial arch is not interrupted in the midline by the heart (Fig. 2–11).

By the late fourth week, nasal placodes develop bilaterally on the lower part of the then-termed "frontonasal process" bordering the oral cavity. Around the nasal placodes, mesenchyme proliferates and produces medial and lateral nasal prominances that enlarge and transform the placodes into nasal pits (nostrils) (Fig. 2–11). Thus, 1 week later, the medial and lateral nasal processes appear as horseshoe-shaped elevations with the open end in contact with the oral cavity (Fig. 2–11). The medial nasal process is that tissue medial to the pit. The lateral nasal process is in close contact with the maxillary process (Fig. 2–12). The point of contact of the epithelia-covered medial nasal and maxillary processes is the fusion point of the upper lip. It is termed the "nasal fin" (Fig. 2–13), and is a vertically positioned epithelia sheet under each nostril that separates the medial nasal and maxillary processes. When the fin disappears, the lip will fuse.

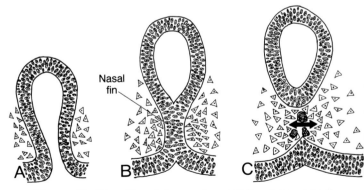

Figure 2–13. Breakdown of nasal fin. Arrows indicate zone of cell intermingling.

During the sixth week, the two medial nasal processes merge in the midline to form the intermaxillary segment (Fig. 2–12). This will give form to the center of the upper lip, which includes the primary palate, which in turn includes the alveolar process carrying the incisor teeth. In the adult face, the center of the upper lip forms the philtrum, which is defined laterally by two vertical ridges under the nostrils. At the lateral boundary of this intermaxillary segment, there initially is a fissure that separates it from the growing maxillary processes that will form the lateral aspects of the upper lip (Fig. 2–12). This fissure is in the floor of the nostril and can result in a cleft lip if the epithelium (Figs. 2–13 and 2–14) covering the adjacent processes does not contact, fuse, and then disintegrate. This allows the tissues of the lip to intermingle. By this development, the upper lip is thus formed from one-third medial nasal and two-thirds maxillary processes. These events occur during the sixth week of intrauterine life. The floor of the nostril at its most posterior deep point then opens into the roof of the oral cavity (Fig. 2–14). The maxillary processes form part of the cheeks vertically (Fig. 2–12) and part of the lateral palatine processes of the secondary palate medially (see Fig. 2–18). The size of the mouth will be determined by the merging of the maxillary and mandibular processes as they close the lateral corners of the mouth (Fig. 2–15).

The eyes develop during the fifth week. The first external sign of eye development is the appearance of the lens placodes positioned between the maxillary and the frontonasal processes at the lateral sides of the face (Fig. 2–11). Growth of the lateral forebrain causes lateral expansion of the face. The broadening of the face in the sixth week also causes the eyes to be positioned more anteriorly on the front of the face, and causes the nasal pits to appear more central in the face (Fig. 2–12). The distance between the nasal pits does not decrease, although it appears to do so when Figures 2–11 and 2–12 are compared. Instead, the width of the face increases by lateral growth during the sixth prenatal week (Fig. 2–15).

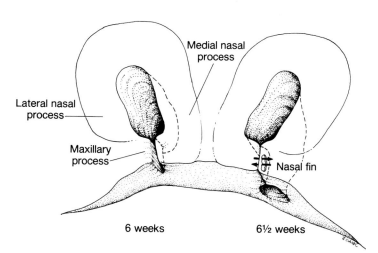

Figure 2–14. Formation of nostril and primary palate. Arrows indicate zone of penetration.

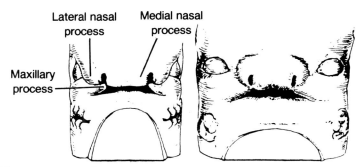

Figure 2–15. Development of face, sixth and seventh weeks.

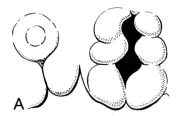

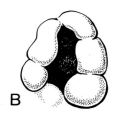

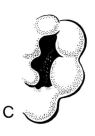

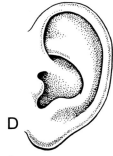

Figure 2–16. Development of ear.

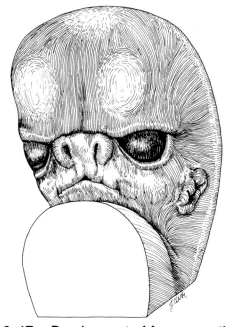

Figure 2–17. Development of face, seventh week.

Ear Development

During the sixth week, the external ear (auricle) develops from six mesenchymal swellings, or hillocks. Three are from the first branchial arch and three are from the second branchial or hyoid arch (Fig. 2–15). These hillocks appear in the upper part of the neck that surrounded the first branchial cleft, which will develop into the external auditory canal. The hillocks will then grow and merge to become the external ear (Fig. 2–16). As the face grows forward and downward, the ears will maintain their position on the lateral face (Fig. 2–17).

Development of Facial Features

The continued development of facial features is the result of differential growth brought about by the increase in breadth of the medial and lateral nasal processes and by the increased growth of the maxillary processes. By the seventh week, the face has acquired a more human appearance (Fig. 2–17). At this time, the medial part of the face increases in an anterior direction, and as vertical height increases, the bridge of the nose will develop, so that the nostrils and eyes will not be on the same plane. The nose is not yet fully developed in the newborn infant and does not acquire its inherited size and shape until puberty. The eyes have moved from the lateral aspects to the front of the head into a position on either side of the nose. In normal development, the distance separating the eyes greatly influences the appearance of the face. A narrow interocular distance (hypotelorism) confers a sharp, foxlike appearance. An increased interocular distance (hypertelorism) causes the face to appear broad. The orbital cavities attain their adult dimensions when the child is about 7 years of age.

During early development, the mandible is at first small in comparison with the upper part of the face. It then grows at a more rapid pace. Later, in utero, however, the mandibular growth again lags behind the growth of the maxilla. The fetus displays a physiologic micrognathia (small mandible), which usually appears at or soon after birth. In the early embryonic period the mouth orifice is very wide, but as the maxillary and mandibular processes merge to form the cheeks, the width of the mouth opening is reduced.

In approximately 2 weeks, from the fifth to the seventh week, the face has emerged from the five unassociated-appearing masses (the frontonasal, paired maxillary, and mandibular processes) and, to a lesser extent, the hyoid arches, to form a human-appearing face.

Clinical Application

Branchial arch syndromes are frequently seen clinically as a group of defects. They occur about the face and neck as cleft lips, malformed ears or eyes, small mandibles or mouths, large tongues, and cleft palates.

Palate Development

The term "palate" refers to the issue that interposes between the oral and nasal cavities. The palate develops from three parts (Fig. 2–18): one medial and two lateral palatine processes. The medial palatine process is also called the "primary palate" because it appears before the secondary palate at the beginning of the sixth week. The primary palate develops as an intermaxillary segment (wedged-shaped mass), as did the lip, between the maxillary processes of the developing upper jaw (Fig. 2–18B). The premaxillary bones, which support the four maxillary incisor teeth, develop in the primary palate.

At the end of the sixth week, the lateral palatine processes that form the secondary palate develop from the medial edges of the maxillary processes that bound the stomodeum. The lateral palatine processes (shelves) first grow medially (Fig. 2–19), then grow downward or vertically on either side of the tongue (Fig. 2–20). At this stage of development, the tongue is narrow and tall, almost completely filling the oronasal cavity, and reaches the nasal septum.

Tongue Development

Because the tongue is believed to take part in palatal closure, it is appropriate to discuss its development at this time. The tongue is composed of the body, the anterior movable oral part, and the posterior firmly attached base or pharyngeal part. The tongue develops from the tissues of the first, second, and third branchial arches, as well as anterior migration of muscles from the occipital myotomes (Fig. 2–21). The body of the tongue develops from three centrally placed elevations on the ventromedial aspects of the first branchial arches: the tuberculum impar (unpaired tubercle) and two adjacent elevations, the lateral lingual swellings (Fig. 2–21). These lateral lingual swellings rapidly enlarge, merge with each other, and overgrow the tuberculum impar to form the oral part of the tongue. A U-shaped sulcus develops in front and on both sides of this oral part, which allows it to be free and highly mobile except at the region of the frenulum linguae, where it remains attached to the floor of the mouth. In this way, the body of the tongue becomes established.

The base of the tongue develops mainly from the third branchial arches (Fig. 2–21). Initially, it is indicated by a midline elevation that appears caudal to the tuberculum impar, which is the large hypobranchial eminence of the third

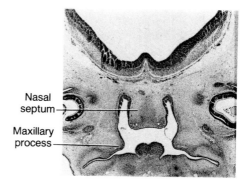

Figure 2–19. Palate at 6 weeks, prenatally.

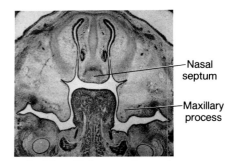

Figure 2–20. Palate at 7 weeks, prenatally.

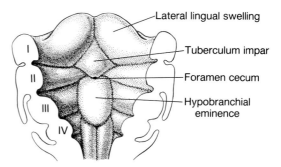

Figure 2–21. Tongue development from three primary masses: two lateral lingual swellings and one tuberculum impar.

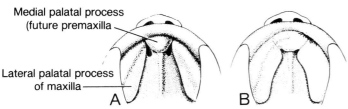

Figure 2–18. Development of palate.

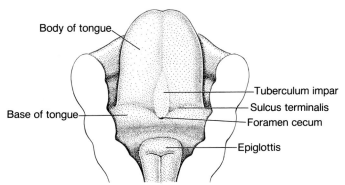

Figure 2–22. Fully formed body and base of tongue.

and fourth arches. Later, this eminence overgrows the second branchial arch to become continuous with the body of the tongue. The site of union between the base and the body of the tongue is delineated by a V-shaped groove called the "sulcus terminalis" (Fig. 2–22). Muscle cells from the occipital myotomes migrate anteriorly into the tongue during the fifth to seventh weeks, a diagram of which will be seen later in this chapter.

In later stages of development, various types of papillae differentiate in the dorsal mucosa of the body of the tongue, whereas lymphatic tissues develop into the pharyngeal part or base of the tongue.

Palatal Shelf Elevation and Closure

At about 8.5 weeks of intrauterine life, the lateral palatal shelves slide or roll over the body of the tongue (Figs. 2–23 and 2–24). The process of shelf elevation occurs when the shelves have developed sufficient strength to slide over the tongue. This process most probably results from the combined action of shelf and tongue movement. As seen in Figure 2–23, the posterior ends of the shelves are above the tongue because the posterior part of the tongue is attached to the floor of the mouth. Palatal shelf elevation thus begins in this posterior region and depresses the tongue downward and forward, which releases the anterior part of the shelves from under the tongue. Whether the tongue is able to move independently after this initial pressure, or whether the shelves exert pressure to move over the tongue, is not known (Fig. 2–24). Shelf elevation occurs as rapidly as swallowing, and is therefore difficult to observe. The important considerations are that shelves ultimately move over the tongue, and

Clinical Application

Severe dietary, chemical, or stress-related factors may cause facial defects, if they affect the mother during the first 8 weeks of gestation.

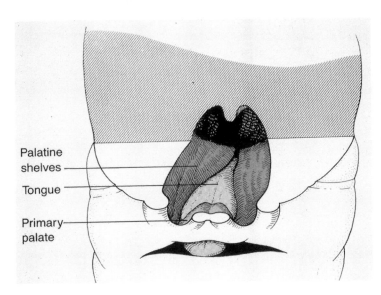

Figure 2–23. Palatine shelves position beside tongue anteriorly and above it posteriorly.

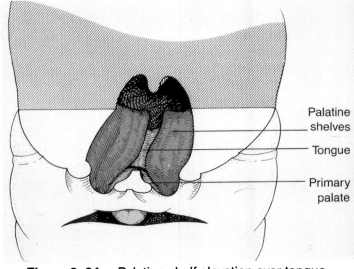

Figure 2–24. Palatine shelf elevation over tongue. Observe tongue's position as palatine shelves move it anteriorly during their elevation process.

that the tongue then broadens to use the lateral space previously occupied by the shelves (Fig. 2–25). The simultaneous events of shelf movement and tongue action are believed to occur. This process is known as palatine shelf elevation and involves all of the movements of the shelves, and probably the tongue, in attaining their relation, as seen in Figure 2–25. It is interesting how highly differentiated the tongue is at this time. None of the tissues in the maxilla or mandible is as differentiated as the tongue. Because the muscles are well differentiated, it is possible that the tongue presses against the overlying shelves and assists in their closure.

After the shelves are in a horizontal position, there is a final growth spurt, and the two shelves contact in the midline (Fig. 2–26). Initial closure or fusion of the lateral palatine shelves first occurs just posterior to the median palatine process (Fig. 2–27). Palatal closure involves the processes of both fusion and merging (Fig. 2–28). When the shelves come in initial contact, the intervening epithelium breaks down and the shelves are then united by intermingling of cells across the midline (Fig. 2–28, Fusion A, B, and C). From the point of initial contact in the anterior palate, the lateral palatine processes fuse with the median palatine process anteriorly (Fig. 2–27). Posteriorly, closure then takes place gradually over the next several weeks and involves merging of the two lateral palatine processes. In merging, the depth of a groove is diminished by growth underlying the groove (Fig. 2–28, merging A to C). Fusion of the lateral palatine processes also occurs with the overlying medial nasal septum (Fig. 2–26), except posteriorly, where the soft palate and uvula remain unattached. At first, palatal fusion is fusion of soft tissues. Later, at about 12 weeks, the palate is invaded by bone anteriorly from the premaxillary, maxillary, and palatal centers to form the hard palate and posteriorly by muscles to form the soft palate.

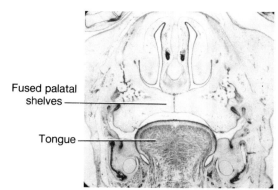

Figure 2–26. Histology of palatal fusion.

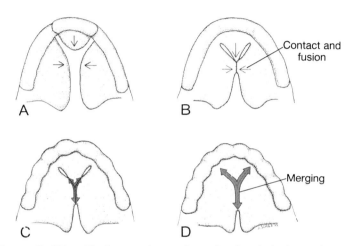

Figure 2–27. Fusion and merging of palatal shelves. Arrows indicate direction of growth.

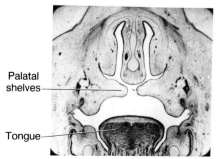

Figure 2–25. Palatal shelves positioned above the tongue.

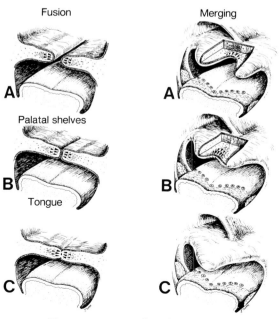

Figure 2–28. Shelf closure.

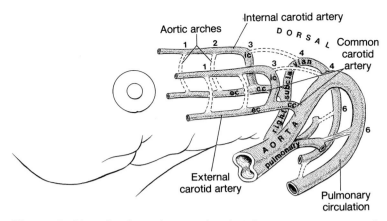

Figure 2–29. Aortic arch vascular development; ec, external carotid; ic, internal carotid.

Vasculature of the Face and Branchial Arches

Each of five (or six) branchial arches ("aortic arches") contains a pair of blood vessels that conduct blood dorsally from the inferiorly located heart through the arch tissue to the brain and the posterior regions. Not all of these paired aortic arches are present at the same time. The anterior right and left aortic arches develop first and, after a week, begin to disappear as more posterior (caudal) arches develop. The more caudal arch vessels then enlarge and mature. The fifth arch vessels disappear next. The third, fourth, and sixth arch vessels do not disappear, but are important in later functions. The third arch vessels become the common carotid arteries that supply the neck, face, and brain. The fourth arch vessels become the dorsal aorta that supplies blood to the entire body, and the vessels of the sixth arch supply blood to the lungs as the pulmonary circulation (Fig. 2–29).

Figure 2–30 illustrates an embryo at 4 weeks; the paired blood vesels (aortic arches) are shown passing through the branchial arch tissue. The heart is ventral to the arches, and the blood passes dorsally through the arches and then to the brain and body. By the fifth week (Fig. 2–31), the first and second branchial arch vessels have disappeared, and then the blood supply to the face is carried by the third branchial arch artery, which becomes the common carotid artery (Fig. 2–31). The common carotid artery gives rise to the external carotid and the internal carotid artery. The external carotid artery supplies blood to the ventral part of the first and second branchial arches. The internal carotid artery supplies blood to the brain (Fig. 2–32). In the region of the ear, the internal carotid artery gives rise to a small vessel, the stapedial artery, which supplies most of the blood to the upper part

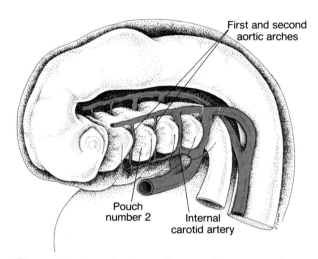

Figure 2–30. Aortic arch vessels at 4 weeks.

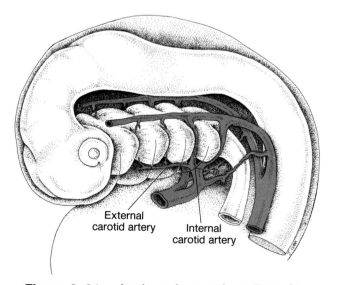

Figure 2–31. Aortic arch vessels at 5 weeks.

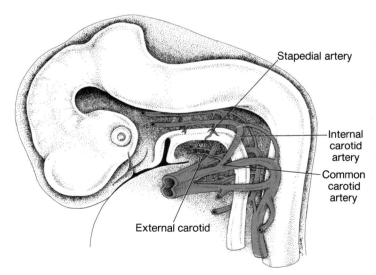

Figure 2–32. Aortic arch vessels at 6 weeks.

of the face and palate (Fig. 2–33). Blood supply to the face by the internal carotid artery is a characteristic of the embryo at 6 and 7 weeks.

An important change in the human embryo takes place during the seventh prenatal week, when the stapedial artery suddenly occludes and separates from the internal carotid artery, which then discontinues its blood supply to the face and palatal tissues (Fig. 2–34). Many of its terminal branches fuse with the peripheral vessels of the external carotid artery. This results in the most unusual shift in the blood supply of the face, from the internal to the external carotid artery, and occurs during the seventh week, an important period of rapid growth expansion and fusion of facial processes. The timing of this transition is very important. The vessels begin to degenerate at one site and rapidly expand at a second site. If timing in the shift is not precise, there will be a period when the face is deprived of oxygen and nutrition carried by this blood supply. This shift in blood supply from the internal carotid to the external carotid artery is shown in Figures 2–33 and 2–34. Because the lip and palate are undergoing maximal developmental changes during the seventh week, a vascular deficiency may result in oxygen and nutritional deficit, which could result in cleft lip, cleft palate, or both.

Development of Cartilages of the Face

The initial skeleton of the branchial arches develops from the mesenchymal tissue as cartilaginous bars. In the first arches, bilateral Meckel's cartilages arise. Meckel's cartilage gradually disappears later, which leaves part of the perichondrium as the sphenomalleolar ligament (anterior ligament of malleus) and part as the sphenomandibular ligament (Fig. 2–35). The malleus and incus develop and ossify at the dorsal end of Meckel's cartilage.

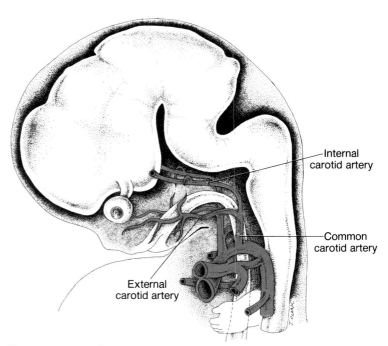

Figure 2–34. Shift of carotid facial blood supply from internal to external carotid artery.

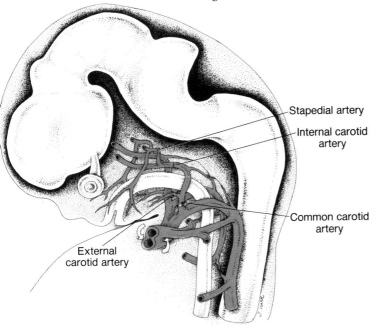

Figure 2–33. Facial blood supply of internal carotid artery by strapedial artery. Note relations of common and external carotid arteries at 7 weeks.

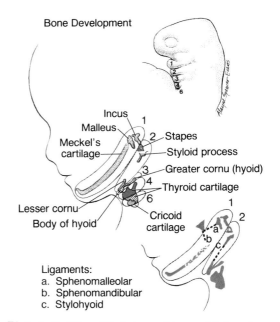

Figure 2–35. Skeleton of branchial arches.

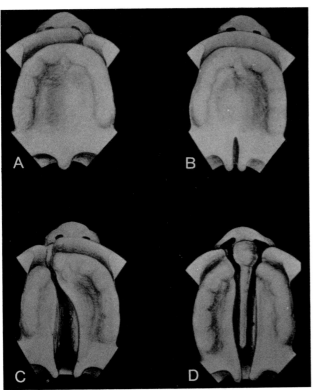

Figure 2-52. Examples of cleft lip and palate. (A). Cleft lip. (B). Cleft of soft palate. (C). Unilateral cleft lip and palate. (D). Bilateral cleft lip and palate.

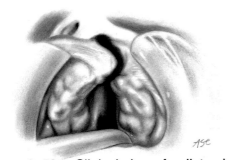

Figure 2-53. Clinical view of unilateral cleft.

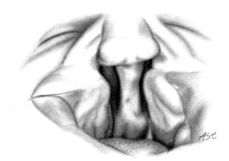

Figure 2-54. Clinical view of bilateral cleft.

Cleft Palate

Cleft palate is less common than cleft lip. It may result from a lack of growth or the failure of fusion between the median and lateral palatine processes and the nasal septum, or it may be due to initial fusion with interruption of growth at any point along its course. It also may be caused by interference with elevation of palatal shelves. Clefts of the palate may be unilateral or bilateral (Fig. 2-52) and are classified as clefts of the primary palate, secondary palate, and both.

Clefts of the primary palate—that is, clefts anterior to the incisive foramen—result from failure of the lateral palatine processes to meet and fuse with the median palatine process or primary palate. The four maxillary incisors develop in the anterior medial palatal segment; cuspids and molars develop in the lateral palatal segment. Clefts of the primary palate are usually associated with missing or malformed teeth adjacent to the clefts, such as lateral incisors and cuspids.

Because fusion of the secondary palate begins in the anterior region and progresses posteriorly, the degree of cleft may vary from the simplest form of bifid uvula to a complete cleft involving both the hard and soft palates. Therefore, clefts of the secondary palate—that is, clefts posterior to the incisive foramen—are the result of partial or complete failure of the lateral palatine processes to meet, fuse, and merge with each other and with the nasal septum (Fig. 2-52B, C, and D).

Clefts of both the primary and the secondary palates or complete palatal clefts are the result of failure of growth or lack of fusion of the three palatine processes with each other and with the nasal septum (Figs. 2-53 and 2-54). Clefts of the palate create many problems; the severity of these problems varies according to the extent of the cleft. Although a bifid uvula causes practically no discomfort and is usually accidentally discovered, a cleft of the soft palate causes varying degrees of speech difficulty and swallowing problems. Clefts of both the hard and soft palates usually produce a severe feeding problem, as food may be aspirated into the lungs. Early correction of this problem should be sought.

Summary

The primitive oral cavity appears during the fourth prenatal week, initially as a pit located between the growing brain cranially and the growing heart ventrally. The branchial arches develop as five or six pairs of mesenchymal bars located laterally and ventrally to the oral pit and surrounding the oropharynx and ventral aspects of the face. The first branchial arch gives rise to the maxillary processes, which in turn form the cheeks. From the mandibular arch, the bony mandible and the masticatory apparatus develops. The upper face arises from the frontonasal process, which develops the forehead, nasal region, and middle of the maxillary lip. Through expansive growth the second, or hyoid, arch gives rise to the muscles of the face and part of the external ear. The lining of the oral cavity gives rise to the pituitary and the thyroid endocrine glands. Each branchial arch gives rise to a specific vascular, neural, and skeletal element. (Contributions of each arch are shown in Table 2–1.) In the area of each pharyngeal pouch, other tissues develop. The tonsils arise from the second pharyngeal pouch, parathyroids from the third and fourth, and thymus from the third.

The roof of the mouth develops from three tissue origins; the median palatine process arises from the frontonasal tissue and the two bilateral palatal shelves arise from the maxillary processes. These lateral shelves initially develop in a horizontal mode and then elevate to position themselves above the tongue. This elevation process is believed to be caused by initial tongue movement anteriorly with a subsequent sliding movement of these shelves over the tongue. The shelves then fuse in the midline posteriorly, and with the primary palate anteriorly.

Malformations may arise from branchial arches in which cervical fistulas or cysts appear laterally in the neck along the anterior margin of the sternocleidomastoid muscle. These are due to abnormal overgrowth of the second to fifth branchial arch tissue. Again, defects may arise in the midline of the anterior neck from the thyroglossal duct as cysts or fistulas. Clefts may arise in the maxillary lip either unilaterally or bilaterally because of a lack of contact and fusion of the maxillary and medial nasal tissues, in the 5-week embryo. Midline clefts of the maxillary or mandibular tissues are rare. Clefts of the palate occur between the primary or medial and secondary or lateral palatine processes. They may occur unilaterally or bilaterally.

Table 2-1.
Contributions of the Branchial Arches

BRANCHIAL GROOVES	BRANCHIAL ARCH STRUCTURES					PHARYNGEAL POUCHES
Adult Derivative	Arch No.	Cranial Nerve	Branchiomeric Muscles	Skeletal Derivative	Aortic Arch	Adult Derivative
Ext. Auditory Meatus 1	I — Mandibular	V — Trigeminal	Muscles of mastication, anterior belly digastric, mylohyoid, tensor tympani, tensor palatini	Malleus, incus, sphenomandibular ligament, sphenomalleolar ligament (Meckel's cartilage)	I	1 Middle ear Eustachian tube
	II — Hyoid	VII — Facial	Muscles of facial expression, stapedius, stylohyoid, posterior belly digastric	Stapes, styloid process, stylohyoid ligament, lesser cornu hyoid, upper part body hyoid	II	2 Palatine tonsil
Cervical Fistula	2 III	IX — Glossopharyngeal	Stylopharyngeus	Greater cornu hyoid, lower part body hyoid	III	3 Thymus, inferior parathyroid
	3 IV	X — Vagus	Laryngeal musculature, pharyngeal constrictors	Laryngeal cartilages	IV	4 Superior parathyroid
	4 V	XI — Spinal Accessory	Sternocleidomastoid / Trapezius		VI	5 Ultimobranchial body

Structures formed from the first branchial groove, the pharyngeal pouches, and the branchial arches.

Self-Evaluation Review

1. Describe the process of the eyes' migration from the sides to the front of the human face.
2. Discuss the origin of the thyroid gland, describing its descent to its location in the adult.
3. Of the five aortic vascular arches, which ones function, and for what purpose, in the adult?
4. Describe the relative timing, function, and importance of the shift from the internal to the external carotid blood supply to the face.
5. What muscles develop from the first and second branchial arches?
6. From what four initial masses does the face arise? What does each contribute?
7. Describe the development of the maxillary lip.
8. Discuss the process, including possible causes, of palate elevation and fusion.
9. What cartilage elements arise from the maxillary and mandibular processes?
10. What are the contributions of each pharyngeal pouch?
11. Describe the origin of the tongue musculature and its innervation.

Acknowledgments

The author acknowledges the original suggestions of Dr. ElNesr to this chapter. Dr. Alfonse Burdi kindly provided Figure 2–47 from research in his laboratory.

Suggested Readings

Diewert VM. The Course of the palatine arteries during secondary palate development in the rat. *J. Dent. Res.* 1973;52:1273–1280.

Gasser RF. The early development of the parotid gland around the facial nerves and its branches in man. *Anat. Rec.* 1970;167:63–78.

Maher WP, Swindle, PF. Submucosal blood vessels of the palate. *Dental Progr.*, 1962;2:167–180.

Millard RD, Williams S. Median lip clefts of the upper lip. *Plastic Reconstr. Surg.* 1968;42:4–14.

Padget DH. The cranial venous system in man in reference to development adult configuration and relation to the arteries. *Amer. J. Anat.* 1956;98:307–356.

Poswillo D. The pathogenesis of the first and second branchial arch syndrome. *Oral Surg.* 1973;35:302–328.

Sadler T, ed. *Langman's Medical Embryology.* 5th ed. Baltimore, Md: Williams and Wilkins; 1985.

Sperber GH. *Craniofacial Embryology.* 4th ed. London, U.K.: Butterworth; 1989.

Sulik KK. Craniofacial defects from genetic and teratogen induced deficiencies in presomite embryos. *Birth Defects* 1984;20:79–98.

Sulik KK, Johnston MC. Embryonic origin of holoprosencephaly. Interrelationship of the developing brain and face *Scan. Elem. Microsc.* 1982;309–322.

Sulik KK, Lauder JM, Dehort DB. Brain malformations in prenatal mice following acute maternal ethanol administration. *Int. J. Devel. Neurosci.* 1984;2:203–214.

Sulik KK, Johnston MC, Smiley SJ, Speight HS, Jarvis BE. Mandibulofacial dystosis (Treacher Collins syndrome), a new proposal for its pathogenesis. *Am. J. Med. Genet.* 1987;27:354–372.

Vander Meulen JC, Mazzola R, Vermey-Keers C, Stricher M, Raphaie B. A morphogenetic classification of craniofacial malformations. *Plastic Reconstr. Surg.* 1983;71:560–572.

3

Development of Cartilages and Bones of the Facial Skeleton

James K. Avery

Introduction

The facial skeleton is derived from both cartilage and bony elements. The centers for hyaline cartilage appear first in the maxillary midline and grow laterally to support the neural tube. As this tube emerges into the brain, bone centers appear to supplant the midline cartilages. These cartilages are gradually replaced by bone through endochondral bone formation. Laterally located and appearing somewhat later in development, ossification centers arise in the connective tissue of the face and in the tissue overlying the brain to become the bony skeleton to which the muscles of the skull and face attach. Cranial bones are frontal, parietal, and occipital, and the facial bones are premaxillae, maxillae, zygomatic, and temporal. In the mandibular arch below the maxillae, the bony mandible develops anteriorly and then grows posteriorly to contact the condyle, which is the cartilage part of the mandible. These condyles are then modified into bone, and these separate anterior and posterior parts next fuse to form the bony mandible. The condyle maintains a cartilage articulating head until it changes to bone in adulthood. Both the right and left temporomandibular joints consist of the condyles and the glenoid fossae. The condyle head is a sliding hinge joint that allows the mandible to function in protrusion, retrusion, and lateral excursion.

Objectives

After reading this chapter, you should be able to describe those skeletal components that form the developing skull and face. You should be able to describe the cartilages and bones of the cranial base, the maxilla, the mandible, and the temporomandibular joint. You should also be able to define the various articulations of the face and palate. Finally, you should be able to describe the abnormal development resulting from a cleft palate.

junction between adjacent bones peculiar to the skull. It functions first as an area of growth and second, as an area that unites and articulates two neighboring bones. As noted previously, the zygomatic arch is important to the growth of the face, as the zygomatic bone has three articulations, which are directed in a downward and forward direction (Fig. 3–18). When the position of these sutures in the fetal and the adult skull are compared, the relation of the sutures is similar, although the bones have increased in size (Figs. 3–18 and 3–19). Histologically, the sutures of the face are composed of a band of fibrous tissue interposed between two bones, called "syndesmoses." The classification of syndesmoses may be subdivided into three types: simple, serrated, and squamosal (plain, denticulate, or beveled). All of these consist of a central zone of proliferating connective tissue cells, with fibrous connective tissue and osteogenic cells appearing along the adjacent bone fronts. Simple sutures are ones in which the bones meet end to end with tissue between them (Fig. 3–20). Serrated sutures are characterized by interdigitating opposing bone fronts, such as the cranial sutures (Fig. 3–21). They exhibit cells and fibers in a relation similar to the simple suture, except they have dense fibrous bands extending across them. Squamous sutures, such as the temporoparietal one, are characterized by the overlap and growth of the opposing bone at an angle to each other (Fig. 3–22). In addition to fibrous connective tissue sutures, there are cartilage junctions between two bones, as was described previously along the midline between ethmoid and sphenoid bones. Such a junction is termed "synchondrosis" (Fig. 3–23). It has the appearance of a cartilaginous epiphyseal plate or "line" on which new cartilage cells have formed in the center of the suture (resting zone). These cells move peripherally as new cells appear in the midline. Laterally, the cartilage mineralizes

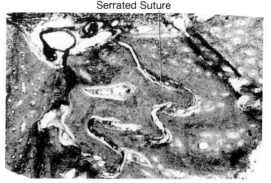

Figure 3–21. Serrated suture.

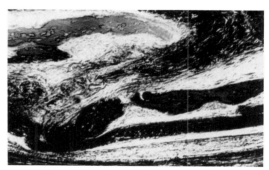

Figure 3–22. Squamous suture.

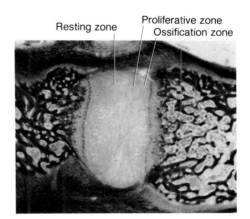

Figure 3–23. Synchondrosis.

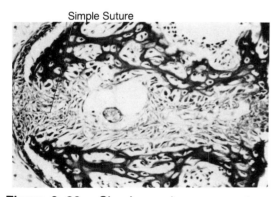

Figure 3–20. Simple syndesmoses suture.

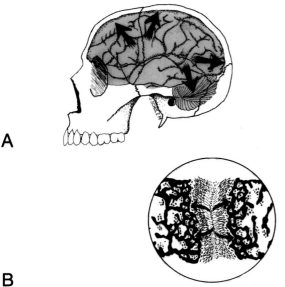

A

B

Figure 3–24. (A). Brain growth promotes skull and suture growth. (B). Growth within suture.

and degenerates, and bone forms on the lateral boundaries. The growth of the two opposing bones along these fronts thus takes place (Figs. 3–23 and 3–24).

The prevalent theory of sutural growth is that growth of underlying or adjacent structures, such as the brain, cause the bones adjacent to the suture to move away from one another (Fig. 3–24A). Thus, sutural growth may compensate for these extrinsic growth forces. The growth at the four significant sutures of the face may therefore be a response to the anterior and downward growth force of the facial tissues as a whole. Another theory is that growth forces reside within the suture (Fig. 3–24B).

Palate Development

In Chapter 2, it was noted that the roof of the oral cavity develops from one medial and two lateral palatine processes (Fig. 3–25), from which appear tiny ossification centers. These centers develop laterally at the junction of the medial and lateral palatine processes (Fig. 3–25A) and are the premaxillary and maxillary ossification centers. The two premaxillary centers will develop within the medial palatine processes on either side of the midline, and this bone will support the central and lateral incisors. The maxillary bone supports the cuspid and molar teeth of the primary dentition and later will provide alveolar bone support to the cuspid, two premolars, and the first, second, and third molars. The palatine bone supports the posterior palate.

These palatal bones grow medially to support the soft tissues of the palate. When the inferior aspect of the palate of a cleared prenatal human skull at 13 weeks is viewed, it appears to be covered with tiny bony trabeculae (Fig. 3–26). In the anterior palate, the premaxilla has lingual and labial plates of bone around the incisor teeth. A suture separates the right and left sides. A posterior suture separates the premaxillary from the maxillary bones (Fig. 3–26). The

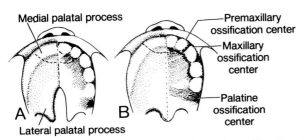

Medial palatal process
Premaxillary ossification center
Maxillary ossification center
Palatine ossification center
Lateral palatal process

Figure 3–25. Palate formation (A) and ossification (B).

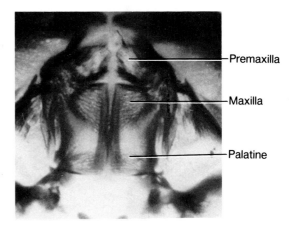

Premaxilla

Maxilla

Palatine

Figure 3–26. Ossification of human palate at 13 weeks.

right and left maxillary bones grow from the periphery to meet at the midline suture. The palatine bones can be seen at the posterior limits of the palate. At this age, the palate is relatively small compared with the cranial skeleton (Fig. 3–26). Later, the palate will be much larger. By the 8th prenatal month, the bony configuration of the palate is well established (Fig. 3–27). The sutures between the premaxillary, maxillary, and palatine bones are still evident, as is the midline suture. Figure 3–27 is a photograph of a cleared human palate at 8 months prenatally, and shows two sutures that provide for anterior growth, the premax-maxillary and the maxillary-palatine. The midline suture provides for lateral growth. Around the periphery of the palate are the crypts of the various developing teeth. Additional growth of the palate occurs around its perimeter, which assures that growth of the palate will keep pace with the growth of the face.

Early Mandibular Development

As the nasal capsule becomes the prominent cartilage in the upper face, Meckel's cartilage bars become apparent in the mandibular arch (Fig. 3–28). The posterior part of each of these bars enlarges to become the malleus, which articulates with a second small cartilage, the incus. These two cartilages become enclosed in the otic capsule. They form a joint that is termed the "malleoincus," or temporomandibular joint (Figs. 3–29 and 3–30). Articulation of these two cartilages continues until they undergo endochondral bone formation during the 18th prenatal week. At that time, the secondary, or permanent temporomandibular joint forms anterior to the middle ear and begins functioning (Fig. 3–31). The shift

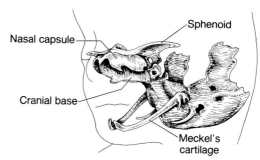

Figure 3–28. Development of cartilage in face and skull.

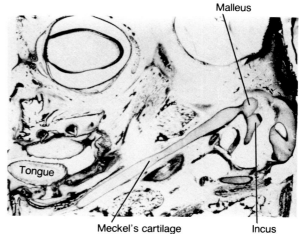

Figure 3–29. Meckel's cartilage and primary temporomandibular joint. Articulation of the joint is between the malleus and incus.

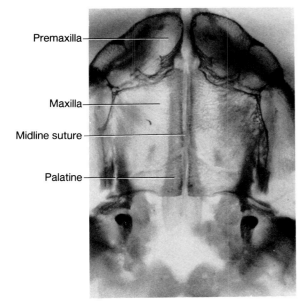

Figure 3–27. Ossification of human palate at 8th prenatal month.

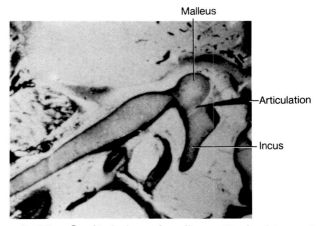

Figure 3–30. Sagittal view of malleus attached to posterior end of Meckel's cartilage. The malleus articulates with the incus as the primary temporomandibular joint.

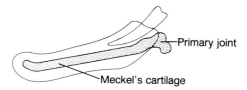

Figure 3–31. Development of mandible.

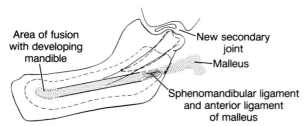

Figure 3–32. Development of secondary temporomandibular joint.

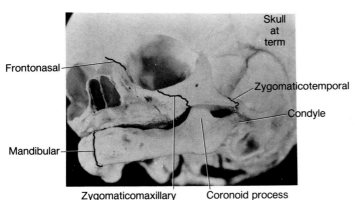

Figure 3–33. Facial sutures at birth.

Clinical Application

Two growth centers in the head of each condyle account for its increase in size. New cartilage cells differentiate under the perichondrium and develop new cartilage matrix, which grows and expands. New bone then forms along the interface of this mature cartilage and the marrow space, again increasing their volume. Both processes take place simultaneously during facial growth.

from the primary to the secondary joint occurs as pressure is relieved from the primary joint and the permanent joint assumes function (Fig. 3–32).

The body of the mandible continues to develop as a rectangular membrane bone (Fig. 3–31). The cartilage condyles develop and are modified into bone by endochondral bone formation. The bone collars that form on the surface of the condyles then fuse to the body of the mandible. The condyles and body of the mandible initially form an angle of 135°, which is maintained during the rest of prenatal life (Fig. 3–32). Bone appears at the angle of the mandible near and after birth as a result of bone depositions at the sites of insertion of the medial pterygoid and masseter muscles. The ramus of the mandible thus remodels by bone addition on the posterior margin and by resorption along the anterior margins of the ramus (Fig. 3–32). This posterior growth lengthens the mandible, which allows space for posterior molar addition. Growth occurs at the head of the condyle, which increases the height of the ramus. Anterior to the condyle, a coronoid process develops in response to the insertion and function of the temporalis muscle. The coronoid process becomes a prominent part of the ramus at birth (Fig. 3–33). At birth, the two halves of the mandible are united at the anterior midline by a suture at the symphysis. Further growth continues at this suture until it ossifies during the first year after birth.

Condylar Cartilage Development and Articular Disc Formation

Between the 8th and the 12th weeks of fetal life, the cartilaginous condyles develop anteriorly to the malleus and incus articulation (Fig. 3–34). The early cone-shaped cartilaginous condyle soon is altered by endochondral bone formation. Figure 3–35, which is a coronal section of a mandible from an 11- to 12-week-old fetus, illustrates the condyle consisting of a large mass of hyaline cartilage covered

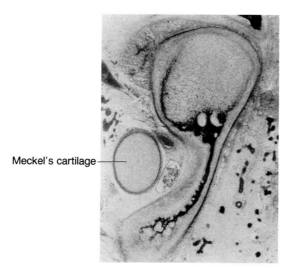

Figure 3–34. Coronal view showing relation of lateral developing condyle to medial Meckel's cartilage.

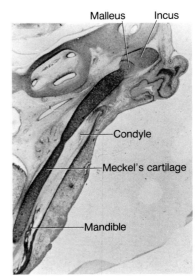

Figure 3–35. Frontal view of condyle and Meckel's cartilage at 11 or 12 prenatal weeks.

by a thin fibrous cap. In this coronal section, the bony ramus is outlined by connective tissue, and a thin core of bone is seen. Meckel's cartilage is seen positioned medially to the ramus and is the functioning TM joint at this time (Fig. 3–35).

The first appearance of a temporomandibular joint cavity is seen in the 12-week-old fetus (Fig. 3–36). The first of the two compartments to form is the inferior, or mandibular compartment. A split first appears in the mesenchyme overlying the condylar head and extends into a small cleft (Fig. 3–36). The precise mechanism of cavitation still remains unknown, although the split outlines the head of the condyle. The process probably is due to programmed cell death (apoptosis) along the path of movement of the condyle and adjacent connective tissue. Within another week, the superior or temporal compartment is formed by the same process (Fig. 3–37).

The gradual formation of the temporal (glenoid) fossa also starts in the 12th prenatal week, when the synovial cavity outlines the condylar head. Then a spicule of the temporal bone develops superior to the forming articular disc (Figs. 3–36 and 3–37). With continued intramembranous bone formation, the small segments soon coalesce to form the glenoid fossa.

Fate of Meckel's Cartilage

When the anterior aspect of Meckel's cartilage fuses to the medial wall of the body of the mandible in the 10th prenatal week, the cartilage then undergoes endochondral bone formation along the medial aspect of the mandible. As the mandible enlarges, the remnants of Meckel's cartilage become relatively smaller, as seen by the remnant anterior to the malleus (Fig. 3–38). By the 16th prenatal week, the malleus and incus have maintained their size and have begun transformation into bones of the middle ear by endochondral bone formation (Fig. 3–38). As Meckel's cartilage degenerates in the area anterior to the ear, two ligaments, the anterior malleus and sphenomandibular, form within its pathway. When the secondary temporomandibular joint becomes functional at 18 to 20 prenatal weeks, Meckel's cartilage loses its function and disappears.

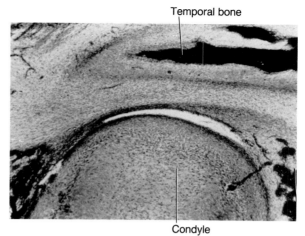

Figure 3–36. Sagittal view of head of condyle and appearance of cleft denote the lower compartment of the joint at the 12th prenatal week.

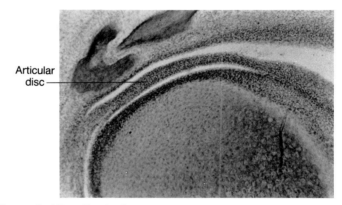

Figure 3–37. Sagittal view of head of condyle and appearance of second cleft outline the articular disc at the 13th prenatal week.

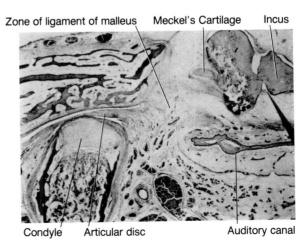

Figure 3–38. Sagittal view of condyle and fossa (left) and malleus and incus (right). Note the endochondral bone formation in the middle ear bones. The arrow indicates articulation of these bones.

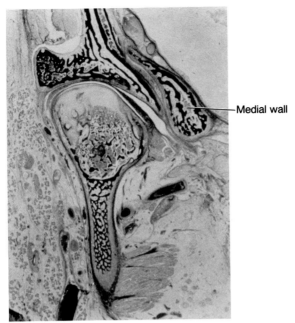

Medial wall

Figure 3–39. Frontal view of temporomandibular joint at 22 prenatal weeks.

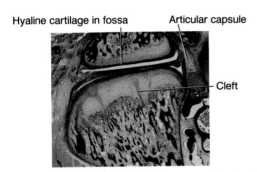

Hyaline cartilage in fossa   Articular capsule

Cleft

Figure 3–40. Frontal view of temporomandibular joint at 26 weeks. Note clefts of connective tissue in condylar cartilage.

Differentiation of Temporomandibular Joint

Once the component parts of the joint have been established, by the 14th prenatal week, no major alterations occur, except in differentiation of the joint tissues and the increase in size of the joint. Compare (Figs. 3–38 and 3–39). The growth of the condyle consists of both interstitial and appositional growth of the condylar cartilage. The apposition of the newly formed cartilage occurs on the surface of the condyle by differentiation of new cells, which grow in size and then form cartilage matrix by interstitial means. This cartilage is then calcified and replaced by bone. The process of cartilage growth and bone replacement helps provide for the enlargement and elongation of the ramus of the mandible.

There is further bone formation in the temporal region, so that at 22 weeks prenatally, the glenoid fossa has developed a superior as well as a medial wall, and muscles have differentiated and attached to the ramus (Fig. 3–39). This joint began function a few weeks before this section was made. Also at this time, the articular plane and eminence has begun to develop.

Late Prenatal Development

The change in structure of the temporomandibular joint after function begins is seen as an increase in size and density of the bone of the condyle and changes in shape and size of the mandible associated with differentiation and function of the muscles of mastication. One noteworthy feature, occurring in the late prenatal life is the appearance of clefts of connective tissue in the condyle head (Figs. 3–40 and 3–41). These connective tissue ingrowths originate from the

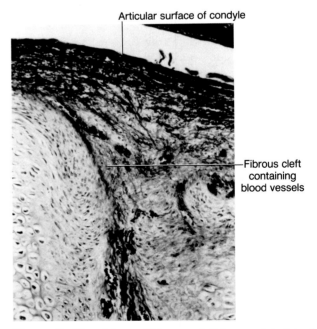

Articular surface of condyle

Fibrous cleft containing blood vessels

Figure 3–41. View of fibrous cleft in condyle head with blood vessels.

fibrous perichondrium covering the cartilaginous condyle head. They carry blood vessels into the rapidly growing cartilage. This is an unusual feature as other cartilages in the human body are considered to be avascular. Some of these vascular ingrowths extend to the endochondral bone front. The connective tissue clefts seem to be related to the rapid increase in size and function of the human temporomandibular joint. Another final, late prenatal change is the general thinning of the cartilage on the condylar head (Fig. 3–42). During the 8th and 9th prenatal months, endochondral bone replaces the cartilage more rapidly than the formation of new cartilage occurs on the condyle surface. This narrow band of cartilage persists, however, in the head of the condyle until approximately the 25th postnatal year of life. In Figure 3–42, the origin of new cartilage cells is seen from the cell reserve zone underlying the periochondrium. These cells enlarge and divide in the multiplication zone, matrix is formed, and the cells mature, further enlarge, and die as the matrix is calcified and bone formation takes place (Fig. 3–42).

Secondary Growth Cartilages

The bony mandible develops by both endochondral bone formation of the condyle and intramembranous development of the mandibular body. This latter statement must be modified to include the appearance of several other cartilage growth centers, known as secondary growth cartilages, in the mandible. These are (1) the coronoid cartilages, (2) some cartilage formation around the tooth follicles, and (3) the symphyseal cartilages that appear in the anterior midline (Fig. 3–43). The cartilage in the coronoid process is a small island that appears between the 14th and 16th prenatal weeks and disappears by the 20th week. Tiny sites of cartilage appear near and around early forming tooth buds, but these cartilage sites soon disappear. Only the symphyseal cartilage persists until birth or later. The two cartilages are separated by the perichondrium in the midline. These cartilages are anterior to, and independent of, the earlier-formed Meckel's cartilages. The symphyseal cartilage undergoes endochondral bone formation throughout prenatal life and contributes to an increase in the growth dimension and width of the mandible. Cessation of growth of these cartilages occurs, but the suture persists in the midline and continues during the 1st postnatal year.

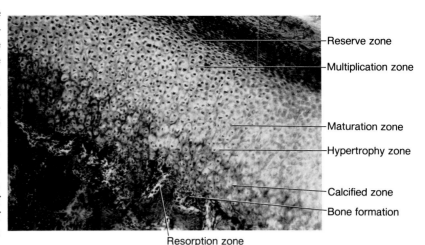

Reserve zone
Multiplication zone
Maturation zone
Hypertrophy zone
Calcified zone
Bone formation
Resorption zone

Figure 3–42. Condylar cartilage with zone of cartilage above and bone formation below.

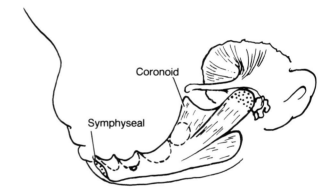

Coronoid
Symphyseal

Figure 3–43. Diagram of mandible and temporomandibular joint at 20 weeks.

Clinical Application

Cartilage and bone function in concert not only in the developing face, but throughout life in the skeletal system of the human to provide strength and flexibility. Cartilage sutures in the cranial base, in the heads of the long bones, and in the vertebrae provide strength and flexibility and are a cooperative effort at sites where growth is needed. Another example is at a fracture site, where a temporary cartilage callus is later replaced by bone.

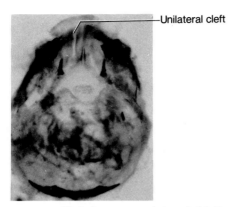

Figure 3-44. Cleft human palate at 11.5 weeks.

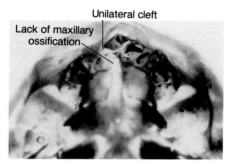

Figure 3-45. Unilateral cleft.

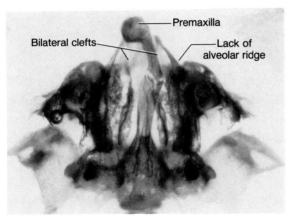

Figure 3-46. Bilateral cleft.

Abnormal Development

Unilateral and bilateral clefts of the palate produce defects in the nasomaxillary skeleton and bones of the human palate. Figure 3-44 shows a cleared human palate at 11.5 weeks. In this figure, a unilateral cleft palate is indicated by the white vertical line through the alveolar ridge and palate. Note the absence of premaxillary ossification on the left side. Compare the size of the maxillary bones. The bone formation on the cleft side is deficient. In the case of a unilateral cleft palate, bone forms appropriately on the normal side; bone deficiency appears along the cleft side (Fig. 3-44). A lack of palatal bone, as well as the absence of the bony alveolar ridge and teeth in the region of the cuspid and lateral incisor is seen on the left of this specimen. Alveolar ridge deficiency occurs where the premaxilla and maxilla join developmentally (Fig. 3-45).

A bilateral cleft usually results in a bony deficiency on both the right and left sides (Fig. 3-46). In this palate there is an absence of bone at the junction of the premaxilla and maxilla, as both of these bones are much smaller than they would be normally. The lateral incisors, cuspids, and primary molar teeth, along with their bony crypts, are also missing. The teeth adjacent to the clefts in the alveolar ridges are usually missing. These most likely would be the lateral incisors and cuspids.

Summary

The initial skeleton of the face is cartilaginous and is composed of the nasal capsule in the upper face and Meckel's cartilage in the mandibular arch (Fig. 3–47). Then the nasal, lacrimal, premaxilla, maxilla, zygomatic, and temporal bones appear in the upper face; the mandible appears in the lower (Fig. 3–48).

The connective tissue sutures between the bones of the face are termed "syndesmoses." Syndesmoses may be further classified as simple, serrated, or squamous, and are located between the frontal and maxillary, the maxillary and zygomatic, the zygomatic and temporal, and the palatine and pterygoid lamina of the sphenoid bones. Other sutures appear in the face between the ethmoid, sphenoid, and basioccipital bones. Cartilage is present between these latter midline bones, whereas connective tissue is present between the membrane bones of the face (Fig. 3–49).

Palatal ossification initiates at the junction of the medial and lateral palatal processes. Bone trabeculae grow medially to the midline from both premaxillary and maxillary centers. Posteriorly, palatine ossification centers appear on both sides and grow to the midline. By the 8th month of intrauterine life, bone covers the palate. Premaxillary–maxillary and maxillary–palatine sutures, as well as a midline suture extending the entire length of the hard palate, are apparent. Further growth at these sutures, as well as at other surfaces, occurs by apposition. The adult skull is seen in Figure 3–50.

Meckel's cartilage is the primary cartilage of the mandible and provides the support for the lower jaw to the first 4.5 months of fetal life. At its superior–posterior surface, the malleus and incus serve as the primary articulation of the mandible (Fig. 3–47) until the true temporomandibular joint becomes functional; then Meckel's cartilage resorbs and disappears. The condyle begins as a cone-shaped cartilage mass at the superior–posterior surface of the bony mandible. The temporal bone is formed by intramembranous bone, although the fossa becomes lined with cartilage. The cartilage gradually transforms to bone. There are several differences in how cartilage in the mandibular condyles and long bones grow as the latter develop secondary ossification centers and exhibit epiphyseal lines. First, the chondrocytes do not form in rows in the condyle, as occurs in long-bone growth; second, a fibrous perichondrium covers the condyle; and third, vascular tracts develop in the condylar cartilage.

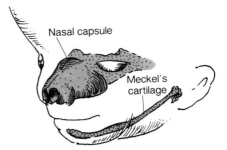

Figure 3–47. Cartilages of face at 8 weeks.

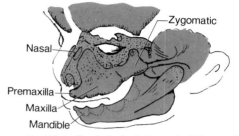

Figure 3–48. Facial skeleton at 4.5 months.

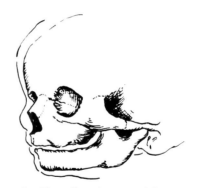

Figure 3–49. Cranium and face at birth.

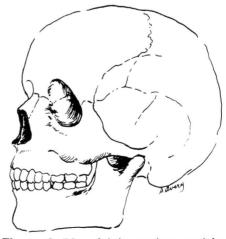

Figure 3–50. Adult cranium and face.

Self-Evaluation Review

1. Define the components of the primary and secondary temporomandibular joints.
2. Name the bones of the palate. What are the ossification centers of the palate?
3. Define and give examples of a synchrondrosis and a syndesmosis suture.
4. Where are nerve endings located in the temporomandibular joint?
5. Describe the differences and similarities in the cartilages and bones of the condyle and long bones.
6. What is the nerve and blood supply of the temporomandibular joint?
7. What is the function of the early-formed cartilages of the craniofacial area?
8. What are the causes of pain in the area of the external ear in temporomandibular joint disfunction?
9. Name the bones of the developing facial skeleton.
10. Name and locate the three supporting ligaments of the temporomandibular joint.

Suggested Readings

Dixon AD, Sarnat BG, eds. *Normal and Abnormal Bone Growth.* New York, NY: Alan Liss Inc; 1985.

DuBrul EL. The craniomandibular articulation. In: *Sicher's Oral Anatomy.* 7th Ed. St. Louis: The C.V. Mosby Co.; 1980:174–210, 527–535.

Enlow DH. Introductory concepts of the growth process. *Handbook of Facial Growth.* Philadelphia, Pa: WB Saunders Co.; 1982: 24–66.

Griffin CJ, Hawthorne, R, Harris, R. Anatomy and histology of the human temporomandibular joint. *Monog. Oral Sci.* 1975;4:1.

Meikie, MC. The role of the condyle in the postnatal growth of the mandible, *Am. J. Ortho.* 1973;64:50–62.

Moore, KL. Articular and skeletal systems. In: *Essentials of Human Embryology.* Toronto, Canada: BC Decker Inc. 1988;137–145.

Ross RB, Johnston MC. Facial development from cleft formation to birth. In: *Cleft Lip and Palate.* New York, NY: Robert Kreiger Pub. 1978;68–87.

Sarnat, BG, Laskin, DM. *Temporomandibular Joint: Biological Basis for Clinical Practice.* Springfield, Ill: Charles C. Thomas; 1979.

Sadler TW. Skeletal system. In: *Langman's Medical Embryology.* 5th ed. Baltimore, Md: Williams and Wilkins; 1985;133–147.

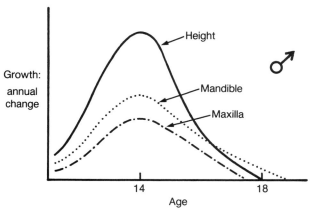

Figure 4-4. Growth curves show average growth increments for height of the maxilla and the mandible in young men. The peak growth rate for the face is believed to occur shortly after the maximum increment in height. Growth ceases at different times, however.

Clinical Application

Relapse of lower anterior dental crowding after orthodontic treatment is a controversal issue in orthodontics. Both late adolescent mandibular growth and third molar eruptive pressures have been blamed.

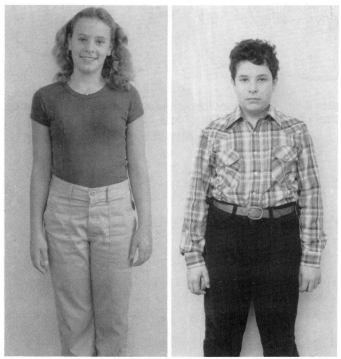

Figure 4-5. As any junior high school teacher will verify, girls tend to reach adolescence earlier than boys. A 13-year old girl may be taller and developmentally more mature than a 13-year-old boy.

Timing of Growth

Individual children differ not only in the amount of growth and their ultimate size, but also in the timing of different phases of their growth.

Growth of the face follows the general timetable of the skeleton, the abdominal and thoracic organs, and the musculature. Periods of rapid growth (dependent on the systemic control of hormones) occur after birth, in midchildhood, and during adolescence. Other tissues have their own timetables: neural tissues (e.g., brain) develop early, the reproductive tissues (e.g., genital organs) develop late, and the lymphoid tissues are variable (e.g., the thymus hypertrophies in childhood and subsequently shrinks). The face is considered to be intermediate in timing, as it follows the somatic growth of the child.

Within a person, considerable variation between growth rates of different body parts occurs. For example, during the adolescent growth spurt in height, the sequence of growth acceleration is foot, calf, thigh, trunk, and finally, weight. The head also demonstrates considerable variation in the growth of its parts. The upper nasal cavities near adult size by 1 year of age, the anterior cranial base is essentially complete in size by 7 years of age, the maxilla finishes growing between 14 and 16 years of age, and the mandible finishes growth at an older age. The maximum growth rate of the face in adolescence is believed to take place a little later than does maximal change in body height. The adolescent growth maxima for the maxilla and mandible occur simultaneously, but growth slows and stops at different times (Fig. 4–4). The mandible continues to increase in length for approximately 2 years after the facial sutures become inactive. The extended period of mandibular growth makes it difficult to predict the final size for surgical correction of mandibular overgrowth and may be responsible for the crowding of lower incisors that is often observed in late adolescence.

The specific growth pattern of the head is influenced by many variables such as gender, ethnic or racial characteristics, physique, illness, and nutritional level. Boys grow "later, longer, and larger" than girls. Consequently, girls mature earlier and pass through the adolescent growth spurt more rapidly than boys (Fig. 4–5). Although black babies generally weigh less than white babies at birth and during childhood, they achieve their developmental milestones earlier. Asian children tend to be smaller than both black and white children. Physique or body build also influences the timing of growth and development. For example, the extremely tall, thin person usually has a later, more prolonged period of growth during adolescence than the shorter, highly muscular individual. The nonmuscular, obese adolescent usually lacks an intense spurt and, instead, gradually increases in size over a long time. Illness or poor nutrition may delay or prevent proper growth. Another factor influencing timing of growth is the so-called "secular trend." Some surveys suggest that in the developed areas of the world, children are maturing at increasingly early ages. However, recent data indicate a leveling-off tendency as good nutrition and preventive health measures become widespread.

The marked variations in growth timing have led to the concept of biologic age, which is determined from the level of maturity rather than chronologic or calendar age. Typically, biologic age is based on developmental milestones in development of the long bones of the skeleton (skeletal age) or in the formation or emergence of the teeth (dental age). Assessments of skeletal maturity are commonly made from hand-wrist radiographs, and dental maturity is best determined from radiographs of the jaws. Readiness for treatment is based on biologic maturity rather than chronologic age.

Growth Processes

Bones of the head grow on surfaces, at synchrondroses, and at stutures, but do not grow by internal expansion. Some basic biologic processes involved in skeletal growth and development are most clearly illustrated by examining the growth of the bones of the cranial vault. In the early period of growth, bone is deposited incrementally on all surfaces of the enlarging bones (Fig. 4–6). This type of growth continues only for a short time. Later growth of a calvarial bone is a complex response to the outward displacement of the bones by the expanding brain (Fig. 4–7). Their enlargement and flattened contour result from both remodeling of the bone as it is displaced and sutural growth at the edges. Remodeling modifies bone structure by the processes of bone deposition and resorption on the bone surface.

Bones also change their position in the growing face by displacement and drift. Displacement involves a change in position of an entire bone as the result of growth at its border or the movement of an adjacent bone. Drift results from apposition on one side and resorption on another. Changes in proportion as well as size are achieved through differential growth, or variations in relative rates and amounts of growth. For example, the mandible grows proportionately more after birth than do other skull bones, and some bone edges on either side of a suture may grow at different rates.

With growth, the changes in the facial soft tissue are not as clearly delineated as are the bony changes. It is known that muscles increase in bulk by an increase in the size of individual muscle cells, not by an increase in the number of cells. Sarcomeres are added to the myofibril at its end (Fig. 4–8). The sheath covering the muscle, however, grows as a result of cell division throughout the length of the muscle. The fact that the muscular pattern of the face is determined very early probably has important consequences in facial development.

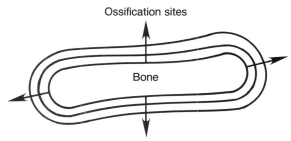

Figure 4–6. In the early period of growth, ossification may occur on all surfaces of a developing cranial bone.

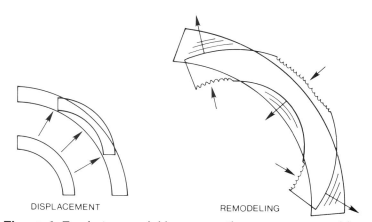

Figure 4–7. Later cranial bone growth occurs as a combination of remodeling and sutural growth.

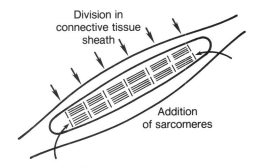

Figure 4–8. Muscle fibers grow by addition of sarcomeres at the ends of the myofibrils. The cells in the connective tissue sheath, however, divide throughout the length of the muscle.

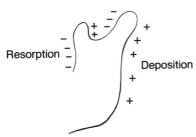

Figure 4-9. Remodeling of mandibular ramus and coronoid process.

Resorption − / + Deposition

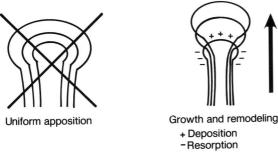

Uniform apposition

Growth and remodeling
+ Deposition
− Resorption

Figure 4-10. The condyle does not grow by the process of uniform apposition but by a complex process of growth and remodeling. +, deposition of bone. −, resorption of bone.

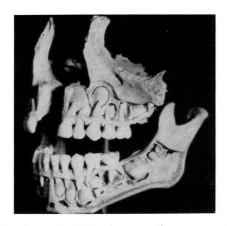

Figure 4-11. As an individual grows, the ramus must remodel to provide adequatae room for eruption of the second and third molars.

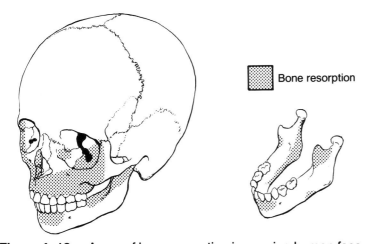

Bone resorption

Figure 4-12. Areas of bone resorption in growing human face.

Specific Areas of Growth

In the mandible, three areas of activity account for the growth changes observed: (1) remodeling of the ramus and coronoid process (Fig. 4–9); (2) growth at the condyle (Fig. 4–10); and (3) alveolar growth and slight growth at the inferior border. Remodeling of the ramus in a growing child provides space for the second and third molars (Fig. 4–11). The condyle grows by proliferation of cartilage in the condylar head and endochondral bone formation. The formed bone is remodeled as it becomes part of the ramus, and the cartilage proliferation continues (Fig. 4–10). Relatively stable areas are located at the inner border of the symphysis, along the mandibular canal, on the chin, and on the contour of tooth germs before root formation. Chin growth is deceptive because the chin "grows" as a result of resorption of bone above the chin rather than deposition of bone at the chin itself (Fig. 4–12).

Clinical Application

That dental arches display only minor changes in transverse and anteroposterior dimensions during childhood is remarkable, especially considering that the teeth erupt several millimeters to maintain dental occlusion as the face grows in height. This allows the clinician to make reasonable predictions about need for treatment even in young children.

The maxilla changes position in the growing face as a result of both drifting by remodeling, and displacement due to growth at the maxillary sutures (Fig. 4–13). The tuberosity increases in length to create space for the molar teeth (Fig. 4–14). The increased height of the palate with maturation is due to the eruption of teeth carryng the alveolar process along. The area of least change is around the nasopalatine foramen. As the maxilla moves forward and downward, the anterior surface is resorbed (Fig. 4–12).

Dental arch relations are usually maintained during the increase in facial height. As the face enlarges, teeth compensate by erupting further. Eruption of teeth continues throughout life to maintain occlusion. An ankylosed primary molar serves as a good marker of eruptive changes because it is fused to the alveolar bone and does not keep pace with the active movements of other teeth.

Both cartilaginous and sutural growth contribute to the growth of the nasal region and upper face. The nasal septum is a cartilaginous remnant of the chondrocranium that ossifies posteriorly as the vomer bone. The anterior part remains as cartilage and continues growing later than most of the rest of the face. The gains in nose length and width are unrelated to other facial measurements. The forward growth of the forehead is due to the development of brow ridges and frontal sinuses. These sinuses are present at birth but are not aerated.

Although the sutures of the upper face are nearly parallel in arrangement, the upper face does not grow in a particular downward and forward direction away from the cranial base. Individual sutures may grow in a vertical, horizontal, or anterior–posterior direction, or permit sliding of bones along the suture line. Moreover, the overall vector of sutural growth is not consistent over time. Changes in direction are fairly common.

Growth Control

Even more important than descriptions of specific growth changes in individual bones and relations of bones is information related to the questions of how and why growth occurs. It is necessary to define the factors controlling growth and to understand growth mechanisms to promote normal facial development and alter deviate growth patterns.

Heredity and Environment

Heredity and environment jointly determine the facial growth pattern. The close resemblance of identical twins shows that the hereditary component is important. However, environmental influences are also active. For example, Eskimos developed a much higher prevalence of malocclusion within a generation of the arrival of modern civilization. Also, human traditions and animal experiments have shown that growth of bones can be altered. Bound Chinese feet and deformed Indian skulls demonstrate the adaptability of skeletal growth to environmental influences.

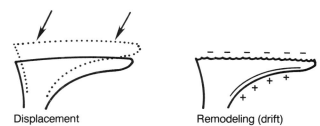

Displacement   Remodeling (drift)

Figure 4–13. In the growing face, the maxilla relative to the cranial base changes position as a result of both displacement and remodeling (drift).

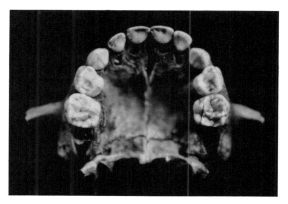

Figure 4–14. The maxillary tuberosity increases in length to create space for the developing second and third molars.

Clinical Application

The proportion of growth determined by heredity or environment is important from the standpoint of tissue receptivity to alteration by such means as the mechanical appliances used during orthodontic treatment. Sutures respond to mechanical stimuli, which makes it possible to inhibit forward maxillary growth or widen a constricted palate. Mandibular growth, however, is much more difficult to control.

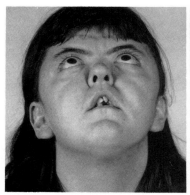
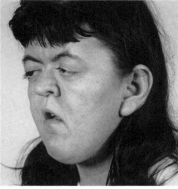

Figure 4–15. An example of Apert syndrome.

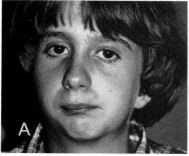
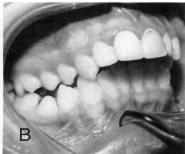

Figure 4–16. Injury to this child's temporomandibular joint has impaired growth, which has resulted in both facial (A) and dental (B) asymmetries.

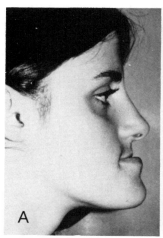
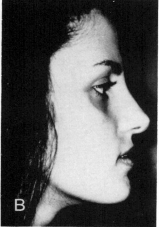

Figure 4–17. An example of mandibular prognathism before (A) and after (B) surgical correction.

Clinical Application

Only about half of young people in the United States have normal jaw and dental relations. The proportion of very severe malocclusions is the same in blacks and whites, approximately 15%. The types of disharmonies, however, differ with race; blacks are more likely that whites to have anterior open bite malocclusions, and whites are more likely than blacks to have severe crowding of teeth.

Abnormal Development

The biologic concepts developed in this chapter can be applied to individuals who have abnormal growth patterns. Knowledge of normal growth processes can be helpful in recognizing aberrant growth and in planning treatment. The gaps in our understanding of deviant growth processes and causes of facial deformity, however, are major and limit preventive and corrective efforts.

Some perplexing growth problems are seen in the genetic syndromes. For example, a patient with Apert syndrome has a peculiarly shaped cranial vault; a retruded midface with the maxilla sometimes fused to the sphenoid bone; abnormalities of the cranial base and upper spine; intraoral abnormalities, including bulbous alveolar processes in the maxilla and crowding of teeth; and fusion of the digits of the hands and feet (Fig. 4–15). Premature fusion of the cranial sutures produces an unusual skull form by preventing skull growth at the fused suture lines. Because the increased presssure produced by the growing brain may lead to severe mental and neurologic handicaps, early release of the fused sutures is a critical step in optimizing brain development. Treatment methods now in use are not effective, however, because osseous bridges between cranial bones soon recur. It is not known whether the sutures are themselves defective or whether the cells function through normal mechanisms but respond to an abnormal environment. Growth abnormalities are not limited to congenital malformations or inherited metabolic defects. Injury to the temporomandibular joint in a child can cause ankylosis or joint damage that leads to asymmetry and underdevelopment of the mandible on the traumatized side (Fig. 4–16). Mobility of the joint should be restored as soon as possible to maximize normal function and growth.

Mandibular prognathism is one of the most common facial deformities (Fig. 4–17A). Unlike many deformities that are congenital, malocclusions become apparent during postnatal development. Many explanations regarding the etiology of mandibular prognathism have been advanced, but no single explanation has proved to be adequate. Although some families seem to have more individuals affected than do other families, the pattern of genetic transmission has been unclear, and in many cases it is found to occur sporadically. The mechanisms of mandibular growth have been explored in animal experiments, but these studies have not progressed to the point of providing a basis for altering human growth. Consequently, the most effective treatment has been surgical reduction of mandibular length (Fig. 4–17B).

Growth is a factor that must be considered in planning treatment of facial deformities. For example, early surgical treatment of mandibular prognathism is often unsuccessful because the mandible continues to grow abnormally. In areas in which growth mechanisms are better understood, however, growth can be used advantageously. One argument in favor of early treatment holds that a primary defect causes secondary deformities in adjacent tissues. For example, lack of appropriate muscle function followed a partial facial nerve palsy and resulted in asymmetries in facial form that included underdevelopment of the mandible on the paralyzed side and deviation of the nasal tip (Fig. 4–18). In more severe deformities, tissues that are initially normal can be distorted even more than those shown in Figure 4–18. If proper relations are achieved at an early age, growth is more likely to proceed along a normal vector. In the development of normal dental relations, normal function of the lips, lip seal, and nasal breathing are thought to be important. Function is also important during remodeling of bone grafts into normal bone structure after surgical reconstruction. A successful mandibular bone graft can be difficult to detect on a radiograph, except for the stabilizing wires that remain (Fig. 4–19). A piece of iliac crest bone from the patient's hip was used to replace the diseased half of the mandible that included the condyle. After remodeling had occurred, not only did the graft assume an appropriate shape, but the bone trabeculations had the appearance of mandibular rather than iliac crest bone.

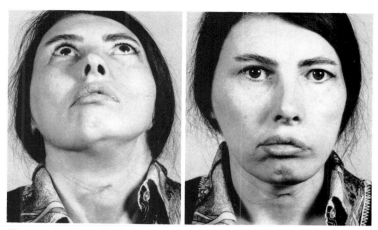

Figure 4–18. Facial asymmetry following partial facial nerve palsy.

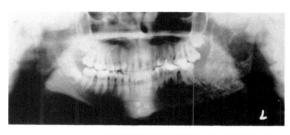
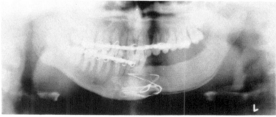

Figure 4–19. A mandible before (upper) and after (lower) placement of successful bone graft.

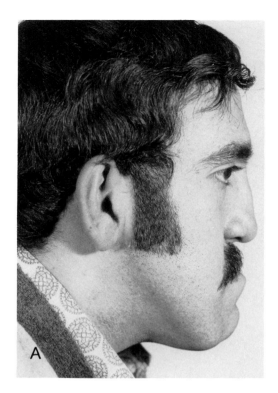

Some attempts to modify abnormal facial structures in children may actually inhibit growth. Surgical repair of clefts of the lip and palate have resulted in extensive scarring that retards forward development of the maxilla, especially when older techniques have been used (Fig. 4–20A). With use of these techniques, a different type of midface deformity is produced that necessitates other operations to advance the midface. If oral clefts are not treated, as has occurred in remote villages in India, even the severe bilateral clefts seen in adults are not accompanied by marked anterior–posterior discrepancies (Fig. 4–20B and C). Despite the devastating functional and cosmetic effects of the untreated oral cleft in the individual seen in Figure 4–20B and C, jaw relations are quite good.

Although many questions regarding growth mechanisms remain, some basic points that recognize the importance of growth can be stated. A program aimed at achieving or maintaining normal facial structure and function should (1) remove inhibitions of normal growth; (2) promote normal function; (3) reduce iatrogenic damage to tissues, such as surgical scars; and (4) consider the effect of growth on the final result when intervention during the growth period is necessary.

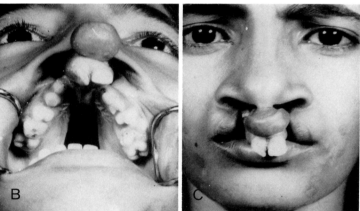

Figure 4–20. (A). Example of midface underdevelopment that resulted from restriction of maxillary growth by excessive scarring after early surgical repair of cleft lip and palate. (B) and (C). Untreated bilateral cleft of lip and palate in adult. Growth of the jaws has not been retarded, and jaw relations are quite good.

Summary

The principles of facial growth and development discussed in this chapter include specific biologic processes, sites of growth, timing, hereditary factors, receptivity to environmental cues, and variations found in abnormal development. Changes in the dental arches and alveolar processes are coordinated with facial growth.

Postnatal growth of the face is complex and varies considerably among children. Growth processes and their timing must be assessed carefully for individual patients to achieve optimal results from clinical treatment. Knowledge of growth concepts is imortant because, in some instances, growth improves the treatment outcome, whereas in other situations, growth interferes with attainment of a successful result.

Self-Evaluation Review

1. When does the face grow with respect to other parts of the body? During the postnatal period, which areas of the face grow proportionately more than other areas?
2. What factors may influence an individual's specific growth pattern?
3. Distinguish between biologic age and chronologic age. Why is maturity so important in determining timing of treatment?
4. How do growing bones change position relative to other bones?
5. Name areas of the mandible and maxilla that change relatively little during growth.
6. Describe the remodeling changes in the growing mandible that create space for the permanent molars.
7. List the cartilaginous structures of the face and identify whether they are primary or secondary in origin.
8. How does scarring affect maxillary growth in patients with cleft lip or palate?
9. Why is growth significant in the treatment of facial deformities?
10. How is the shape of bones influenced by function?

Acknowledgments

Figures 4–15, 4–18, and 4–20 were provided courtesy of Dr. Joseph Murray. Figures 4–16 and 4–17 were provided courtesy of Dr. Walter Guralnick.

Suggested Readings

Bjork A. *The Face in Profile*. Lund: Berlingska Boktryckeriet; 1947.

Enlow DH. *Facial Growth*. Philadelphia, Pa: WB Saunders Co; 1990.

Horowitz SL, Hixon E. H. *The Nature of Orthodontic Diagnosis*. St. Louis, Mo: CV Mosby; 1966.

Lundstrom A. Dental genetics. In: *Orofacial Growth and Development*. Dahlberg AA, Graber TM, eds. The Hague: Mouton Publishers; 1977.

Marshall WA, Tanner JM. Puberty. In: Davis JA, Dobbing J, eds. *Scientific Foundations of Paediatrics*. Philadelphia, Pa: WB Saunders; 1974.

Moore WJ, Lavelle CLB. *Growth of the Facial Skeleton in the Hominoidea*. London: Academic Press; 1974.

Moorrees CFA, Gron AM, Lebret LML, Yen PKJ, Frohlich FJ. Growth studies on the dentition: a review. *Am. J. Orthod.* 1969;44:600.

Tanner JM. *Growth at Adolescence*. Oxford: Blackwell Scientific Publications; 1962.

SECTION II

Development of the Teeth and Supporting Structures

CHAPTERS 5–8

Development of Teeth: Crown Formation

Nicholas P. Piesco and James K. Avery

Introduction
Overview of Dental Tissues

Prior to acquiring an understanding of tooth development, it is important to briefly review the structure of a fully developed tooth. Detailed descriptions of tooth anatomy are found in dental anatomy texts. Observing the gross features and low power microscopic view of a longitudinal section of the developed tooth provide important landmarks for understanding the process of odontogenesis or tooth formation.

Under gross inspection, the tooth consists of two parts, a crown and a root (roots) (Fig. 5–1). The crown provides the chewing or biting (occlusal or incisal) surface of the tooth and the root, with the alveolar bone and periodontal ligament, provides support for the tooth. The crown of a healthy tooth is covered with enamel. The part of the tooth exposed to the oral cavity is the clinical crown. That part covered with enamel is the anatomical crown. In young individuals, the gingiva covers part of the anatomical crown and the clinical crown may be smaller than the anatomical crown. In older individuals with gingival recession, part of the root may be exposed to the oral cavity and in this case the clinical crown will be larger than the anatomical crown since it would include some anatomical root structure. In this chapter, the term crown will refer to the anatomical crown. The root(s) of the tooth are covered with cementum. The junction between cementum and enamel, cementum-enamel junction, lies at the cervix (neck) of the tooth and is an important anatomical and embryological landmark.

Both the root and the crown consist primarily of dentin. On closer inspection, it is seen that dentin is tubular in nature and that the enamel consists of enamel rods or prisms. In both enamel and dentin, landmarks can be seen which indicate the incremental nature of matrix deposition. These are the incremental lines, stria or Retzius in enamel and incremental lines of von Ebner in dentin. The junction between the enamel and dentin (dentin-enamel junction) is another important embryological landmark.

The cementum is composed of mineralized matrix in which fibers of the periodontal ligament are embedded. It invests the root of the tooth which is surrounded by alveolar bone. Alveolar bone serves as the second attachment site for the fibers of the periodontal ligament.

The crown encloses a mass of soft tissue, the dental pulp, which resides in the central pulp chamber. This pulp chamber also has an extension into the root, the root canal. The outermost cells of the pulp form the protein matrix of dentin (mostly type I collagen) and are responsible for its mineralization. Between these dentin forming cells (odontoblasts) and the calcified dentin is a layer of predentin, a matrix which has not yet been mineralized. The junction between the dentin and predentin is the dentin mineralization front or dentin-predentin junction. At the apex of the root there is an opening, the apical foramen. This foramen functions as a passage for blood vessels, lymphatics and nerves to enter and exit the pulp chamber.

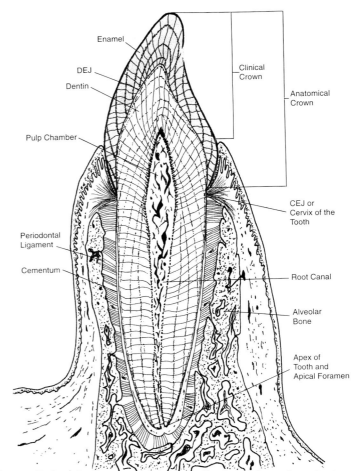

Figure 5–1. A diagram of longitudinal section of an incisor in situ. Note the anatomical boundaries between the mineralized tissues. DEJ, dentin-enamel junction. Observe the incremental lines in enamel and dentin.

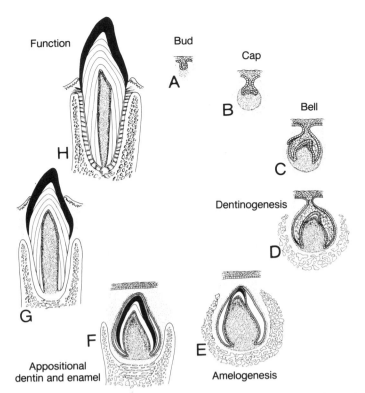

Figure 5-2. (A-H). Diagram depicting the stages of tooth development beginning with the bud stage (A).

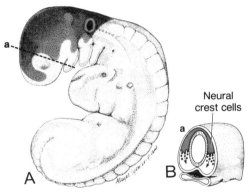

Figure 5-3. (A). Map of neural crest cell migration in a 4 week embryo. (B). Frontal section representing plane of section "a" in A and illustrating neural crest migration.

Clinical Application

The size of the tooth is dependent upon both the proliferative and secretory activities of the cells. Macrodontia, large teeth, and microdontia, small teeth, are the result of factors affecting the growth of the tooth germ at the cap and bell stages. In true macro- and microdontia all teeth are affected. In false macro- and microdontia individual teeth are affected. True macro- and microdontia may be the result of over- and undersecretion of pituitary hormones (gigantism and dwarfism).

Overview of Tooth Development

Teeth develop as a result of the interaction between oral epithelium and underlying mesenchymal tissue. Twenty primary tooth germs develop initially, with 32 additional tooth germs differentiating to form the permanent dentition. Although each tooth germ develops as an anatomically distinct unit, the fundamental developmental process is similar for all teeth. Each tooth develops through successive bud, cap, and bell stages (Fig. 5-2A, B, and C). During the early stages, tooth germs grow and expand, and cells that will form the hard components of the teeth differentiate. Once the formative cells of the tooth germ differentiate, formation and mineralization of dentin and enamel matrices take place (Fig. 5-2D, E, and F). Subsequently, the completed tooth erupts into the oral cavity (Fig. 5-2G). As eruption occurs, tooth roots surrounded by the periodontal ligament and supporting alveolar bone develop (Fig. 5-2G and H). Root formation proceeds until a functional tooth and its supporting apparatus are fully developed (Fig. 5-2H).

Objectives

The overall objectives of this chapter are to enable the student to: 1) describe, in detail, the origin of the tooth formative cells and the role of induction in tooth formation; 2) describe each stage of tooth formation, including the details of mineralization of the dentin and enamel in the crown; 3) explain the developmental processes which are responsible for crown growth and the distinct junctions between dissimilar dental tissues.

Origin of Dental Tissues

Neural crest cells constitute the ectomesenchyme of the head and neck and induce the formation of many connective tissues of the face, which include the dental structures. The role of ectomesenchyme in the development of teeth and their supporting structures, however, is not completely understood. Ectomesenchyme arises from the neural folds. As these folds close, neural crest cells migrate down the sides of the head along pathways underlying the skin (Fig. 5.3A and B). Some investigators consider these to be a fourth germ layer, cytologically; others consider these to be a merging of two cell types, ectodermal and mesodermal, which in turn, form cells that resemble both types.

During the sixth week in utero, the ectoderm covering the oral cavity is composed of an epithelial layer, two to three cells thick. In the region of the future alveolar processes, the oral epithelium proliferates and forms the dental laminae (Fig. 5–4A and B). These are horseshoe-shaped bands that traverse the circumference of the lower and upper jaws, and give rise to the ectodermally-derived portions of the teeth (Fig. 5–5). The dental laminae undergo further proliferation at sites corresponding to the positions of the 20 primary teeth, which results in rounded or ovoid tooth buds or tooth germs that protrude into the mesenchyme (Fig. 5–5). The maxillary and mandibular dental laminae give rise to 52 such buds, 20 for the primary teeth, which arise between the sixth and eighth prenatal week and 32 for the permanent teeth, which appear at later prenatal periods (Fig. 5–5). Successional tooth buds of the permanent dentition develop lingual to the tooth buds of their deciduous predecessors. This occurs in utero at 5 months of age for the central incisors and 10 months of age for the premolars. The lingual extension of the dental lamina that gives rise to the successional teeth is therefore, called the successional lamina (Fig. 5–5).

The permanent molars develop posterior to the deciduous molars. The posterior growth of the dental lamina gives rise to the first permanent molar buds during the fourth prenatal month and the second permanent molars at 4 years of age. A second lamina, the vestibular lamina, develops simultaneously and in association with the dental lamina. The vestibular lamina first forms a wedge of epithelial cells, facial or buccal to the dental lamina (Fig. 5–5 and 5–6). It will form the oral vestibule or the space between the teeth and lips or cheeks. Teeth develop anteroposteriorly, which means that anterior teeth develop slightly ahead, temporally, of posterior teeth. Each is of a different type (Figs. 5–5 and 5–6).

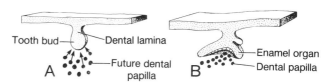

Figure 5–4. (A). Induction of tooth primordia. (B). Further induction of the enamel organ.

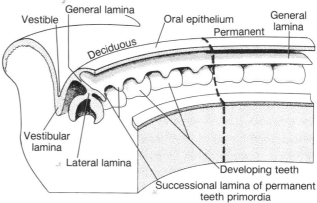

Figure 5–5. Stylized diagram depicting the continuity of the dental lamina system for deciduous and permanent teeth. Note the permanent molars arise from the general lamina and not the successional lamina.

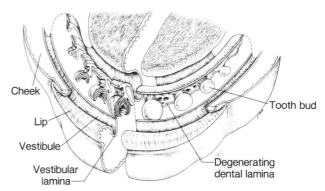

Figure 5–6. Development of tooth buds in developing alveolar processes.

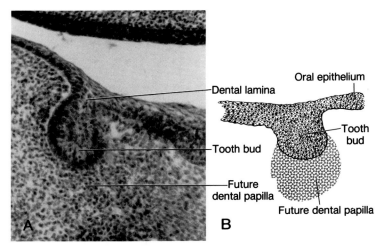

Figure 5–7. (A). Histology of tooth development at the bud stage. (B). Diagram of tooth development at the bud stage.

Bud, Cap, and Bell Stages

Although tooth formation is a continuous process, it may be characterized by a series of distinguishable stages referred to as the bud, cap and bell. These developmental stages are named according to the shape of the epithelial portion of the tooth during transition (Figs. 5–7, 5–8, and 5–9).

The *bud stage* is the initial stage of tooth development. The bud stage designates the rounded, localized growth of the epithelial cells of the dental lamina (Fig. 5.7A and B) and is also defined as the proliferative stage because it is the stage in which the initial proliferation of oral epithelial cells and adjacent mesenchymal cells is occurring. The result is a bud-shaped enamel organ. The mesenchymal cells then form the dental papilla. Gradually, the epithelial bud gains a concave surface, and the developing tooth is then considered to be in the cap stage (Fig. 5–8A and B). The cells which surround the enamel organ and the cells of the adjacent dental papilla further divide and grow around the enamel organ to form an additional ectomesenchymal condensation, the dental follicle or sac.

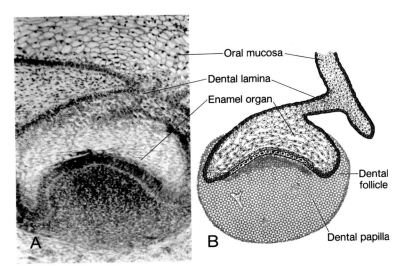

Figure 5–8. (A). Histology of tooth development at the cap stage. (B). Diagram of tooth development at the cap stage.

Clinical Application

Absence of teeth, partial or total anodontia (missing some or all teeth), is due to factors that disrupt tooth development at the initiation stage (at the dental lamina or bud stage). In the genetic disorder ectodermal dysplasia there is total anodontia. Other ectodermal derivatives are affected as well. For example, hair, sebaceous, and sweat glands are missing. In partial anodontia the most common missing teeth are maxillary and mandibular third molars. Canines are the teeth least likely to be missing.

All three structures, enamel organ, dental papilla and dental follicle, are seen in the *cap stage*. These constitute the tooth germ and give rise to teeth supporting structures (Fig. 5–8A and B). The epithelial enamel organ gives rise to enamel. The dental papilla gives rise to the dentin and pulp. The dental follicle forms the cementum, periodontal ligament, and adjacent alveolar bone. The enamel organ in the cap stage consists of four types of cells: (1) those cells that cover the convex surface, which are the outer enamel epithelial cells (OEE); (2) those cells that line the concavity of the enamel *organ*, which are called the inner enamel epithelial cells (IEE); (3) a layer of cells adjacent to the IEE, are referred to as the stratum intermedium (SI); and those cells that fill the remainder of the enamel organ, are termed the stellate reticulum (SR). The area of the enamel organ where the inner and outer enamel epithelial cells join one another is called the cervical loop. It is an area of active cell proliferation and lies in an area which will become the cervix of the tooth. Following the formation of the crown this area will give rise to the epithelial root sheath and epithelial diagram. During the cap stage another localized area of cell proliferation forms a relatively dense mass of cells near the center of the enamel organ adjacent to the stratum intermedium. This area is known as the enamel knot. Its function is unknown but it may serve as a source of epithelial cells during the ensuing stages of development or eruption.

After further increase in the size of the enamel organ and adjacent dental papilla, the tooth germ proceeds from the cap stage to the bell stage or differentiation stage (Fig. 5–9). This stage has two characteristics: (1) the shape of the future tooth crown is defined by the junction between the inner enamel epithelium and dental papilla. (This process, a change from an undifferentiated cap stage tooth to a differentiated adult-looking bell stage tooth is also called morphodifferentiation.); and (2) the inner enamel epithelial cells elongate and differentiate into ameloblasts which become the future enamel-forming cells. Adjacent to the ameloblasts, the layer of cells of the dental papilla differentiate into odontoblasts. In the enamel organ, the cells adjacent to the opposite side of the ameloblasts make up the stratum intermedium, these cells become spindle-shaped and lie in an axis at 90° to the ameloblasts. These cells are connected to the ameloblasts by desmosomes and gap junctions. The stratum intermedium cells, are thought to function with ameloblasts in the mineralization of the enamel. The cells of the stellate reticulum constitute the bulk of the enamel organ at this stage. They are star-shaped (stellate) and are connected to one another by numerous desmosomes. The extracellular matrix in the large extracellular spaces between these cells is thought to be filled with proteoglycans. Although the cells of the stellate reticulum are metabolically active, their role in amelogenesis has not been entirely determined. The large spaces within the stellate reticulum are thought to provide a protective "cushion" for the developing crown, and provide space into which the ameloblasts move during matrix formation. The outer enamel epithelial cells then become

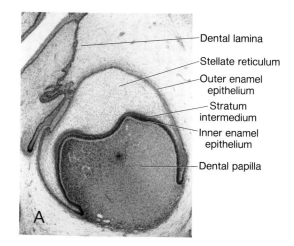

Dental lamina
Stellate reticulum
Outer enamel epithelium
Stratum intermedium
Inner enamel epithelium
Dental papilla

A

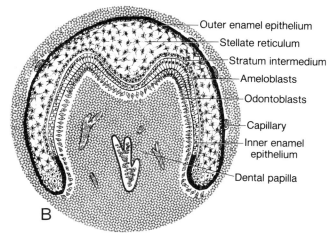

Outer enamel epithelium
Stellate reticulum
Stratum intermedium
Ameloblasts
Odontoblasts
Capillary
Inner enamel epithelium
Dental papilla

B

Figure 5–9. (A). Histology of tooth development at the bell stage. (B). Diagram of tooth development at the bell stage.

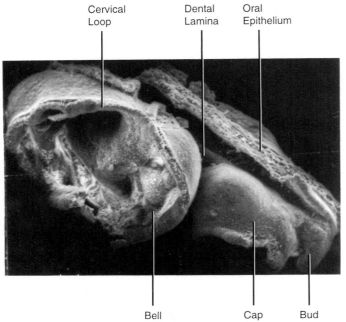

Figure 5–10. Scanning electron micrograph of the dental lamina with attached enamel organs at the bud cap and bell stage of development. Epithelium was separated from dental mesenchyme by enzyme treatment and gentle mechanical force.

associated with a capillary plexus, which will function to bring nutritional substances and oxygen to ameloblasts and other enamel organ cells (Fig. 5–9A).

The enamel organ during the *bell stage* consists of four well-defined types of cells: (1) those cells that cover the outer convex surface, which are the outer dental or enamel epithelial cells (ODE or OEE); (2) these cells that line the concavity of the enamel organ, which are called the inner dental or enamel epithelial cells (IDE or IEE); (3) a layer of cells adjacent to the IDE which are referred to as the stratum intermedium (SI); and (4) those that fill the remainder of the enamel organ which are termed the stellate reticulum (SR). This process, differentiation of the cells of the enamel organ and dental papilla, is called cytodifferentiation. The position of the inner enamel organ cells, at the bell stage defines the shape of the crown, and is called the morphodifferentiation stage (Fig. 5–10).

During the late bell stage, the general and lateral dental laminae begin to degenerate. The tooth bud has differentiated and is independent of the oral epithelium. In this process, the epithelial cells of the dental lamina undergo lysis until the lamina disappears (Fig. 5–11). The general lamina is maintained more posteriorly in the mouth, however, where other teeth are less advanced in development (Fig. 5–11).

Development of the Pulp Organ

The young dental papilla is more densely packed with cells than are tissues surrounding the teeth. In Figure 5–12, two primary maxillary tooth buds are seen above two mandibular molars in the lower jaw. Both are in the bell and dentinogenesis stages. The high cell density in the papillae is an indication of cell division in the papilla which will keep pace with growth of the enamel organ.

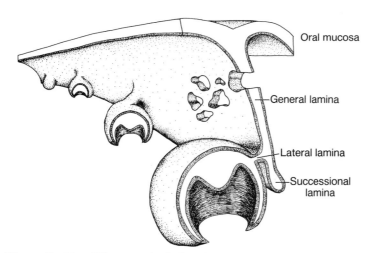

Figure 5–11. Diagram depicting the general and lateral lamina as well as the beginning of the dissolution of the dental lamina.

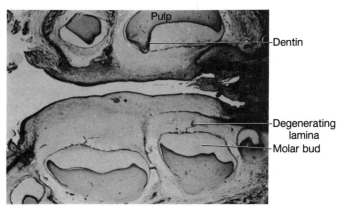

Figure 5–12. Sagittal section of the jaws of an embryo illustrating developing teeth.

As peripheral dental papilla cells transform into columnar-shaped odontoblasts they develop cell processes (Fig. 5–13). The odontoblasts then begin dentin formation, which is termed dentinogenesis, (Fig. 5–13A). During dentinogenesis, the dental papilla becomes surrounded (except at the apical area) by dentin and it is then termed the pulp organ (Fig. 5–13A). The pulp organ and dentin are closely related. The dentin-forming odontoblasts reside in the periphery of the pulp and recede as they form the dentin matrix. These cells maintain cell processes in dentin.

In Figure 5–13B the majority of the cells of the pulp organ are seen to be fibroblasts and appear as a delicate reticulum. A few larger blood vessels traverse the central area of the pulp; and smaller ones appear in its periphery. Although large nerve trunks are located near the developing young teeth, only those associated with blood vessels enter the young pulps. Later as the teeth erupt and come into function, the larger myelinated nerves become more abundant throughout the pulp organ.

Interaction of the Epithelium and Mesenchyme in Tooth Development

Experiments designed to determine the role of epithelium and mesenchyme in the initiation of tooth development make use of epithelial-mesenchymal recombinations. In these experiments, the epithelium and mesenchyme of developing teeth or other organs are experimentally separated with the aid of matrix digesting enzymes and some gentle mechanical force (Fig. 5–10). This tissue is allowed to grow in culture. These experiments determine whether the interaction between mesenchyme and epithelium is necessary for induction. Furthermore, it provides the distinction between instructive and permissive interactions.

When the enamel organ and dental papilla are separated from one another and grown independently both will proliferate, but no recognizable tooth structures are formed. At best, the epithelium may keratinize and the papilla may form bone. This shows that the interaction of the two cell types are necessary and that neither tissue can continue along a path of differentiation independent of the other.

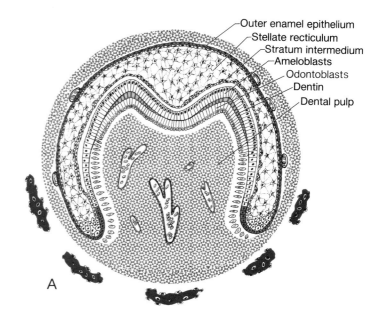

Outer enamel epithelium
Stellate recticulum
Stratum intermedium
Ameloblasts
Odontoblasts
Dentin
Dental pulp

A

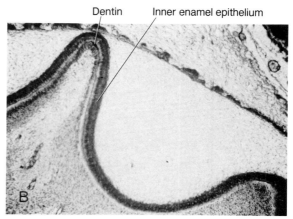

Dentin   Inner enamel epithelium

B

Figure 5–13. (A). Diagram of tooth development and initial dentinogenesis. (B). Light micrograph demonstrating the histology of initial dentinogenesis and the beginning of the appositional stage.

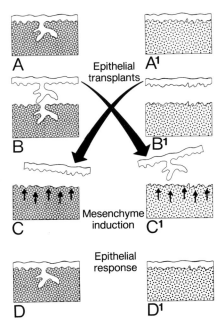

Figure 5–14. Induction of tooth primordia by neural crest cells in mesenchyme. (A). Indicates transplantation of enamel organ epithelium from the site of the alveolar process to lip or check mesenchyme; the result is a lack of continued induction of tooth primordia (C¹, D¹). (A¹). Indicates the transplantation of epithelium from lip or cheek to mesenchyme of dental alveolar process; the result is the induction of tooth primordia at C and D.

When cap-derived dental mesenchyme from molar teeth is recombined with epithelium from an incisor a molar tooth will result. Furthermore, when recombined with epithelium from the diastema (a toothless region in the jaw) or nonoral epithelium a complete tooth will result. Dental epithelium (enamel organ) when recombined with nondental mesenchyme does not result in the formation of tooth structures (Fig. 5–14). These experiments indicate that the mesenchyme, at the cap stage of development and beyond, determines tooth type and can induce dental development from nondental epithelium (secretion of enamel). The mesenchyme exerts an instructive influence on the epithelium, because it can change the fate of the epithelium (from the original stratified squamous keratinizing or nonkeratinizing epithelium to an enamel organ which secretes enamel). On the other hand, the epithelium exerts a permissive influence on the dental mesenchyme, because only its presence is necessary for dental development.

These recombination experiments are true for interactions occurring during the morphogenesis and proliferative stages. A somewhat different image emerges when looking at similar experiments performed during the period in which the patterning or positioning of teeth occur, i.e., prior to the bud stage of development. Recombinations have been performed in which premigratory neural crest and early oral epithelium or early first arch (maxillary) mesenchyme and epithelium were recombined with second arch (hyoid) epithelium and mesenchyme. In these circumstances, tooth development would only proceed if oral (first arch) epithelium was included in the recombination. This indicates that the epithelium provides an instructional role during the earliest stage of tooth formation and that the fate of the neural crest cells are not determined prior to migration. It appears that these reciprocal cell interactions occur in two stages. The first specifies the "dental nature" of the mesenchyme, and the second specifies the tooth type and nature of products produced by the epithelium and mesenchyme. Recent research indicates that the proliferation of epithelium and possibility the patterning of teeth (incisor and molar fields) at the earliest stage of tooth formation may be controlled by the local production of retinoids and/or growth factors.

In order to determine the mechanism of induction at later stages, during the differentiation of dental tissues, dental papilla and enamel organ have been cultured on opposite sides of a porous membrane. These transfilter experiments test the hypothesis of whether cell-cell contact or diffusible molecules are involved in the signaling process. Filters which had pore sizes less than 0.2 μm prevented differentiation. Pores of this size would not prevent the diffusion of molecules but do prevent cell processes from either the mesenchyme or epithelium from reaching one another. This rules out the existence of a diffusible molecule as the signal. Since inhibitors of matrix synthesis inhibit tooth development and processes of dental mesenchyme have been seen reaching the epithelial basement membrane, it has been concluded that contact with the basal lamina and its associated matrix is the trigger for odontoblastic differentiation. This would be an example of a short range matrix-mediated interaction. It is now known that the basement membrane contains molecules which have growth factor capabilities as well as growth factors themselves. Furthermore, basement membrane proteoglycan is capable of binding many growth factors with high affinity. These may be active during the early stages of differentiation. Another matrix molecule in the basement membrane, fibronectin, with cell adhesion molecules has been implicated in contributing to initiation of odontoblastic polarization. Tenascin, a matrix protein not associated with the basement membrane, has been implicated as being involved in mesenchymal condensation during the early development of numerous organs including teeth.

Direct cell-cell contact, without the formation of specialized junctions, between preameloblasts and preodontoblasts has been seen with the electron microscope. During this period the basal lamina, between preodontoblasts and preameloblasts, is penetrated by epithelial processes. It becomes discontinuous and is eventually eliminated. Some epithelial processes come close to the processes from preodontoblasts, and some preodontoblast processes encroach into epithelial territory and may extend between epithelial cells. The eventual deposition of enamel around these preodontoblast processes results in the formation of enamel spindles. These heterotypic contacts are not believed to be involved in induction, because they occur following the initiation of polarization of odontoblasts and ameloblasts (see Fig. 5–15). Furthermore, these heterotypic contacts form at a time when the first enamel and dentin are being deposited prior to the full differentiation odontoblasts and ameloblasts.

Dentinogenesis

Oval or polygonal cells located near the basal lamina that separates the enamel organ from the dental papilla are the preodontoblasts. These cells elongate and become young odontoblasts. With further elongation and the formation of an apical process, they are termed odontoblasts. As the odontoblasts secrete matrix materials consisting of collagen fibrils and other organic materials (predentin), they migrate towards the center of the pulp and away from the basal lamina (Fig. 5–15A and D).

In the process of differentiation, odontoblasts become columnar polarized cells having a secretary or apical pole and a nonsecretory or basal pole. This polarization distinguishes odontoblasts from other collagen-producing cells. Odontoblasts, joined to one another by extensive gap junctions and junctional complexes, form a well defined layer of cells on the periphery of the pulp. An extensively developed endoplasmic reticulum and Golgi apparatus, hallmarks of protein secreting cells, are characteristic of the active secretory odontoblast. The odontoblast process, also known as Tomes' fiber, becomes embedded in the extracellular matrix of the

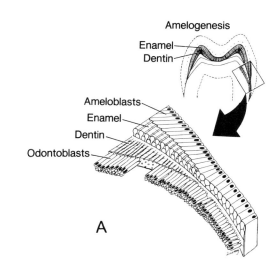

Figure 5–15. Diagram of histodifferentiation within the developing tooth. (A). Sites of initial dentin and enamel formation. (Figure continued on next page).

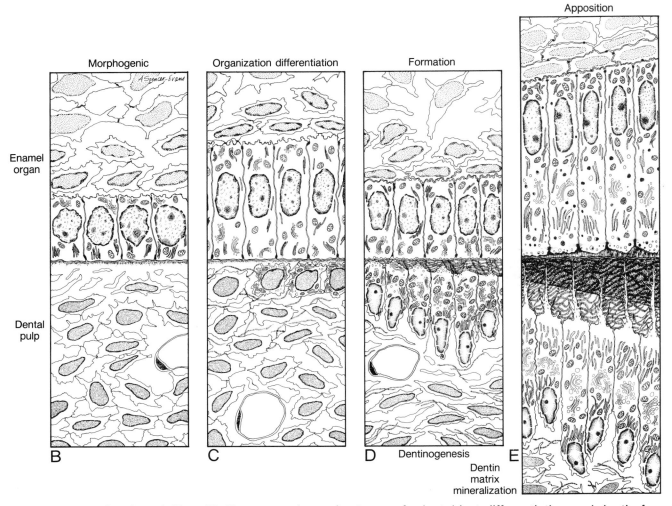

Figure 5–15. *Continued.* (B to D). Represent the early stages of odontoblast differentiation and dentin formation. (B to I). Represent important stages of ameloblast differentiation and the formation of enamel. Note in G and H the ameloblast differentiation and the formation of enamel. Note in G and H that the ameloblasts modulate alternating these forms during amelogenesis.

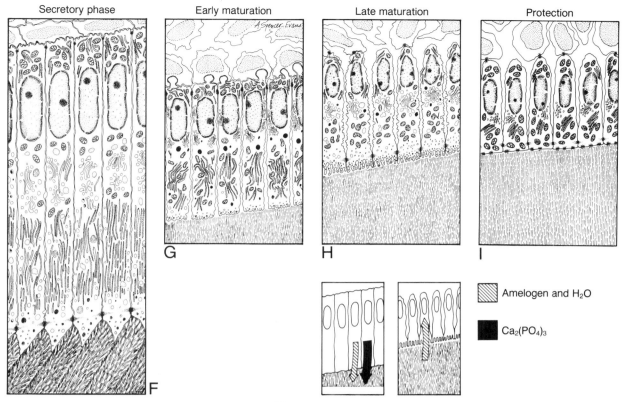

| Secretory phase | Early maturation | Late maturation | Protection |

F

G

H

I

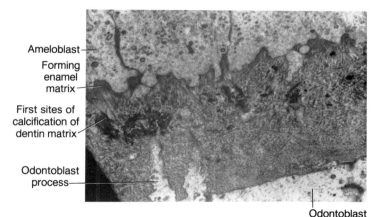

Amelogen and H₂O

Ca₂(PO₄)₃

Figure 5–15. *Continued.*

predentin and elongates as the odontoblast retreats from the ameloblast layer of the enamel organ. Observe the first-formed predentin matrix in Figures 5–15 and 5–16. As the odontoblasts elongate, their nuclei occupy a basal position in the cell, and the organelles become more evident toward the apical ends of the cells (Fig. 5–15D). The appearance of the granular endoplasmic reticulum, Golgi complex, and mitochondria indicates the protein-synthesizing nature of these cells (Figs. 5–15D and E). The odontoblasts immediately begin forming the precursors of collagen on the ribosomes of the granular endoplasmic reticulum, and the protein is concentrated in the Golgi complex. The cells then secrete the protein externally via transport vesicles at the apical part of the cell and along its process. The collagenous dentin matrix is not mineralized when it is first deposited and is therefore termed predentin.

During differentiation, some of the first formed collagen fibers pass between the differentiating odontoblasts and extend toward the basal lamina where they appear to end in a fan-like arrangement. These fibers, Korff's fibers, stain with silver salts and are visible at the light microscopic level. However, electron microscopy has revealed that these thick fibers are mostly made of proteoglycans. Ultrastructural evidence has shown that some fine collagen fibers pass between odontoblasts and appear to have their origin deeper in the papilla.

Ameloblast

Forming enamel matrix

First sites of calcification of dentin matrix

Odontoblast process

Odontoblast

Figure 5–16. Transmission electron micrograph of initial mineralization of dentin which appear in small vesicles.

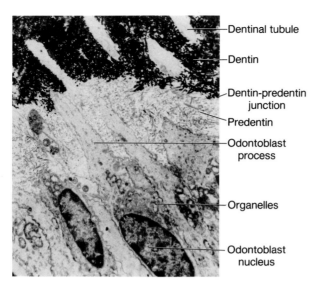

Figure 5–17. Transmission electron micrograph of the mineralization front or dentin-predentin junction.

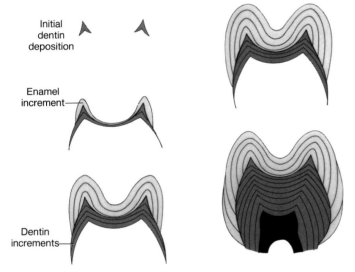

Figure 5–18. Diagram depicting the incremental deposition of dentin and enamel.

As this collagen matrix formation proceeds, the odontoblasts move further away (inwardly) from what will become the dentin-enamel junction (DEJ). The ends of odontoblastic processes maintain their positions (Figs. 5–15D and E and 5–16 and 5–17) and as a result the odontoblast process lengthens. The dentin-enamel junction lies at the former junction between the inner enamel epithelium and dental mesenchyme or basement membrane. The matrix which forms around the elongated cell processes eventually mineralizes (Fig. 5–15E) and the odontoblastic process will lie within a dentinal tubule.

Mineralization of the first-formed predentin is thought to occur in one of two ways: (1) Small mineral crystals appear in extracellular vesicles, matrix vesicles, and mineralization spreads from these sites throughout the first-formed predentin. (2) Small mineral crystals are nucleated in spaces which exist in collagen fibrils (due to the staggered arrangement of tropocollagen molecules). Crystals are oriented along the long axis of these fibrils. These minute crystals grow and spread throughout the predentin, until only the newly formed band of collagen along the pulp is uncalcified (Fig. 5–16). The average crystal attains a size of 425 nm in length and 65 nm in width and 25 nm in thickness. The process of matrix formation and mineralization, therefore, are closely related. Mineralization proceeds by a gradual increase in mineral density of the dentin (Fig. 5–17). As each daily increment of predentin forms along the pulpal boundary, the more peripheral adjacent predentin, which formed during the previous day, mineralizes and becomes dentin (Fig. 5–18). As the predentin calcifies and becomes dentin the mineralization front or dentin-predentin junction becomes established. Following the establishment of the dentin-predentin junction, the dental papilla becomes the dental pulp. Predentin is continuously formed along the pulpal border during crown formation and following eruption, and is calcified along the predentin-dentin junction (Figs. 5–16 and 5–17). This results in a decrease in the volume of the pulp cavity.

During the period of crown development and during eruption, approximately 4 μm of dentin is laid down daily (Fig. 5–18). After the teeth reach occlusion, the deposition rate decreases to a level of less than 1 μm per day. The amount of predentin formed each day along the pulpal boundary is termed an increment. "Increment" means an increase in number or size, and the daily incremental deposition is demarcated by microscopically visible lines in either the teeth or hard tissue of the teeth or bones. These lines are appropriately termed incremental lines (Fig. 5–18) and are believed to result from hesitation in matrix formation and subsequently altered mineralization. This may occur when the basal metabolism is lowest each day. Incremental deposition and mineralization of dentin begins at the tips of the pulp horns at the DEJ and proceeds by the rhythmic deposition of conical layers in the cusps until the crowns are completely formed (Fig. 5–18). Dentinogenesis is thus continued until the entire crown is complete and long after the tooth begins to erupt. Root development continues during and after tooth eruption. These details are described in detail in other chapters.

The odontoblastic process contributes an important role in maintaining the vitality and the distribution of matrix proteins (for example, dentin phosphoproteins are only found in mineralized dentin and at the mineralization front), the secretion and removal of matrix components as well as the mineralization of dentin.

Amelogenesis

As the premeloblast differentiates to become a secretory ameloblast it also polarizes (Fig. 5–15F–H). Intracellular changes involve a lengthening of the cell, proliferation of ER, and redistribution of cellular organelles (basal migration of the nucleus and apical migration of the Golgi apparatus). As enamel matrix is deposited, the ameloblast migrates in an outward direction and acquires a set of apical and basal terminal bars, as well as a specialized apical process, Tomes' process. Tomes' process can be defined as that part of the ameloblast, apical (or distal) to the apical terminal bars. The process contains numerous secretion granules and is usually devoid of endoplasmic reticulum and mitochondria. The Tomes' process can be divided into two portions, a proximal and distal part. The proximal part of Tomes' process contacts adjacent ameloblasts. The distal part, also called the interdigitating part, is surrounded by (or interdigitates with) the enamel matrix (Fig. 5–19A and B).

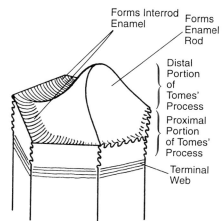

Figure 5–19. (B). Diagram of the Tomes' process of a secretory ameloblast. The distal part projects into the enamel (see also Fig. 5–22) and forms the enamel rod. The proximal part rests on the enamel surface forming interrod enamel.

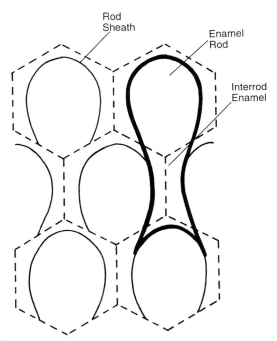

Figure 5–19. (A). Diagram depicting enamel rods. The arcades represent the rod sheaths and a line connecting the open ends encloses an enamel rod; the rest is interrod enamel. The hexagonal profile represents the secretory territory of one ameloblast. Note that it takes 4 ameloblasts to form the outlined keyhole structure but only one forms an enamel rod.

The supranuclear cytoplasm of the ameloblast contains a cylindrical Golgi apparatus. Its trans (maturing) face is more centrally located. Mitochondria are scattered throughout the cytoplasm. Laterally, ameloblasts are connected to one another by gap junctions, tight junctions and desmosomes. The part of the ameloblast which lies basal to the basal terminal web is called the basal bulge. Numerous blunt processes extend from the basal bulge which contact neighboring stratum intermedium cells. Ameloblasts and cells of the stratum intermedium are connected to one another by desmosomes and gap junctions. The gap junctions between adjacent ameloblasts and the ameloblasts and the cells of the stratum intermedium provide the basis for cell-cell communication and enable these cells to function as a unit.

The secretary ameloblast (Fig. 5–19B and C) like the odontoblast is a polarized cell having a secretory or apical end and a nonsecretory or basal end. It migrates in an outward direction away from the dentin-enamel junction and secretes enamel. The initial or first-formed enamel is aprismatic. As the ameloblast develops and acquires a Tomes' process enamel prisms are formed. Unlike dentin, enamel matrix is partially mineralized as soon as it is secreted. Two major types of proteins, the amelogenins and the enamelins have been found in the enamel matrix. These proteins are believed to provide important roles in the orientation and growth of enamel crystals. Amelogenins have been detected in secretory ameloblasts by immunocytochemical staining and are ameloblast secretory products. The nature of enamelins is controversial. They have not yet been proven to be the products of cells of the enamel organ, but are similar to serum albumins in amino acid composition. Therefore, the possibility exists that they are serum-derived. Recently, a new enamel protein with the characteristics of enamelin, tuftulin, has been found in enamel. Enamelins bind tightly to hydroxyapatite and may in some way regulate crystal growth. Unlike dentin, enamel crystals are arranged in a pattern and are much larger than those of dentin.

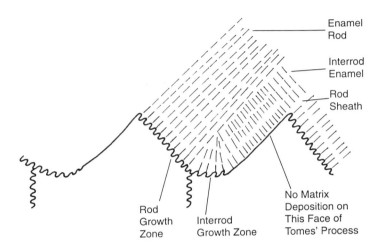

Figure 5–19. (C). Diagram depicting a longitudinal section through Tomes' process. Note that there are 2 growth sites, one for the rod and one for interrod enamel. The smooth face of the distal Tomes' process slides along the enamel matrix as the ameloblast retreats. Lines represent the orientation of enamel crystallites which grow perpendicular to the forming membrane. Observe the abrupt change in direction at the tip of the Tomes process (see Fig. 5–20).

Concept of the Enamel Rod

The structure of fully developed enamel will be explained in another chapter. However, a general understanding of the enamel rod provides an important foundation for the understanding of its development. Mature enamel, when sectioned perpendicularly to its free (external) surface is seen to consist of arch-like structures, rod sheaths or arcades which serve as the boundaries of the enamel rod (Fig. 5–19A). The alternate arrangement of these arcades in rows roughly outlines a keyhole-, fish- or paddle-like pattern (see Fig. 5–19A). This pattern is not seen near the dentin-enamel junction nor near the enamel surface. These areas represent areas of prismless enamel. The formation of enamel into rods or prisms is due to the staggered secretory front created by the orientation of the distal end of the secretory ameloblast (Tomes' process). When enamel secretion occurs along a flat secretory front, during the initial and final secretion of enamel (see below), there are no prisms in the enamel. When enamel secretion occurs by fully developed secretory ameloblasts in the presence of a Tomes' process enamel rods are formed.

There are two different concepts of an enamel rod. One definition holds that the keyhole- or paddle-like structures referred to above represent the enamel rod. If one projects the secretory territory of an ameloblast over these keyhole-shaped rods we can see that 4 different ameloblasts contribute to the synthesis of one enamel rod or keyhole (Fig. 5–19A). With this view there can be no interrod enamel.

Other investigators hold the view "one enamel rod—one ameloblast." With the "one rod—one ameloblast view" an enamel rod is defined as the enamel bounded by the rod sheaths (arcades) and a line connecting the two ends of the arcades. This corresponds to the head of the keyhole and it is made by one ameloblast. The "tail" would then represent interrod enamel, enamel which lies between the enamel rods (Fig. 5–19A, B, C). The difference between rod and interrod enamel is not chemical, but in the orientation of the hydroxyapatite crystals (Figs. 5–20 and 5–21). Initial enamel is formed when the basal lamina is being eliminated and lacks enamel rods and is aprismatic. The bulk of the enamel, inner enamel, is secreted during the secretion stage of amelogenesis when the ameloblasts have a fully developed Tomes' process. Enamel rods are formed at this time. The enamel rod represents the path an ameloblast took during its outward migration from the DEJ. Final enamel is produced during the time the Tomes' processes are regressing, and the ameloblasts are in the stage of postsecretory transition and maturation. During the formation of initial and final enamel layers only the proximal, or noninterdigitating portion of Tomes' process is present. Since this is the portion of Tomes' process responsible for forming interrod enamel, the initial and final enamel layers would resemble one another because of their similar origin. With the "one ameloblast—one rod" theory the enamel rods can be thought of as being bound by interrod enamel on their sides, and capped by aprismatic initial and final enamel. The initial and final enamel would be continuous with interrod enamel, and could be considered as interrod enamel. While neither concept of the enamel rod is "wrong," the "one ameloblast—one rod" approach better correlates the formation of the enamel rod during development and with other species which have very different prismatic arrangement.

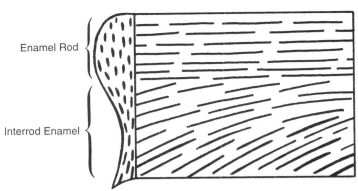

Figure 5-20. Diagrammatical representation of the orientation of crystals in rod and interrod enamel.

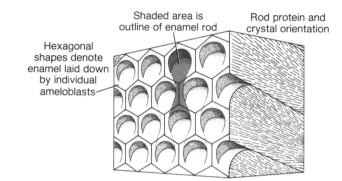

Figure 5–21. Diagram of the emeloblast-enamel rod interface.

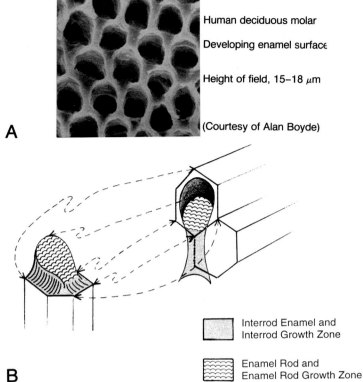

Human deciduous molar

Developing enamel surface

Height of field, 15–18 μm

(Courtesy of Alan Boyde)

A

B

☐ Interrod Enamel and Interrod Growth Zone

〰 Enamel Rod and Enamel Rod Growth Zone

Figure 5–22. (A). Scanning electron micrograph of the forming enamel rod-ameloblast interface. (B). Diagram of the relationship of the Tomes' process to the interface in A. Note the edge of the Tomes' process corresponds to the rod sheath.

Relationship of Tomes' Process to the Enamel Rod

Figures 5–19B and 5–22B are diagrammatical representations of a Tomes' process which might be seen in human enamel. The interdigitating portion of Tomes' process, also called the distal portion of Tomes' process, is surrounded by enamel. It has a sloping surface which faces the newly forming enamel rod (the formative face) and an opposing face (nonformative face) lying adjacent to interrod enamel. As can also be seen in the diagram, the Tomes' process has at its base a ''trough.'' The interrod enamel is formed in this area. The trough represents the face of the proximal portion of Tomes' process and can be thought of as a formative face. However, it forms the interrod enamel while the formative face of the interdigitating portion of Tomes' process forms the enamel rod.

When the Tomes' processes are removed from developing enamel, the exposed enamel surface consists of ''pits'' in which the Tomes' processes resided (Figs. 5–21 and 5–22A and B). These pits have three relatively steep ''walls'' and one gently sloping ''floor.'' The ''floor'' of the pit represents the enamel rod, and is formed by the sloping formative face of the interdigitating or distal portion of Tomes' process. The walls of the pit represent interrod enamel, formed by the formative face of the proximal portion of Tomes' process. Since the floor is sloped, the enamel of the floor blends with the wall or interrod enamel. It should be obvious that the enamel formed at the ''deeper regions'' of the floor of the pit, the enamel rod, is developmentally younger than the adjacent walls or interrod enamel.

When examined in section, triangular profiles of the ameloblasts are seen in the surrounding enamel (Fig. 5–15F and 5–19C). The appearance is somewhat deceiving in that the outline of the Tomes' process is not triangular but really consists of the apex of the triangle, one side being the formative and the other the nonformative face of Tomes' process, which is an extension from the side of an adjacent triangle (Fig. 5–19C).

The crystals in enamel tend to grow with their long axis perpendicular to the membrane, which produces the matrix. It can be observed that the orientation of the crystals change in conjunction with the orientation of the membrane. Sharp changes in crystal direction can be seen at the boundary of the rod sheaths, and more subtle changes occur from the "open end" (the line joining the ends of the arcade or sheath) of the rod to interrod enamel (Fig. 5–19C).

Post Secretory Transition

The stage of post secretory transition occurs toward the end of enamel secretion, and is marked by two developmental events which are a change in the ameloblast's morphology and cell death. Following the deposition of the majority of the enamel matrix, ameloblasts lose their Tomes' process, they become shorter and many (up to 25%) of the ameloblasts die. A basal lamina and associated hemidesmosomes, which provide attachment to the enamel surface is formed between the enamel matrix and ameloblasts.

Changes have also taken place in the stellate reticulum. These cells, which were once stellate and separated by extracellular spaces, are now compact. The stratum intermedium and outer enamel epithelium cells will form a papillary layer of cells beneath the ameloblasts.

Maturation Stage

During the process of maturation, enamel becomes fully mineralized. The organic and water content of enamel becomes reduced and the inorganic component (principally hydroxyapatite) increases. The process of maturation is really an ongoing process, which begins early in the secretion stage. Enamel matrix becomes mineralized as soon as formed and continues to mature until completely developed (Fig. 5–15G–I). This feature distinguishes it from dentin and bone. Unlike dentin and bone there is no "preenamel," as predentin or osteoid exist as unmineralized matrices in dentin and bone, respectively. During the secretion stage, enamel nearest the DEJ, being developmentally older, is more mineralized or mature. Maturation is a continuous process (Fig. 15G and H). However, it is most pronounced during the stage of maturation. This stage is first recognized by the formation of a ruffled apical border in ameloblasts (Fig. 5–15H).

Hydrolytic enzymes have been found in the enamel matrix. These enzymes are responsible for the degradation of the enamel matrix proteins, amelogenins and enamelins. More mature enamel is "enamelin-rich" because it appears that the amelogenins are removed more readily than the enamelins. Enamelins are also more intimately associated with the mineral element of enamel.

During the stage of maturation, ameloblasts have been found to modulate. Modulation is a reversible change in cell activity and morphology. Two types of ameloblasts, as well as transitional forms, have been seen in this stage. They are the ruffle-ended and smooth-ended ameloblasts. Ruffle-ended ameloblasts possess a ruffled distal border. This

Clinical Application

In intercuspal areas, during enamel secretion, the ameloblasts may become strangulated when their bases begin to touch one another. These areas become pits and fissures in the erupted tooth. They are extremely difficult to clean. Pit and fissure sealants are used to keep bacteria out of these areas.

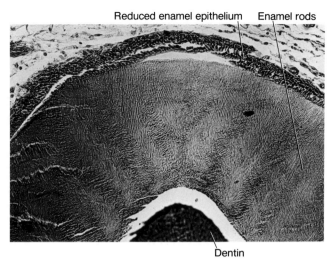

Figure 5–23. Histological section through developing partially mineralized enamel. Note the wavy appearance of the enamel rods.

Micrographs

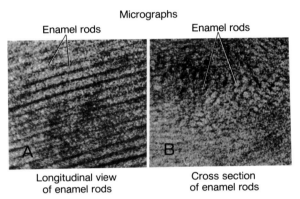

Figure 5–24. High magnification view of microradiographs of forming enamel with rods cut in longitudinal A and cross-section B.

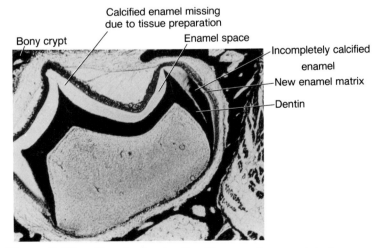

Figure 5–25. Developing tooth with a neatly completed crown residing in a bony crypt.

specialization resembles that of intestinal villi, but is more irregular (thus the term ruffled instead of striated, (Fig. 5–15H). Because of their superficial resemblance to resorptive cells these cells may be responsible for the uptake of peptides and amino acids from the matrix. Smooth-ended ameloblasts have a relatively smooth apical border. However, their apical cytoplasm contains many vesicles. During the modulation process changes in the junctions between ameloblasts also occur. Ruffle-ended ameloblasts have well developed distal junctional complexes but lack proximal junctions. Smooth-ended ameloblasts loose their distal junctions, but acquire proximal junctional complexes. The exact functions of these two different cell types is only beginning to be understood. It is known that the chemistry of the enamel overlying smooth and ruffle-ended ameloblasts differs. This indicates that functional differences occur during modulation.

The net result of the activity of maturation stage is a gain in the mineral content (mostly calcium and phosphate) of the enamel and a loss of protein and water. Spaces between enamel crystals diminish in size with an increase in crystal diameter and length. The enamel rod core or head of the rod appears to contain the most mineral in later maturation. The rod periphery or rod tails (interrod enamel) still contain sufficient mineral to be seen (Fig. 5–23). A Grenz x-ray illustrates spaces between rods, which indicates a lower mineral content (Fig. 5–24A and B).

Measurements of these rods indicate that they are less than the $5 \times 9 \ \mu m$ mature rod size. Therefore, the final increase in mineral content to 96% + probably takes place in the rod periphery. There is evidence this final process of mineralization occurs shortly before eruption.

Final enamel thickness (from 2 mm to 2.5 mm over the cusps) is attained after the ameloblast completes enamel formation. The cervical region of the crown and the central grooves are the last zones to mineralize, and thus rarely reach the hardness of the cusps. Ameloblasts in these regions may lose functional ability before mineralization is complete. Figure 5–25 illustrates the incompletely mineralized enamel matrix at the cervical region. Lack of complete mineralization of the central grooves or cervical areas is believed to be a reason for caries in these areas.

In summary, enamel mineralization (Fig. 5–26) follows the pattern of matrix formation from the dentin-enamel junction peripherally. The extent of mineralization is indicated by the dark-to-light shaded zones proceeding from the DEJ peripherally. The very dark zones are the most highly mineralized and the white areas, the least mineralized. The final stage of mineralization of the enamel rod may be in its periphery, and at a time just prior to eruption of the crown into the oral cavity.

Crown Growth and Completion

Crowns of the teeth increase in size by incremental deposition of enamel matrix (Fig. 5.27). The first area of the crown to completely form is the cusp tip, and the last, the cervical region. Crowns increase in height or length by differentiation of new ameloblasts, followed by enamel formation at the cervical aspects of the enamel organ (Fig. 5.27). Crowns also increase in size by cell division of the inner enamel epithelial cells between the cusps. This results in a slight separation of the cusps with a resultant slight increase in crown size. From the inception of dentinogenesis to the completion of amelogenesis, the crowns increase in size about four times. This is primarily due to cell division at the cervical region and the deposition of enamel to the thickness of 2.5 mm. As soon as the ameloblasts differentiate (in any area), they can no longer divide. The last areas to differentiate, therefore, are the intercuspal and cervical areas (Fig. 5.27). After cell differentiation, crown size is dependent upon incremental growth.

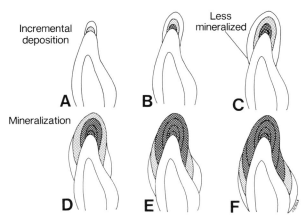

Figure 5–26. Summary of the stages of enamel mineralization. Initial enamel is formed in A and becomes more mature (more calcified) in B as further matrix is formed. (C). Further increments are formed. (D). Mineralization and matrix deposition increases. (E). Enamel matrix is formed on the side of the cusps. (F). Final matrix is formed and progresses cervically.

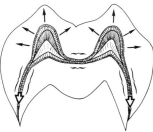

Figure 5–27. Diagram depicting the growth of the developing crown at cuspal, intercuspal and cervical sites.

Clinical Application

Certain antibiotics, like the tetracyclines, have an affinity for calcified tissues. They may become incorporated within the mineral phase during maturation, and cause discoloration of the enamel and underlying dentin.

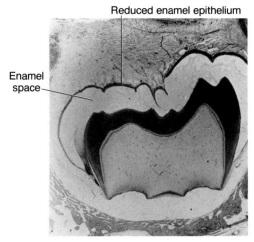

Figure 5–28. Enamel formation is near completion. Mineralization is not complete at the cervical region. The enamel organ is now in the form of a reduced enamel epithelium.

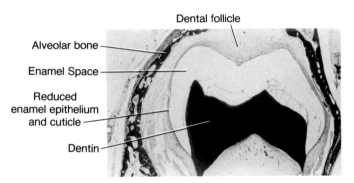

Figure 5–29. Completed crown residing in a crypt with a cuticle formed on the surface of the enamel.

Enamel completion is signaled, not only by attainment of crown size, but also by mineral content. At the final stage of mineralization, the flattened ameloblasts and their basement membrane along with the remainder of the cells of the enamel organ (reduced enamel epithelium) for a membrane on the surface of the enamel (Figs. 5.28 and 5.29). This membrane is termed the primary or developmental cuticle.

Crown and Surrounding Tooth Crypt

Mesenchymal cells immediately surrounding the crown appear as a capsule known as the dental follicle (Fig. 5.30). Those follicular cells of ectomesenchymal origin which are adjacent to the young enamel organ in the cap and bell stages migrate away from their origin into the follicle, and induce formation of the surrounding alveolar bone and periodontal ligament. The future periodontal ligament is a connective

> *Clinical Application*
>
> The enamel cuticle may remain adherent to the tooth after eruption appearing as a reddish or brown spot on the crown which may cause undue concern for parents. However, this layer is soon shed.

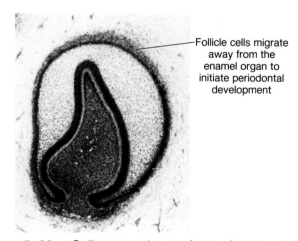

Figure 5–30. Cells near the surface of the outer dental epithelium at the bell stage migrate outward to induce the formation of surrounding periodontal structures.

tissue zone that surrounds the tooth, and is positioned between the protective thin shell of alveolar bone and the developing tooth. Later, as the tooth erupts, root formation occurs and the periodontal ligament matures (Fig. 5.31).

Summary

Tooth development is the result of the inductive interactions which occur between the oral epithelium and the cells of the neural crest. The oral epithelium develops a dental laminar system from which 20 primary and 32 permanent enamel organs originate.

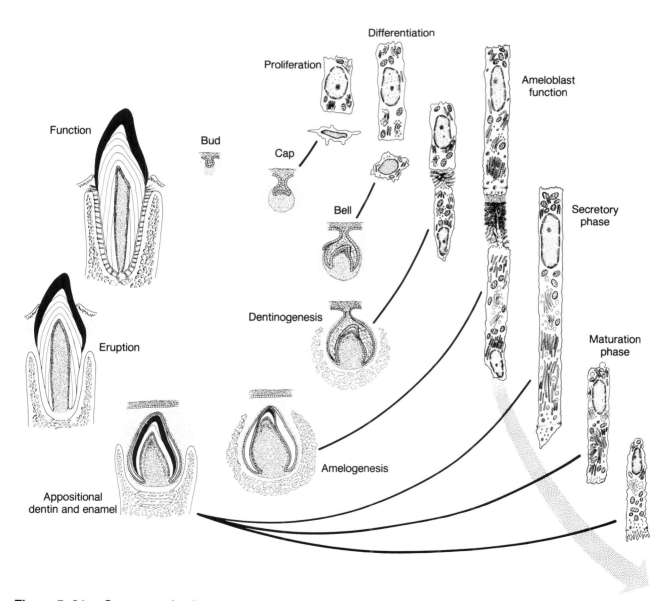

Figure 5–31. Summary of cell activities correlated to early stages of tooth formation which are important to the development, eruption, and function of teeth. Ameloblast and odontoblast differentiation and function are seen on the right and tooth development stages on the left.

All enamel organs pass through the same bud, cap and bell stages. The proliferating cells differentiate into the tooth formative cells during the bell stage. Ameloblasts arise from the inner enamel epithelial cells and induce the adjacent cells of the dental papilla to differentiate into odontoblasts, which form dentin. The formation of enamel and dentin matrices occurs nearly simultaneously. Following the deposition of a layer of aprismatic enamel, ameloblasts deposit enamel in the form of rods or prisms which become highly mineralized. During enamel maturation, ameloblasts function to resorb much of the water and organic matrix from enamel to provide space for the growing enamel crystals. Enamel and dentin matrices form by the incremental deposition of about 4 μ of matrix daily.

Odontoblasts first form an increment of collagenous matrix called predentin which is later minearlized. As daily increments of predentin form, the adjacent earlier-formed increment minearlizes as dentin. The odontoblastic process grows in length as more matrix is deposited, and is instrumental in controlling the environment at the mineralization front between dentin and predentin. Dentin consists of 70% mineral 10% organic material and 20% water by weight.

The hydroxyapatite crystals in enamel increase in size, which results in enamel being 96% mineral and 4% organic material and water. The arrangement of ameloblasts with their Tomes' process results in the formation of enamel rods. The process of amelogenesis is a series of successive stages of proliferation, differentiation, secretion, and maturation (Fig. 5.31). A four-fold increase in the size of the crowns occurs from time of initiation until the completion of hard tissue formation. This increase is accomplished by an increase in cell number (cell division) between cusps and also incremental deposition. The tooth follicle develops around the tooth and eventually gives rise to supporting structures.

Self-Evaluation Review

1. Describe the stages of tooth development.
2. What components make up the tooth bud? What structures do they form?
3. What cell types comprise the bell stage enamel organ?
4. Define the terms morphodifferentiation and cytodifferentiation as they relate to tooth development.
5. What is meant by the terms instructive and permissive as they relate to epithelial-mesenchymal interactions?
6. Describe the changes which occur during odontoblast differentiation.
7. Describe the changes in the inner enamel epithelium during the process of ameloblast differentiation. What is Tomes' process?

8. Describe the distribution of prismatic and aprismatic enamel in the crown.
9. What is meant by the term modulation? At which stage in amelogenesis do ameloblasts modulate? What is happening to the enamel matrix during this stage?
10. Compare and contrast the mineral and organic matrix of enamel and dentin.

Acknowledgments

Figure 1 is modified after Figure 21–5 in *Histology* (8th ed.) by Arthur W. Ham and David H. Cormack (Philadelphia: JB Lippincott). Figure 5.22A was provided courtesy of Alan Boyde, London.

Suggested Readings

Bhussry BR, Sharawy M. Development and growth of teeth. In: *Orban's Oral Histology and Embryology.* St. Louis, Mo: The C.V. Mosby Co.; 1986:28–48.

Boyde A. The structure of developing mammalian dental enamel. In: *Tooth Enamel: Its Composition, Properties and Fundamental Structure.* Bristol, England: John Wright and Sons; 1964.

Boyde A. The development of enamel structure. *Proc. R. Soc. Med.* 1967;60:923–928.

Deutsch d, Palmon A, Fisher LW, Kolodny N, Termine JD, Young MF. Sequencing of bovine enamelin ("tuftulin"), a novel acidic enamel protein. *J. Biol. Chem.* 1991;24:16021–16028.

Kronmiller JE, Upholt WB, Kollar EJ. Alteration of murine odontogenic patterning and prolongation of expression of epidermal growth factor mRNA by retinol in vitro. *Arch. Oral Biol.* 1992; 37:129–138.

Kallenbach E. Fine structure of ameloblasts in the kitten. *Am. J. Anat.* 1977;148:479–511.

Kallenbach E, Piesco NP. The changing morphology of the epithelium-mesenchyme interface in the differentiation zone of growing teeth of selected vertebrates and its relationship to possible mechanisms of differentiation. *J. Biol. Buccale* 1978;6:229–240.

Josephson K, Fejerskov O. Ameloblast modulation in the maturation zone of the rat incisor enamel organ. *J. Anat.* 1977; 124:45–70.

McKee MD, Wedlich L, Pompura JR, Nanci A, Smith CE, Warshawsky H. Demonstration by staining and radioautography of cyclical distributions of protein at the enamel surface in rat incisors. *Arch. Oral Biol.* 1988;33:413–423.

Nanci A, Smith CE. Development and calcification of enamel. In: *Calcification in Biological Systems.* Boca Raton, Fla: CRC Press; pp 313–343.

Robinson C, Kirkham J. Dynamics of amelogenesis as revealed by protein compositional studies. In: *The Chemistry and Biology of Mineralized Tissues.* Birmingham, Ala: Ebsco Media Inc; 1985;248–263.

Sasaki T. *Cell Biology of Tooth Enamel Formation: Functional Electron Microscopic Monographs.* Basel, Switzerland: Karger; 1990.

Schroeder H. *Oral Structural Biology: Embryology, Structure and Function of Normal Hard and Soft Tissues of the Oral Cavity and the Temporomandibular Joints.* New York: Thieme; 1991.

Thesleff I, Vaahtokari A. The role of growth factors in the determination and differentiation of odontoblastic cell lineage. *Proc. Finn. Dent. Soc.* 1992;88(S1):357–368.

Warshawsky H, Josephsen K, Thylstrup A, Fejerskov O. The development of enamel structure in rat incisors as compared to the teeth of monkey and man. *Anat. Rec.* 299:371.

6

Development of Teeth: Root and Supporting Structures

Nagat M. ElNesr and James K. Avery

Introduction

Root development is initiated through the contributions of the cells originating from the (1) enamel organ, (2) dental papilla, and (3) dental follicle. The cells of the outer enamel epithelium contact the inner enamel epithelium at the base of the enamel organ, the *cervical loop* (Fig. 6–1). During crown formation, cervical loop cells continue to divide, which results in growth of the enamel organ at the cervical region of the crown (Fig. 6–1; the cervical loop is seen in higher magnification in Fig. 6–2A). Later, with crown completion, the cells of the cervical loop continue to grow away from the

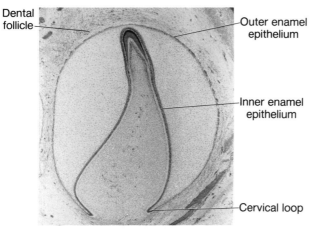

Dental follicle
Outer enamel epithelium
Inner enamel epithelium
Cervical loop

Figure 6–1. Formation of cervical loop.

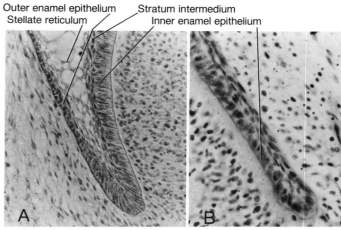

Outer enamel epithelium
Stellate reticulum
Stratum intermedium
Inner enamel epithelium

Figure 6–2. Higher magnification of cervical loop (A) and root sheath (B).

crown and become *root sheath cells* (Figs. 6–2B and 6–3). The inner root sheath cells cause root formation by inducing the adjacent cells of the dental papilla to become odontoblasts, which in turn will form root dentin. The root sheath will further dictate whether the tooth will have single or multiple roots. The remainder of the cells of the dental papilla become the cells of the root pulp.

The third component in root formation, the dental follicle, is the tissue that surrounds the enamel organ and the dental papilla. It will give rise to cells that form the supporting structures of the tooth—that is, the cementum that forms on the surface of the root, the periodontal ligament, and the inner layer of the alveolar bone. This bone initially encloses the developing crown of the tooth and later surrounds the roots (Fig. 6–3). It attaches to the periodontal ligament fibers, which also attach to the root by means of the cementum.

Objectives

After this chapter is studied, the following topics should be understood: details of root formation including origin, and functions of the root sheath in initiation of root dentin and intermediate cement formation; and details of the development of cementum and the periodontal ligament, and formation of alveolar bone.

Root Sheath Development

During crown formation, the enamel organ enlarges by cell division. Cell proliferation occurs, in part, at the cervical region or base of the organ. The remainder of the cells of the enamel organ have already differentiated, and these cells have formed enamel. The proliferating zone is thus termed the *cervical loop* (Fig. 6–1). After the crown is completed, the outer and inner enamel epithelial cells come together, with minimal inclusion of the stratum intermedium and stellate reticulum (Fig. 6–2). The cervical loop cells continue to proliferate and form a bilayer of cells called the *root sheath* (Hertwig's) (Figs. 6–2B and 6–3). The crown is defined as that area of the tooth covered by enamel and supported by dentin (Fig. 6–3). Below the crown, on its interior surface, the root sheath encloses the cells of the dental papilla; on its exterior it is surrounded by the cells of the dental follicle (Fig. 6–4A). The root sheath is the architect of the root; the length, curvature, thickness, and number of roots are dependent on this cell layer and the adjacent mesenchymal or ectomesenchymal cells. As the root sheath continues to grow away from the crown, it bends at its extremity, pulpward almost 45° to form a disclike structure. This bent portion of the root sheath is termed the *epithelial diaphragm* (Fig. 6–4A). The epithelial diaphragm surrounds the apical opening to the pulp. This opening will become the *apical foramen*. The epithelial diaphragm maintains a constant size during root development because the root sheath grows in length at the angle of the diaphragm (Fig. 6–4A and B). With increased root length, the crown begins to move

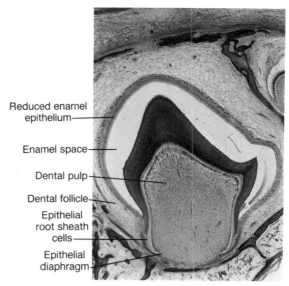

Figure 6–3. Beginning of root development.

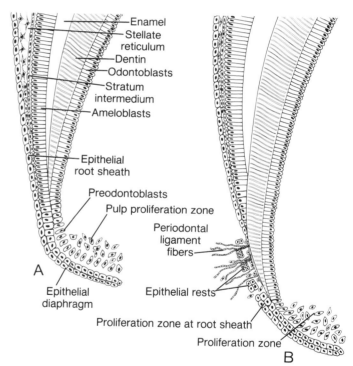

Figure 6–4. Formation of epithelial diaphragm. (A). Initial root formation. (B). Later root formation.

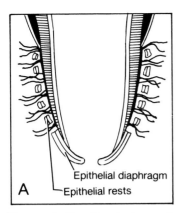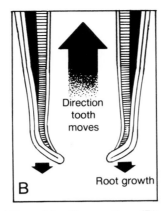

Epithelial diaphragm
Epithelial rests

A

Direction
tooth
moves

B

Root growth

Figure 6–5. Root elongation (A) and tooth eruption (B).

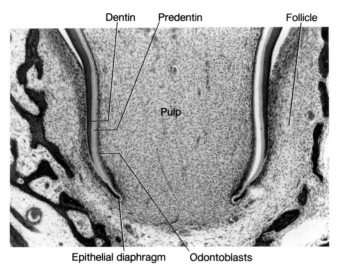

Dentin Predentin Follicle

Pulp

Epithelial diaphragm Odontoblasts

Figure 6–6. Root sheath and epithelial diaphragm.

Clinical Application

The presence of the root sheath initiates development of the root and determines the size and shape of the root, its length, and whether the root will be curved or straight. Before root formation occurs, the root sheath must be present. Its interruption may result in root deformities.

away from the base of the crypt. This uplifting of the tooth provides space needed for continued root growth. As a result, the epithelial diaphragm maintains its position in relation to the base of the crypt. The root thus lengthens at the same rate as the tooth moves occlusally (Fig. 6–5A and B).

Single-Root Formation

Formation of single-rooted teeth occurs by the growth of the root sheath, like a cuff or tube, around the cells of the dental pulp (Fig. 6–4A), followed by development of the root dentin (Fig. 6–4B). Cells of the inner layer of the root sheath induce adjacent cells of the dental pulp to differentiate into odontoblasts, which in turn form dentin. The odontoblasts secrete the dentin matrix in consecutive layers or increments. As the first layer of dentin matrix mineralizes, the epithelial root sheath cells separate from the root dentin and breaks occur in its continuity (Fig. 6–4B). The breaks are due to the degeneration of some epithelial cells. The separated root sheath cells then begin migrating away from the root surface, deeper into the follicular area. Mesenchymal or ecto-mesenchymal cells of the dental follicle then migrate between the remaining epithelial cell groups to contact the root surface. At this surface, they differentiate into cementoblasts and secrete cementum matrix (cementoid), which subsequently mineralizes to form cementum. As root cementum forms the remaining cells of the root sheath in that area migrate farther away from the root surface. They persist in the developing periodontal ligament as *epithelial rests* (Malassez) (Figs. 6–4B and 6–5A). Root elongation continues progressively, with proliferation of the remaining root sheath cells at the base of the angle of the epithelial diaphragm (Fig. 6–6). This is accompanied by proliferation of the adjacent cells of the dental pulp and the dental follicle (Fig. 6–6). As the root lengthens the compensatory movement of eruption provides space for further root development (Fig. 6–5B).

The root sheath is never seen as a continuous layer because it breaks down rapidly once root dentin begins to form. The zone of the epithelial diaphragm, however, remains constant and is the last part of the root sheath to degenerate after root completion. The process of root development continues after the tooth has erupted into the oral cavity.

Multiple-Root Formation

Human multirooted teeth have in common a *root trunk*, which is the area of common root base located between the cervical enamel and the area at which root division occurs (Figs. 6–7 and 6–10). Development of multirooted teeth proceeds in much the same manner as development of single-rooted teeth, until the furcation zone is complete (Figs. 6–7 and 6–10). Division of the root takes place through differential growth of the root sheath. In the region of the epithelial diaphragm, tonguelike extensions develop (Fig. 6–7) and grow until contact is made with one or two opposing extensions, which fuse with each other. This divides the original single opening of the root trunk into two or three openings. The epithelium then continues to proliferate at an equal rate at the perimeter of each of the openings and forms epithelial diaphragms and cuffs that grow farther from the crown and form the elongating roots. The areas of contact of the tonguelike extensions form epithelial bridges at the furcation zone (Fig. 6–8). A view of a section through the future bifurcation zone at higher magnification (Fig. 6–9) shows this to be an island of epithelial cells. These cells are not an island, however, but the tip of a tonguelike extension from the root trunk. At each bridge, the inner cells of the epithelial root sheath induce formation of odontoblasts, which in turn will produce a "span" of dentin between and around each root (Fig. 6–10). Odontoblasts continue to differentiate along

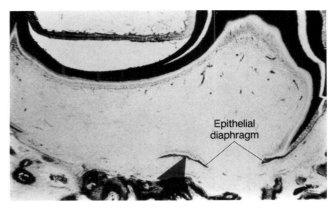

Figure 6–8. Development of furcation zone.

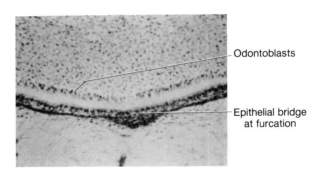

Figure 6–9. Odontoblast differentiation at bifurcation zone.

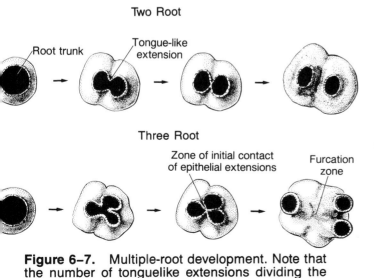

Figure 6–7. Multiple-root development. Note that the number of tonguelike extensions dividing the single root on left is equal to the number of roots to be formed on the right.

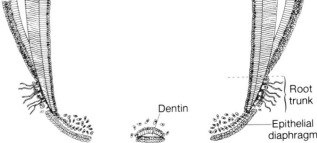

Figure 6–10. Formation of root trunk.

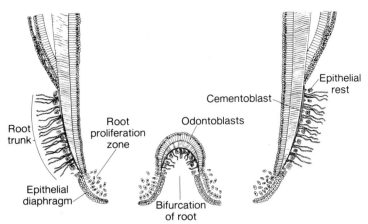

Figure 6–11. Development of individual root.

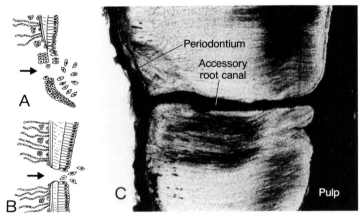

Figure 6–12. (A). Formation of defective root sheath. (B). Lack of odontoblast differentiation and formation of dentin. (C). Resulting accessory canal in mature tooth.

the coronal pulpal floor. Dentin formation will then follow the root sheath and produce multiple roots (Fig. 6–11). Some root sheath cells will then degenerate in the same manner as seen in single-root formation (Fig. 6–11), which will provide space for cementoblasts to deposit cementum on the root surface.

Root Formation Anomalies

The continuity of the epithelial root sheath and the timing of its proliferation and degeneration are believed to be essential to normal root formation. If the continuity of the root sheath were broken before dentin formation, the result could be missing or defective epithelial cells. Then odontoblasts would not differentiate, and dentin would not form opposite the defect in the root sheath (Fig. 6–12A). The result would be a small lateral canal connecting the periodontal ligament with the main root canal. Such a supplemental canal is called an *accessory root canal* and may occur anywhere along the root, particularly in the apical third (Fig. 6–12B and C). Defects also are seen in the furcation area of multirooted teeth. Defects in this location may be due to incomplete fusion of the tonguelike extensions of the epithelial diaphragm dividing the root trunk. Accessory root canals are not an uncommon finding at this site.

If, on the other hand, the epithelial root sheath does not degenerate at the proper time and remains adherent to the root dentin surface, mesenchymal cells of the dental follicle will not come into contact with the dentin. Then there would be no differentiation into cementoblasts and no formation of cementum. This would result in areas of the root being devoid of cementum (Fig. 6–13A and B). Areas of *exposed root dentin* may be found in any area of the root surface, particularly in the cervical zone (Fig. 6–13B), and may be the cause of cervical sensitivity later in life when gingival recession takes place.

Clinical Application

Accessory root canals can spread infection from one site to another. Infection may occur initially in the tooth pulp and be transmitted to the periodontal space or from infection in the periodontium to the pulp tissue.

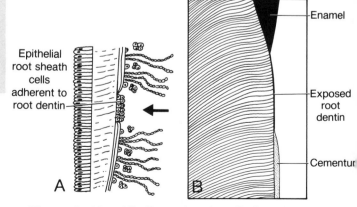

Figure 6–13. (A). Root sheath cells fused to dentin. (B). Area of exposed dentin.

The epithelial root sheath may also remain adherent to the dentin in the cervical area near the furcation zone. In this case, the inner cells of the root sheath may differentiate into functional ameloblasts and produce enamel droplets known as *enamel pearls*. Enamel pearls often are found lodged between the roots of the permanent molars (Fig. 6–14).

Epithelial Root Sheath (Hertwig's)

After dentin formation the epithelial root sheath breaks down, and its remnants migrate away from the dentinal surface. These remnants come to lie some distance from the root, in the periodontal ligament. They then become known as the epithelial rests of Malassez. These cells persist in the periodontal ligament throughout life. They are often found near the apical zone in young individuals up to 20 years of age. Later, these cells tend to be seen more in the cervical areas of the tooth. This could be because the epithelial cells have an inherent characteristic of moving toward the surface and exfoliate. In humans, some of the epithelial cell remnants of the root sheath may become trapped in baylike depressions between the dentin and cellular cementum, forming what is known as enameloid or intermediate cementum.

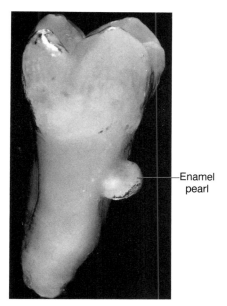

Enamel pearl

Figure 6–14. Enamel pearl on tooth root.

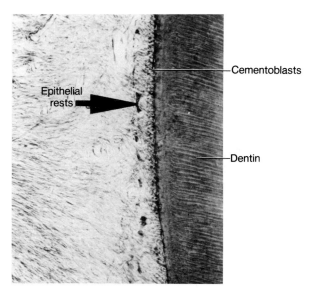

Figure 6–15. Development of epithelial rests.

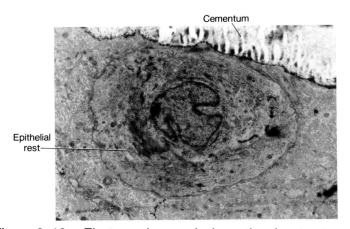

Figure 6–16. Electron micrograph shows the ultrastructure of an epithelial rest, with desmosomes between adjacent cells.

Microscopically, epithelial rests appear as a network of epithelial strands along the root surface, as isolated islands of cells surrounded by connective tissue (Fig. 6–15), or as isolated cells in close contact with the cementum. Three types of epithelial tests develop: proliferating, resting, and degenerating. This description is dependent on whether they are in the process of dividing or inactive or undergoing cell lysis. Ultrastructurally, the epithelial cells are surrounded by basal lamina and hemidesmosomes. Each cluster is composed of a few irregularly shaped cells with ovoid, oblong, or indented nuclei (Fig. 6–16). The cytoplasm is rather dense with mitochondria, ribosomes, and tonofilaments appearing singly or in bundles. These are seen anchored to attachment plaques at sites of desmosomes and hemidesmosomes. Dense granules are also seen in the cytoplasm. When singly present, the epithelial cell has a uniform shape surrounded by a basal lamina with a smooth and round nucleus outline. When chronic inflammation or other pathologic conditions occur, the epithelial rests may proliferate into cysts or tumors. Degenerated epithelial cells, however, may form a nidus for calcified bodies contributing to the formation of a cementicle in the periodontal ligament.

Currently, the physiological role of epithelial rests is unknown. The behavior of these cells is said to be species dependent. In teeth of persistent growth, such as a rat incisor, where collagen turnover is rapid, the epithelial rests are reported to degrade collagen by phagocytosis. In vitro studies have also shown procine epithelial rests to phagocytose collagen.

Dental Follicle

The *dental follicle (sac)* is the mesenchymal condensation that initially surrounds the enamel organ and the enclosed dental papilla (Fig. 6–17). Later, it surrounds the crown and eventually the tooth root. Cells of the dental sac initiate the development of the supporting tissues of the tooth (Fig. 6–17). They arise from the area near the outer enamel epithelium and migrate peripherally. Cells of the sac will therefore give rise to cells that produce cementum, the periodontal ligament, and the alveolar bone (crypt or alveolus). Dental follicular cells thus control the formation of future periodontal structures and are first apparent in very early developmental stages.

At all stages of development, teeth are protected and stabilized by follicular tissue. When the tooth germs of the permanent (successional) teeth first appear, they are in the same dental sac as their decisuous predecessors (Fig. 6–18A). This relationship is maintained until the deciduous teeth begin to erupt. The permanent tooth germs then develop separate sacs within separate crypts (Fig. 6–18B). A *crypt* is the bony cavity enclosing a developing tooth and is formed by the dental sac. Each crypt has an opening in its roof through which dental sac fibers extend for communication with the oral mucosa. The fibrous extension of the dental sac, which connects the permanent tooth germ to the oral

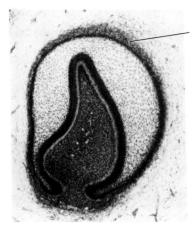

Sac cells migrate away from the enamel organ to initiate periodontal development

Figure 6–17. Dental follicle in developing tooth.

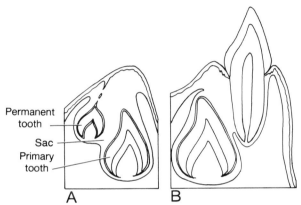

Permanent tooth

Sac

Primary tooth

A B

Figure 6–18. Development of bony crypt. (A). Relationship of primary and permanent tooth buds in early development. (B). Relationship of primary and permanent tooth buds in later development.

Clinical Application

The dental follicle is important because it contributes to each of the supporting tissues of the tooth root, the periodontal ligament, cementum, and alveolar bone. The formative cells of these structures are important in the initiation, formation, and maintenance of these tissues.

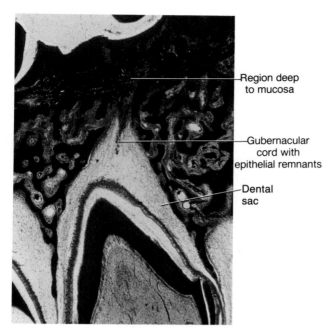

Figure 6–19. Eruption pathway.

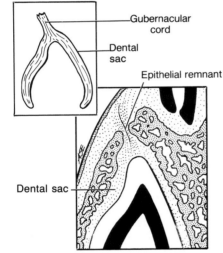

Figure 6–20. Gubernacular development.

mucosa, is called the *gubernacular cord* (Figs. 6–19 and 6–20). Some authorities believe that after the eruption of the deciduous teeth the gubernacular cords lie in bony canals known as gubernacular canals, which are extensions of the bony crypts of the successional teeth. Although the gubernacular cord is formed of fibrous tissue (extension of the tooth sac), it may contain epithelial cells, possibly remnants of the dental lamina (Fig. 6–20). Some of these remnants proliferate and form small epithelial masses composed of keratinized material and known as *epithelial pearls*, epithelial cell nests, or cysts. The dental sac (follicle) initially surrounds the young tooth (Fig. 6–21). As the root forms and the tooth erupts, the follicular tissue becomes the supportive tissue of the teeth: the cementum, the periodontal ligament, and the supporting alveolar bone. Therefore, the functions of the dental sac are (1) to protect and stabilize the tooth during formation and later eruption, (2) to provide nutrition and nerve supply to the developing tooth, and (3) to give rise to the cells that form the cementum, the periodontal ligament, and the inner wall of the bony crypt or alveolus.

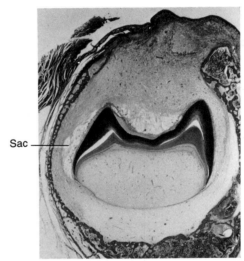

Figure 6–21. Tooth in crypt.

Development of Cementum (Cementogenesis)

Just before the degeneration of the epithelial root sheath after root dentin has been deposited adjacent to it, a thin amorphous structureless and highly mineralized secretion appears on the surface of the root dentin. This substance is devoid of collagen but contains tryptophane, an amino acid found in the enamel matrix. Its consistency is thus like that thin layer of peripheral enamel, aprismatic enamel. This secretion is more evident in the apical region of the root and averages some 10 to 20 μm in thickness. This deposit is believed to be formed by the root sheath cells just before they break up and begin migration from the root surface. Therefore, its origin, like that of ameloblasts, would be from the enamel organ. It probably functions to attach the next-to-be-deposited cementum to the dentin of the root surface as it is interposed between the dentin and the cementum (Fig. 6–22). It has recently been reported that this substance may contain occasional epithelial cells. The root sheath cells have an odontoblast-stimulating ability as well as possible secretory functions in producing the intermediate cementum. After root sheath cells begin migration, the mesenchyme cells from the dental follicle then contact the surface of the intermediate cementum and begin formation of the cellular cementum, which covers the roots and functions to attach the periodontal ligament fiber bundles.

Cementogenesis proceeds at a slower pace than that of the adjacent root dentin (Figs. 6–23 and 6–24). The cementoblasts exhibit features characteristic of cells capable of protein synthesis and secretion. They have a well-developed rough endoplasmic reticulum, a notable Golgi apparatus, numerous mitochondria, a large nucleus that contains prominent nucleoli, and abundant cytoplasm (Fig. 6–25). They are markedly different from the adjacent epithelial rest cells (see Fig. 6–16). The newly differentiated cementoblasts first

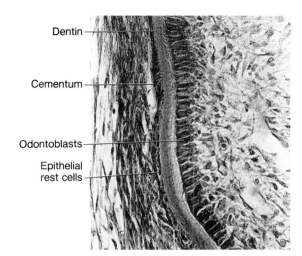

Figure 6–23. Histology of early cementum and dentin formation.

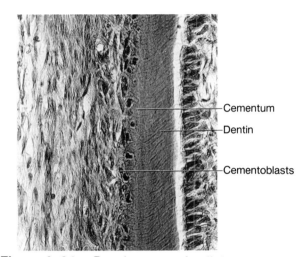

Figure 6–24. Development of cellular cementum.

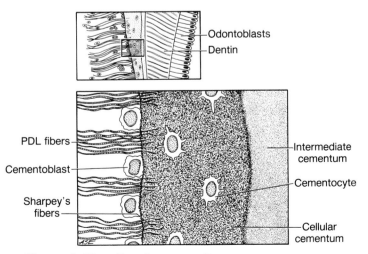

Figure 6–22. Development of intermediate cementum. PDL, periodontal ligament fibers.

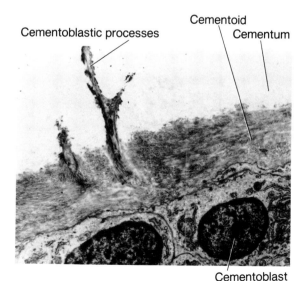

Figure 6–25. Ultrastructure of early cementum.

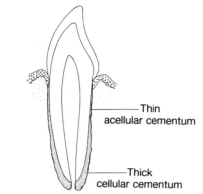

Figure 6–26. Cemental deposition pattern.

Thin
acellular cementum

Thick
cellular cementum

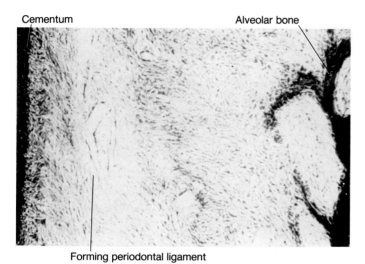

Cementum

Alveolar bone

Forming periodontal ligament

Figure 6–27. Differentiation of periodontal ligament.

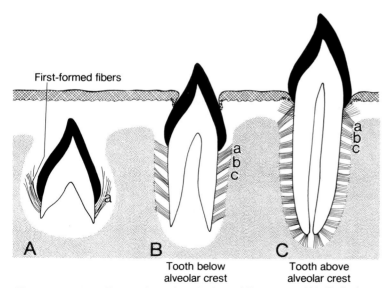

First-formed fibers

Tooth below
alveolar crest

Tooth above
alveolar crest

Figure 6–28. Formation of periodontal ligament. (A). Relations of periodontal fibers on unerupted crown. (B). Relation of periodontal fibers during intraoral eruption. (C). Relation of fibers in the adult tooth. Note the orientation of the first-formed fibers in A, B, and C.

elaborate the organic matrix or cementoid. This matrix consists of collagen fibers and a ground substance composed of protein polysaccharides (proteoglycans). The collagen fibers produced by the cementoblasts are called the intrinsic fibers. They run parallel to the cementum surface in an irregular manner. Then the organic matrix mineralizes, and cementum is laid down in successive layers or increments until its full thickness is reached. Thereafter, the cementoblasts enter a quiescent state near the cementum front, ready to function according to need, whether for further growth or for repair. Adjacent fibroblasts elaborate collagen fibers, which become embedded in the cementum matrix, to provide attachment of the tooth to the surrounding bone. The embedded portions of the periodontal ligament fibers in the cementum are known as *perforating fibers* (Sharpey's) (Fig. 6–22). These are the extrinsic fibers of the cementum and run at right angles to the root surface (Fig. 6–28).

Cementum is described as either cellular or acellular, depending on whether it contains cells in its matrix. The behavior of cementoblasts during matrix formation determines the type of cementum to be formed. Cellular cementum develops when some of the cementoblasts elaborating the matrix become embedded in it as cementocytes (see Fig. 6–28). Acellular cementum, on the other hand, develops when all the cementoblasts retreat into the periodontal ligament, leaving no trapped cells behind. Generally, acellular cementum covers the cervical half of the root dentin whereas cellular cementum is found on the apical half. However, layers of acellular and cellular cementum may alternate at any site (Fig. 6–26). In cellular cementum trapped cementoblasts develop cytoplasmic processes which reside in the cementum matrix to become cementocytes. The difference between intermediate and acellular cementum is the absence of collagenous fibers in the former.

Development of Periodontal Ligament

The periodontal ligament originates from the dental follicle and is the specialized, soft, connective tissue ligament that provides the attachment for the teeth to the adjacent alveolar bone. Its fibers are embedded in the cementum on the tooth's surface and in the alveolar bone at the other end.

Some delicate fiber bundles of the forming periodontal ligament first appear as root formation begins. At this time, the follicular cells show increased proliferative activity. The innermost cells near the forming root differentiate into cementoblasts and lay down cementum. The outermost cells differentiate into osteoblasts and furnish the lining of the bony socket (Fig. 6–27). The more centrally located cells in the ligament differentiate into fibroblasts that produce collagen fibers that will become embedded in both forming cementum and bone. At first, all the developing fibers of the periodontal ligament run obliquely in a coronal direction, from tooth to bone (Fig. 6–28A). The apical fibroblasts are the stem cells that proliferate and migrate cervically to form the first group of collagen fibers. As tooth eruption proceeds, the obliquity of the fibers gradually decreases and the position of the cementoenamel junction, which was originally apical to the crest of the crypt (Fig. 6–28A) becomes level and then coronal to the alveolar crest (Fig. 6–28B and C). This change between the cementoenamel junction and alveolar crest may relate to their functional role during tooth eruption. It also brings about the final arrangement of the principal fiber groups of the mature periodontal ligament.

The periodontal ligament is in a continuous state of remodeling, both during development and throughout the life-span of the tooth. The ligament persistently maintains support of an erupting or functioning tooth (Fig. 6–29). Remodeling is achieved by fibroblasts that rapidly synthesize and secrete collagen. Rapid *turnover* of collagen takes place throughout the whole thickness of the ligament, from bone to cementum. Turnover is not restricted to the metabolically active middle zone, which was sometimes referred to as the *intermediate plexus*. There is a differential rate of collagen turnover in the ligament, in an apicocervical direction. The highest turnover is in the apical region, and the lowest, in the cervical region of the ligament. Maturation and thickening of the fiber bundles of the periodontal ligament occur as the teeth reach functional occlusion.

Development of Alveolar Process

The alveolar bone develops as the tooth develops. Initially, this bone forms a thin eggshell of support, the tooth crypt, around each tooth germ (Fig. 6–30). Gradually, as the roots grow and lengthen, the alveolar bone keeps pace with the elongating and erupting tooth and maintains a relation with each tooth root (Figs. 6–27 and 6–31).

Development of the alveolar process begins in the eighth week in utero. At that time, within the maxilla and the mandible, the forming alveolar bone develops a horseshoe-shaped groove that opens toward the oral cavity. The bony groove, or canal, is formed by growth of the facial and lingual plates of the body of the maxillae or mandible and contains the developing tooth germs together with the alveolar vessels and nerves (Fig. 6–30). At first, the developing tooth germs lie free in the groove. Gradually, bony septa develop between teeth, so that each tooth is eventually contained in a separate crypt (Fig. 6–30). The actual alveolar process develops during the eruption of the teeth (Figs. 6–28).

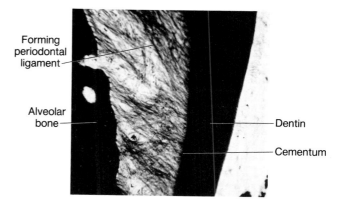

Figure 6–29. Differentiation of periodontal ligament fibers.

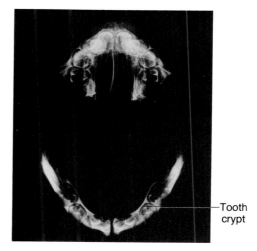

Figure 6–30. Formation of alveolar bone.

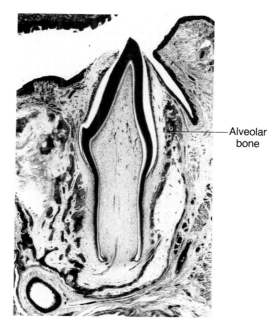

Figure 6–31. Bone development around erupting tooth.

During uterine life, the dental alveolus, like the rest of the skeleton, is formed from an embryonic type of bone composed of bony spicules (Fig. 6–30 and 6–31). This embryonic bone, a variety of coarse-fibered or woven bone, is gradually replaced by compact and spongy bone. Both compact and spongy bones initially are composed of layers (lamellae) arranged in an orderly manner.

The bone between the roots of adjacent single-rooted or multirooted teeth is termed the *interdental septum*. The bone between the roots of a multirooted tooth is known as *interradicular bone* or *septum* (Fig. 6–32).

In its mature form, the alveolar bone is composed of two parts, the *alveolar bone proper* and the *supporting bone* (Fig. 6–33). The alveolar bone proper is a thin lamella of compact bone that lines the root socket, and in which the periodontal fibers are embedded. It is known radiographically as the *lamina dura*. The supporting bone consists of both spongy and dense (compact) bone and functions in support of the alveolar bone proper. The cortical plate, or covering of the mandible or maxilla, furnishes the compact portion of the supporting alveolar bone (Fig. 6–33).

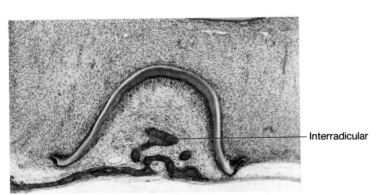

Interradicular

Figure 6–32. Development of interradicular bone.

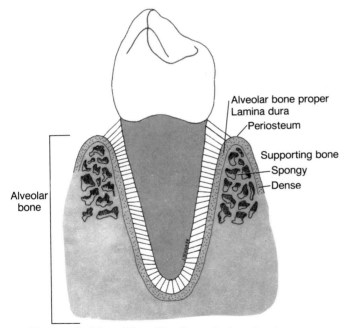

Alveolar bone proper
Lamina dura
Periosteum

Supporting bone
Spongy
Dense

Alveolar bone

Figure 6–33. Classification of alveolar bone.

The alveolar bone proper is a specialized type of dense bone composed of bundle bone and haversian bone that appears radiopaque on X-ray and is therefore called the *lamina dura*. The bundle bone is so named because it is penetrated by periodontal ligament fibers (Fig. 6–34). The alveolar bone proper is formed by the outermost cells of the dental follicle, which differentiate into osteoblasts and lay down the bone matrix or osteoid in which some osteoblasts become embedded as osteocytes. The matrix then calcifies to form mature bone.

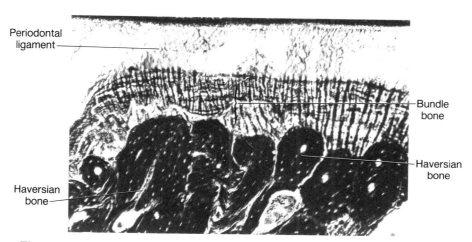

Figure 6–34. Histology of alveolar bone proper: Haversian and bundle.

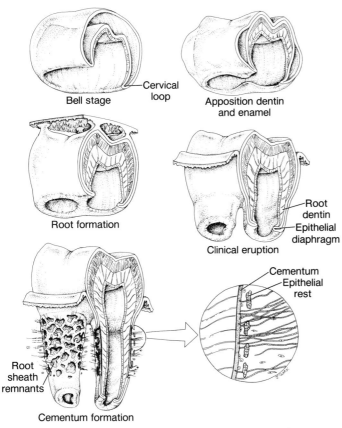

Figure 6–35. Summary of development of root.

Bell stage — Cervical loop

Apposition dentin and enamel

Root formation

Clinical eruption — Root dentin — Epithelial diaphragm

Cementum — Epithelial rest

Root sheath remnants

Cementum formation

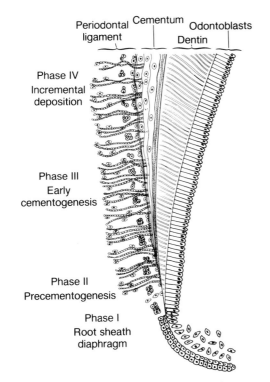

Periodontal ligament — Cementum — Odontoblasts — Dentin

Phase IV Incremental deposition

Phase III Early cementogenesis

Phase II Precementogenesis

Phase I Root sheath diaphragm

Figure 6–36. Summary of formation of cementum.

Summary

Root development begins after enamel formation nears completion and has reached the cementoenamel junction. An extension of the enamel organ has an important role in root development by forming the epithelial root sheath, which consists of an epithelial extension of the cervical loop (Fig. 6–35).

The inner cells of the sheath induce the adjacent mesenchymal cells to differentiate into odontoblasts, which form the root dentin. The cells of the root sheath also form a thin, structureless layer of cementum on the dentin and then begin to degenerate. As a result, three types of epithelial rests develop: proliferating, resting, and degenerating rests. These rests are present in the periodontal ligament along the root surface throughout life.

Development of the supporting tissues of the tooth takes place simultaneously with root development. The cementum, periodontal ligament, and bone of the inside of the crypts or alveoli have a common origin, the cells of the dental follicle.

Root and cementum development may be divided into four phases (see Fig. 6–36). Phase I is the formation of root sheath. In phase II, as the dentin is formed internal to the root sheath, a layer of intermediate cementum is deposited. The sheath then breaks up into rests. In phase III, mesenchymal cells appear and differentiate into cementoblasts that lay down the first layer of cementum. Periodontal ligament fibers, which are termed perforating or Sharpey's fibers, become enmeshed in the cementum along the root surface. They will become the means of attachment of the principal fibers of the periodontal ligament. In phase IV, further layers of cementum are deposited. Finally, the epithelial rests move farther from the root, into the periodontal ligament.

Self-Evaluation Review

1. Describe two differences in the cervical loop and epithelial diaphragm.
2. Define the reduced enamel epithelium.
3. What cells are responsible for the initiation of root formation?
4. How does eruption compensate for root growth?
5. Define the root trunk.
6. What causes the development of an accessory root canal?
7. Describe the arrangement of the developing principal fiber bundles.
8. Define and describe the furcation zone.
9. What are the multiple functions of the dental follicle?
10. What is the origin of the thin layer of intermediate cementum?

Suggested Readings

Davidson D, McCulloch CAG. Proliferative behavior of periodontal ligament cell populations. *J. Periodont. Res.* 1986;21:444.

Gemonov VV. Histological characteristics of the rests of Malassez in the human periodontium. *Stomatology.* 1980;59:-9.

Lindskog S. Formation of intermediate cementum I: early mineralization of aprismatic enamel and intermediate cementum in monkey. *J. Craniofac. Genet. Dev. Biol.* 1982;2:147–160.

Lindskog S. Formation of intermediate cementum II: a scanning electron microscope study of the epithelial root sheath of Hertwig in monkey. *J. Craniofac. Genet. Dev. Biol.* 1982;2:161–169.

Lindskog, S. Formation of intermediate cementum III: 3 H Tryptophan and 3 H proline uptake into the epithelial root sheath of hertwig in vivo. *J. Craniofac. Genet. Dev. Biol.* 1982;2:171–177.

Melcher AH, Bowen WH, eds. *The Biology of the Periodontium.* New York, NY: New York Press Inc.; 1969.

Owens PDA. A light and electron microscope study of the early stages of root surface formation in molar teeth in the rat. *Arch. Oral Biol.* 1982;24:901–907.

Sims MR. Ultrastructural analyses of the microfibril components of mouse and human periodontial oxytalan fibers. *Connec. Tissue Res.* 1984;13:59–67.

Stern IB. Current concepts of the dentogingival junction: the epithelial and connective tissue attachment to the tooth. *J. periodont.* 1981,9:465–475.

Van der Linden FPGM, Duterloo HS. *Development of the Human Dentition.* New York, NY. Harper and Row; 1976.

Yamasaki A, Rose GG, Pinero G, Mahan CJ. Microfilaments in human cementoblasts and periodontal fibroblasts. *J. Periodont.* 1987;58:40–45.

7

Tooth Eruption and Shedding

Nagat M. ElNesr and James K. Avery

Introduction

Eruption is the movement of the teeth within and through the bone of the jaws and the overlying mucosa to appear in the oral cavity and contact the opposing teeth. Eruptive movements begin with the onset of root formation, well before the teeth are seen in the oral cavity. The emergence of the tooth through the gingiva is the first clinical sign or eruption. Following emergence the teeth erupt at a maximum rate to reach occlusal contact, and then they continue to erupt at a slower rate to compensate for jaw growth and occlusal wear.

Movements leading to tooth eruption can be divided into three phases: (1) the preeruptive phase, (2) the prefunctional eruptive or emergence phase, and (3) the functional eruptive or posteruptive phase. All three phases of eruption can usually be seen going on at the same time in a dentition.

Objectives

The objective of this chapter is to familarize you with tooth eruption by describing its three phases: preeruptive, prefunctional, and functional stages. You will obtain information as to how initial growth of the tooth occurs relating to compensating changes in the crypt and how the supporting fiber system develops. Later, during functional occlusion, minute changes taking place apically and elsewhere in the support system are described.

Movements Leading to Tooth Eruption
Preeruptive Phase

The preeruptive phase of tooth movement is preparatory to the eruptive phases. It consists of the movements of the developing and growing tooth germs within the alveolar process before root formation (Fig. 7–1). During this phase, the growing teeth move in various directions to maintain their position in the expanding jaws. This is accomplished by both *bodily movement* and *eccentric growth*. Bodily movement is a shift of the entire tooth germ, which causes bone resorption in the direction of tooth movement and bone apposition

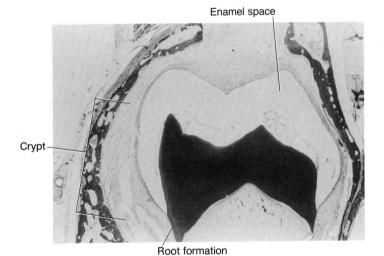

Enamel space

Crypt

Root formation

Figure 7–1. Preeruptive phase of tooth eruption.

behind it (Fig. 7–2A–C). This movement occurs continuously as the jaws grow. Eccentric growth refers to relative growth in one part of the tooth while the rest of the tooth remains constant. For example, the root elongates, yet the crown does not increase in size. As a result, the center of the tooth changes. Note that because the tooth has not yet begun to erupt, the crown maintains a constant relation to the surrounding alveolus whereas an increase in alveolar height compensates for root growth (Fig. 7–2D and E). These movements relate to the adjustments that each crown must make in relation to its neighbor and to the jaws as they increase in width, height, and length. The primary teeth in the alveolar processes therefore move in a facial and occlusal direction or in the direction of the growth of the face. At the same time, there is some mesial as well as distal movement. The permanent teeth also move within the jaws to adjust their position in the growing alveolar process.

Early in the preeruptive phase, the successional permanent teeth develop lingual to, and near the incisal or occlusal level of, their primary predecessors (Figs. 7–3A and 7–4A). At the end of this phase, the developing anterior permanent teeth are positioned lingually and near the apical third of the primary anterior teeth (Fig. 7–3B). The premolars are located under the roots of the primary molars (Fig. 7–4B). The change in the position of the permanent tooth germs is mainly the result of the eruption of the primary teeth and the coincident increase in height of the supporting tissues, not to the apical movement of the permanent tooth germs. The permanent molars, having no primary predecessors, develop without this kind of relation. The upper molars develop in the tuberosities of the maxilla, with their occlusal surfaces slanting distally (Fig. 7–5). The lower molars develop in the base of the mandibular rami, and their occlusal surfaces slant mesially (Fig. 7–5). The permanent molars undergo considerable eccentric movement, adjusting their positions as the jaws and the alveolar processes grow. Note that all movements in this phase take place within the crypts of the developing and growing crowns before root formation. The preeruptive and prefunctional phases overlap to some extent, but proceed in the following order: preeruptive, prefunctional, functional.

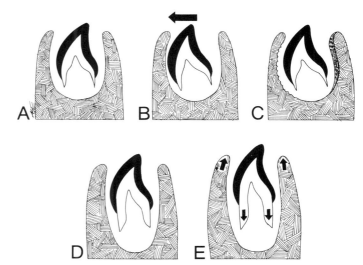

Figure 7–2. (A–C). Bodily movement of crown during preeruptive phase. (D) and (E). Eccentric growth of crown during preeruptive phase.

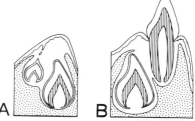

Figure 7–3. Relative position of primary and permanent teeth in (A) preeruptive and (B) eruptive phases.

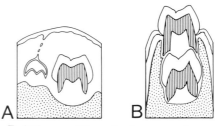

Figure 7–4. Relative position of primary molar and permanent premolar teeth in (A) preeruptive and (B) eruptive phases.

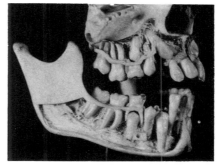

Figure 7–5. Human jaws during mixed dentition period. Permanent maxillary molar in tuberosity.

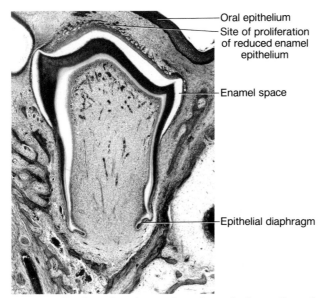

Figure 7–6. Prefunctional eruptive phase in formation of root.

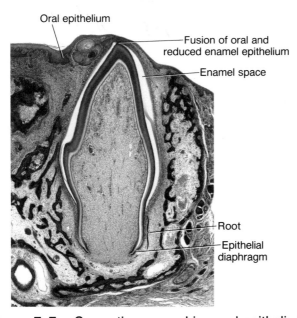

Figure 7–7. Crown tip approaching oral epithelium.

Prefunctional Eruptive Phase

The eruptive phase begins with the initiation of root formation and ends when the teeth reach occlusal contact (emergence phase). Five major events take place during this phase.

1. The secretory phase of amelogenesis is completed just before the onset of root formation and prefunctional eruption. There is a relation between the cessation of mineral and activation of the epithelial cells behind the enamel forming area.
2. The intraosseous stage occurs when the roots begin their formation as a result of the proliferation of both the epithelial root sheath and the mesenchymal tissue of the dental papilla and the dental follicle (Fig. 7–6).
3. The supraosseous stage begins when the erupting tooth moves occlusally through the bone of the crypt and the connective tissue of the oral mucosa, so that the reduced enamel epithelium covering the crown comes into contact with the oral epithelium (Fig. 7–7). As this occurs, the reduced epithelium of the crown proliferates and forms a firm attachment with the oral epithelium. A fused, double epithelial layer over the erupting crown is thus formed (Fig. 7–8).

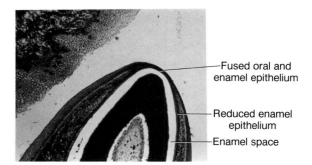

Figure 7–8. Contact and fusion of reduced enamel epithelium and oral mucosa.

4. The tip of the crown enters the oral cavity by breaking through the center of the double-layered epithelial cells. This breakthrough is accomplished by the cusp tip causing degeneration of the membrane, and is the beginning stage of *clinical eruption*. The crown erupts further, and the lateral borders of the oral mucosa become the *dentogingival junction* (Fig. 7–9). The reduced enamel epithelium, now surrounding the crown like a cuff, becomes known as the *junctional* or *attachment* epithelium. When the tip of the crown appears in the oral cavity, about one half to three quarters of the roots are formed (Fig. 7–9).

5. The erupting tooth continues to move occlusally at a maximum rate, and there is gradual exposure of more of the clinical crown (Fig. 7–10). Occlusal movement is the result of active eruption. As the tooth moves occlusally, gradual exposure of the clinical crown is accomplished through separation of the attachment epithelium from the crown and the resulting apical shift of the gingiva. The *clinical crown* is the part of the tooth (coronal to the attachment epithelium) exposed in the oral cavity, and differs from the *anatomical crown*, which is the part of the tooth covered by enamel. The prefunctional eruptive or emergence phase is also characterized by significant changes in the tissues overlying the teeth, around the teeth, and underlying the teeth.

Changes in Tissues Overlying Teeth. The initial change seen in the tissues overlying the teeth before eruption of the crown is the alteration of the connective tissue of the dental follicle to form a pathway for the erupting tooth. Usually, this is more prominent in erupting permanent teeth. Histologically, the coronal part of the dental follicle becomes heavily populated by numerous monocytes in parallel with osteoclasts to participate in bone resorption and formation of the eruption pathway. The future eruption pathway appears as a zone in which connective tissue fibers have disappeared, cells have degenerated and decreased in number, blood vessels have become fewer, and terminal nerves have broken up and degenerated. These changes are probably the partial result of the loss of blood supply to this area, as well as the release of enzymes that aid in degradation of these tissues. Clinically, tooth eruption may be accompanied by discomfort or pain, irritability, and/or a slight temperature increase. An altered tissue space or compartment overlying the tooth becomes visible as an inverted, funnel-shaped area (Fig. 7–11). In the periphery of this zone, the follicle fibers

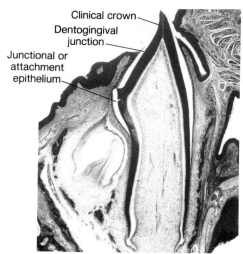

Figure 7–9. Clinical appearance of crown.

Clinical crown
Dentogingival junction
Junctional or attachment epithelium

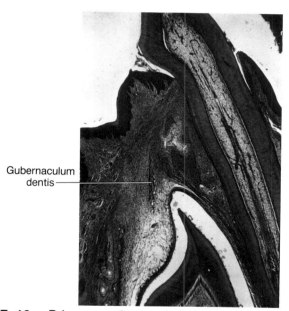

Gubernaculum dentis

Figure 7–10. Primary tooth at end of eruptive phase. Permanent successor in preeruptive phase.

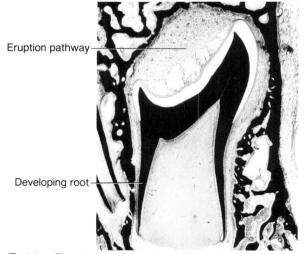

Eruption pathway

Developing root

Figure 7–11. Development of eruptive pathway overlying crown.

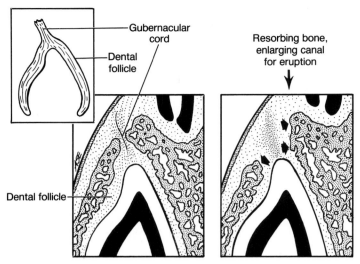

Figure 7-12. Developing eruption pathway and gubernaculum dentis.

Gubernacular cord

Dental follicle

Resorbing bone, enlarging canal for eruption

Dental follicle

Clinical Application

Eruption of the teeth is determined genetically rather than by factors such as environment. Only cases of severe malnutrition, for example, cause delayed eruption.

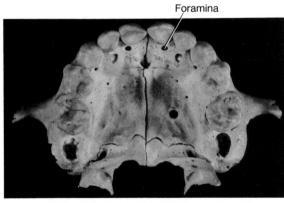

Foramina

Figure 7-13. Eruption sites of permanent teeth (gubernacular foramina) lingual to primary crowns. Note the tip of the lateral incisor in the foramen.

direct themselves toward the mucosa and are defined as the *gubernaculum dentis* or gubernacular cord (Figs. 7-10 and 7-12). Some authors believe that this structure guides the tooth in its eruptive movements.

For successful tooth eruption, there must be some resorption of the overlying bony crypt (Fig. 7-12), which is in a constant state of remodeling as the tooth germ enlarges and the face grows anteriorly and laterally. The eruptive process can be considered part of this remodeling growth. Osteoclasts differentiate and resorb a portion of the bony crypt overlying the erupting tooth. The eruption pathway, which at first is small, increases in dimension, allowing movement of the tooth to the oral mucosa (Fig. 7-12). Although the eruption of most permanent teeth is similar to that of primary teeth, the overlying primary teeth are an additional complication. The eruptive pathway of permanent incisors and cuspids is lingual to the corresponding primary teeth. This area shows a pronounced enlargement to accommodate the advancing crown.

Small foramina in the mandible and maxilla are evidence of eruption pathways of the anterior permanent teeth. These openings, the gubernacular foramina, are found lingual to the anterior primary teeth and are the sites of the gubernacular cords (Fig. 7-13). The premolars are between the roots of the primary molars. Root resorption in primary teeth proceeds in much the same manner as bone resorption (Fig. 7-14). When the roots are fully resorbed, the attachment of the primary crown is lessened and the crown is shed. This produces an eruption pathway for the premolars. Most roots resorb completely; the primary pulps degenerate as well. During the period of *mixed dentition* (around 6 to 12 years of age), when both primary and permanent teeth are in the mouth, the phenomena of root resorption and tooth formation proceed side by side (Fig. 7-14). These changes occur while the teeth still maintain chewing efficiency.

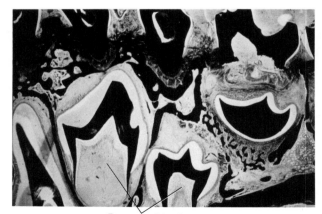

Permanent teeth

Figure 7-14. Microscopic appearance of relation of primary and permanent teeth.

When the tooth nears the oral mucosa, the reduced enamel epithelium comes into contact with the overlying mucosa (Figs. 7–7, 7–8, and 7–15B). Simultaneously, the oral epithelial cells and reduced enamel epithelial cells proliferate and fuse into one membrane (Fig. 7–15C). Further movement of the tooth stretches and thins the membrane over the crown tip (Fig. 7–15D). At this stage the mucosa become blanched because of a lack of blood supply to the area. Very soon, the tips of the teeth penetrate the area and appear in the oral cavity (Fig. 7–15E). Eruption is a gradual, as well as an intermittent, process. The tooth will erupt slightly, remain stationary for some time, and then erupt again. In this manner, the supporting tissues are able to make adjustments to the eruptive movements. Each eruptive movement results in more of the crown appearing in the oral cavity and further separation of the attachment epithelium from the enamel surface (Fig. 7–15F and G). Recent observations of human premolar eruption revealed eruptive activity occurred mostly at night with a marked slowing or cessation during the day.

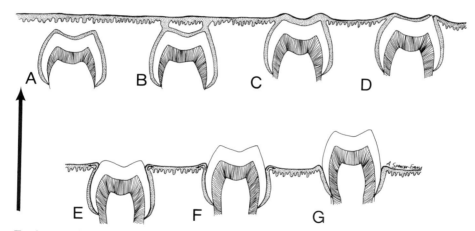

Figure 7–15. Fusion and rupture of reduced enamel epithelium and oral epithelium in tooth eruption.

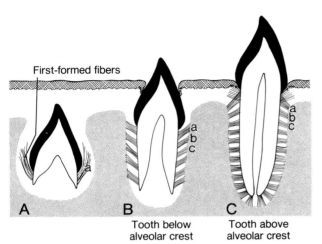

Figure 7–16. Development of periodontal fibers and modification of alveolar bone during tooth eruption (A). Early fiber formation. (B). Bone changes. (C). Further fiber development, near occlusion, with fibers more dense.

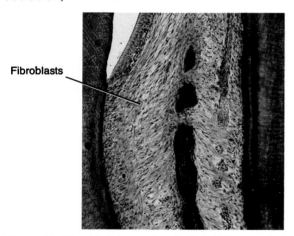

Figure 7–17. Histology of periodontal ligament of erupting tooth.

Changes in Tissues around Teeth. The tissues around the teeth also undergo change during tooth eruption. Initially, the dental follicle is composed of delicate connective tissue. Gradually, as eruptive movements commence, collagen fibers become prominent, extending between the forming root and the alveolar bone surface. The first noticeable periodontal fiber bundles appear at the cervical area of the root and extend at an angle coronal to the alveolar process (Fig. 7–16A). At the same time, the alveolar bone of the crypt is remodeled to accommodate the forming root. As the large crown moves occlusally, the bone fills in to conform to the smaller root diameter (Fig. 7–16B–D). As eruption, proceeds, other collagen fiber bundles become visible along the forming root (Fig. 7–16B–D). The area becomes more densely populated with fibroblasts (Fig. 7–17). A special type of fibroblast, the myofibroblast, is said to have contractile capabilities. It has been reported to be present in the periodontal ligament. If present, the myofibroblast could aid in the force needed in tooth eruption. All ligament cells and fibers are currently believed to be important in the eruptive process. During eruptive movements, collagen formation and fiber turnover are very rapid (possibly 24 hours). Very early in the eruptive process, perforating fibers attach to the cementum on the root surface and to the alveolar bone. Some fibers release as the tooth moves, then reattach to stabilize the tooth. In this manner, the tooth-stabilizing process is performed by the same groups of fibers throughout tooth eruption. The fibroblasts are the cells active in formation and degeneration of collagen fibers. Alveolar bone remodeling is continuous during eruption. As the tooth moves occlusally, the alveolar bone increases in height and changes shape to accommodate passage of the crown (Fig. 7–18). The tooth crown, as seen in Figure 7–18, has migrated occlusally, which results in new bone being deposited around the root to reduce the size of the crypt. Above and around the crown, osteoclastic and osteoblastic action occurs. These actions are coordinated during the entire eruption process, as well as throughout life.

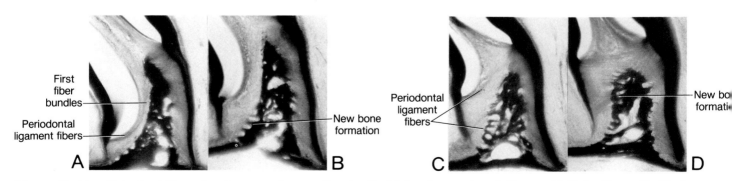

Figure 7–18. Principal fiber development in erupting teeth. Note change in relations of follicle fibers (A–D), from tooth to bone.

Changes in Tissues Underlying Teeth. Changes also occur in the follicular tissue underlying the developing tooth. These changes take place in the soft tissue and the *fundic bone* (bone surrounding the apex of the root). As the tooth erupts, space is provided for the root to lengthen, primarily because of the crown moving occlusally and the increase in height of the alveolar bone. Changes in the fundic region are thus believed to be largely compensatory to the lengthening of the root. During the preeruptive and early eruptive phases, the follicular fibroblasts and fibers lie in a plane parallel to the base of the root (Fig. 7–19). The tooth moves more rapidly in the socket during prefunctional eruption than at any other period. Fine bony trabeculae appear in the fundic area. They compensate for tooth eruption and provide some support to the apical tissues (Fig. 7–19). Some authors describe this as a bony ladder. The ladder becomes more dense as alternate layers of bone plates and connective tissue are laid down (Fig. 7–20). At the end of the prefunctional eruptive phase, when the tooth comes into occlusion, about one third of the enamel remains covered by the gingiva (Fig. 7–21D), and the root is incomplete. At this time, the bony ladder is gradually resorbed, one plate at a time, to make space for the developing root tip. Root completion continues for a considerable time after the teeth have been in function; this process takes from 1 to 1.5 years in primary teeth and from 2 to 3 years in permanent teeth.

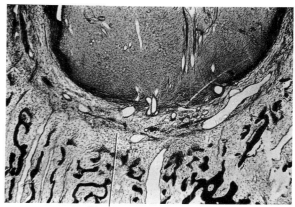

Proliferating cells and new bone formation

Figure 7–19. Changes in fundic bone during eruptive movement.

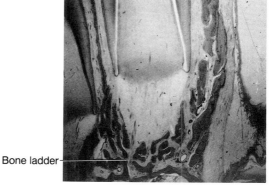

Bone ladder

Figure 7–20. Formation of bone ladder in fundic region.

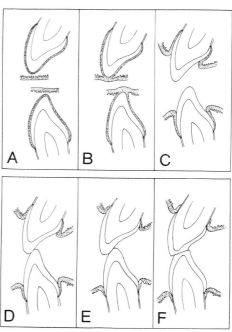

A B C D E F

Figure 7–21. Changes in relation of epithelial tissue during tooth eruption. Formation of junctional epithelium. (A, B). Preeruptive. (C). Prefunctional. (D–F). Functional.

Functional Eruptive Phase (Posteruptive Phase)

The final eruptive phase, the functional eruptive phase, begins when the teeth reach occlusion, and continues for as long as each tooth remains in the oral cavity. During the early phase of this period, the alveolar processes increase in height and the roots continue to grow. The teeth continue to move occlusally, which accommodates jaw growth and allows for root elongation. The most marked changes occur as occlusion is established. Alveolar bone density increases, and the principal fibers of the periodontal ligament establish themselves into separate groups oriented about the gingiva, the alveolar crest, and the alveolar surface around the root.

The diameter of the fiber bundles increases from delicate, fine groups of fibers to heavy, securely stabilized bundles (Fig. 7–22). Arteries are established circumferentially and longitudinally in the central zone of the periodontal ligament. Figure 7–23 is a photomicrograph of a developing root. India ink outlines each of the blood vessels in the pulp, as well as in the periodontal ligament. Observe the numerous vessels that enter the ligament from the alveolar bone. Nerves for sensing pain, heat, cold, proprioception, and pressure organize in the periodontal ligament and course alongside these vessels. From apex to gingiva, both myelinated and nonmyelinated nerves traverse the central region of the ligament along with the blood vessels (Fig. 7–24). When the root canal narrows, as a result of root tip maturation, apical fibers develop to help cushion the forces of occlusal impact (Fig. 7–22). Later in life, attrition may wear down the occlusal surfaces of the teeth. The teeth erupt slightly to compensate for loss of tooth structure and to prevent occlusal overclosure (Fig. 7–21F). If the occlusal wear is excessive, cementum

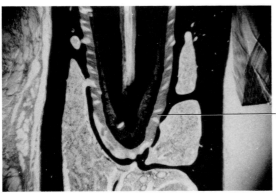

Figure 7–22. Increased density of periodontal ligament fibers during eruption.

Periodontal fiber bundles

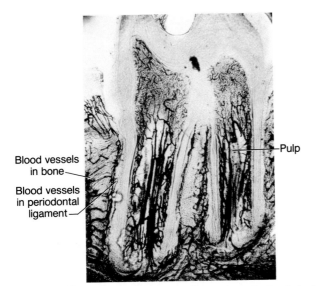

Figure 7–23. Vascularization or pulp and periodontal structures during tooth eruption.

Blood vessels in bone

Blood vessels in periodontal ligament

Pulp

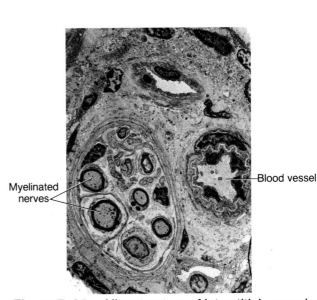

Figure 7–24. Ultrastructure of interstitial space in periodontal ligament along with nerves and blood vessels.

Myelinated nerves

Blood vessel

is deposited on the apical third of the root (Fig. 7–25); it is deposited in the furcation region to compensate for hypereruption of the teeth. Some bone apposition occurs at the alveolar crests. In addition to slight occlusal movement, the teeth tend to move anteriorly. This is termed *mesial drift*, and results in bone resorption on the mesial wall of the socket and bone apposition on the distal wall.

Theories of Tooth Eruption

Many factors related to tooth eruption have been studied, and several appear to be important to the eruptive process. It was once thought that root growth and pulpal pressure were fundamental factors, until cases of eruption of rootless teeth were reported. The idea that the fundic bone area and bony ladder formation were causes was discounted as measurements of the eruption pathway and the timing of its appearance revealed that these factors are more likely a result, rather than a cause of eruption. Vascularity has long been considered to have a role in tooth eruption. For example, resection of the sympathetic nerves causes vasodilation and results in earlier eruption of teeth. Localized hyperemia, as a result of periodontitis, also causes increased vascularity of periodontal tissues and increased eruption of adjacent teeth. Many other factors, such as hypopituitarism, decrease vascularity and also retard eruption.

Important to the discussion of causes of tooth eruption is the tooth at the cap and bell stage. It has been shown that follicular cells migrate from near the surface of the enamel organs and dental papillae to give rise to the cementum, periodontal ligament, and alveolar bone. Because these cells affect the resorption of bone in eccentric growth and bodily movement of the teeth, they probably have a role in tooth eruption. These cells may cause enzymatic degeneration of the tissues overlying the teeth and may contribute to the formation of tissues surrounding and underlying the teeth. Recent studies have shown the dental follicle to be of prime importance in tooth eruption. Removal of the dental follicle causes cessation of eruption. The main role of the dental follicle in tooth eruption is the formation of the eruption pathway ahead of the advancing tooth. The folicle also provides the osteoblasts that form the bone trabeculae apical to the tooth. These events all take place at precise times during tooth eruption.

There are many unanswered questions concerning the biochemistry of the follicle tissue, such as the role of epidermal growth factor, prostaglandins, transforming growth factor, and other influencing factors. What the biologic basis of directionality of tooth eruption is, remains unanswered.

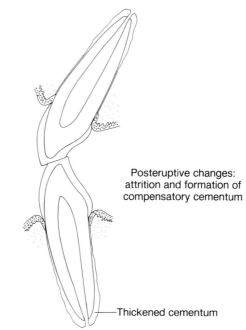

Posteruptive changes: attrition and formation of compensatory cementum

Thickened cementum

Figure 7–25. Posteruptive changes: attrition and compensative formation of cementum.

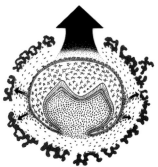

Figure 7–26. Cells lying near the outer enamel epithelium migrate into the follicle and aid in periodontal development and eruption of the tooth.

Decreased pressure overlying a tooth and increased pressure around and under it are major factors in tooth eruption. First, the eruption pathway begins development when root formation commences (Fig. 7–26). In fact, several investigators have shown that this pathway will develop even when the tooth is mechanically prevented from eruption. Second, remodeling of tissues surrounding the teeth occurs during both prefunctional and functional eruptive periods. As the periodontal ligament fibers increase in number and change position, the alveolar bone remodels and thus limits the soft-tissue space around the teeth. At the same time, the periodontal fibroblasts proliferate and the vascular supply increases (Fig. 7–27). All these changes bring about increased pressure around and under the erupting teeth.

Degeneration of epithelium overyling cusps

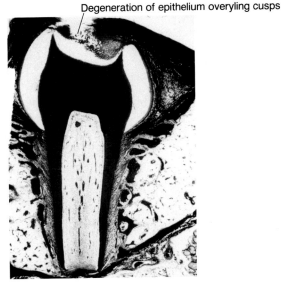

Figure 7–27. Increase in cell activity in periodontal ligament during eruption.

Clinical Application

The "six/four" rule for primary tooth emergence means that from birth, four teeth will emerge for each 6 months of age. Thus, age 6 months = 4 teeth, 12 months = 8 teeth; 18 months = 12 teeth; 24 months = 16 teeth; and 30 months = 20 teeth.

Chronology of Tooth Eruption

The eruption sequence of the primary dentition is presented in Figure 7–28 and Table 7–1; the eruption sequence of the permanent dentition is shown in Figure 7–29 and Table 7–2. In the *primary* dentition, eruption occurs earlier in boys than in girls. In the permanent dentition, however, eruption in girls usually precedes that in boys. There are no sex differences in the eruption *sequence* of the *primary* teeth.

Clinical Application

The pattern and sequence of eruption of the primary teeth affects the eruption, and therefore occlusion, of the permanent teeth. This is significant because it is essential to accurate treatment planning.

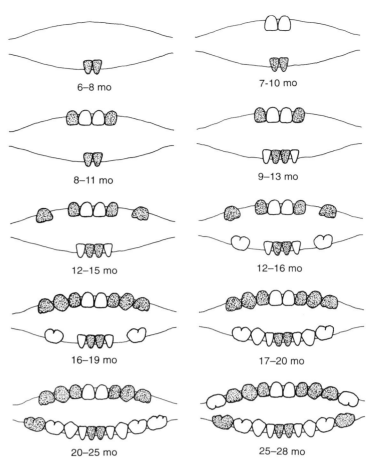

Figure 7–28. Eruption time and sequence of the primary dentition. Shaded teeth erupt earlier than the corresponding teeth in the opposing arch (see Table 7–1).

Table 7–1.
Chronology of Development of the Primary Dentition

Primary Teeth in Order of Eruption (Sequence)	Beginning Calcification (mo In Utero)	Crown Completed Postnatally (mo)	Appearance in the Oral Cavity (Eruption Time) (mo)	Root Completed Time (y)
Lower central incisor	3–4	2–3	6–8	1–2
Upper central incisor	3–4	2	7–10	1–2
Upper lateral incisor	4	2–3	8–11	2
Lower lateral incisor	4	3	9–13	1–2
Upper first molar	4	6	12–15	2–3
Lower first molar	4	6	12–16	2–3
Upper canine	4–5	9	16–19	3
Lower canine	4–5	9	17–20	3
Lower second molar	5	10	20–26	3
Upper second molar	5	11	25–28	3

The normal range of eruption times indicates a wide variation in eruption times. A difference of 1 or 2 months on either side of the normal range would not necessarily mean that a child's eruption time schedule is abnormal. Only deviations considerably outside this range should be considered abnormal.

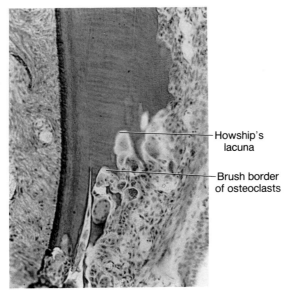

Figure 7–33. Osteoclasts on surface of tooth root.

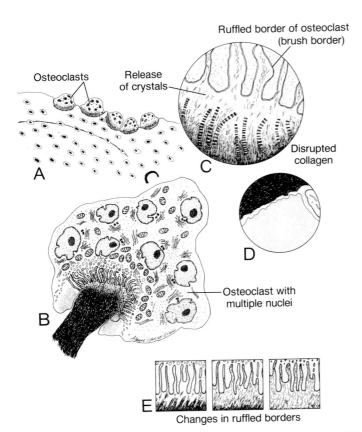

Figure 7–34. Osteoclast activity in Howship's lacunae. (A). Osteoclasts in lacunae. (B). Multinucleated osteoclast with brush border contacting spicule. (C). Ruffled border of osteoclasts with mineral intracellularly and collagen extracellularly. (D). "Clear zone" of osteoclast. (E). Constant flux of ruffled border during resorption process.

2. Loss of bone: Weakening of the supporting tissues of the primary teeth occurs as a result of root resorption and modifications of the alveolar bone. Supporting structures are weakened also by facial growth of the alveolar bone, which occurs to provide sufficient space for the positioning of the permanent teeth (Fig. 7–30).

3. Increased force: Increased masticatory forces on the weakened teeth are a result of muscular growth. This amplifies compression of the periodontal ligament and promotes resorption of teeth and alveolar bone (Fig. 7–33).

Root and Bone Resorption

The process of resorption is initiated by osteoclasts or odontoclasts thought to originate from the fusion of circulating blood monocytes. Osteoclasts are generally large, multinucleated cells that appear in cup-shaped depressions of the resorbing front of any hard tissue (Fig. 7–32). The cup-shaped depressions are called *Howship's lacunae* (Fig. 7–33). Under the light microscope, the osteoclast appears as a large cell containing 6 to 12 nuclei. It has a vacuolated cytoplasm and a striated or brush border adjacent to the resorbing hard tissue (Fig. 7–34). The electron microscope reveals a ruffled border consisting of deep invaginations of the cell membrane forming numerous intermingled villuslike processes. These differ in diameter not only from one another but also along the course of individual villi. The cytoplasm of the ruffled border is almost devoid of organelles. Between the ruffled border and the nuclei the cytoplasm is extremely rich in mitochondria (Fig. 7–34). Still deeper and closer to the nuclei many Golgi stacks are present surrounded by electron-dense granules and smooth and coated vesicles. The electron-dense granules are membrane-bound granules with a central electron-dense core surrounded by a pale halo. They are specific granules characteristic of osteoclasts and their precursors. They appear spherical or elongated and are found in monocytes as well. Acid phosphatase has been demonstrated in them. As for the nuclei, their ultrastructural appearance differs according to whether the osteoclast is young or old. In young osteoclasts the nuclei are ovoid and euchromatic (pale) with smooth nuclear membranes. In older osteoclasts the nuclei become heterochromatic (dark) showing wrinkled outlines and may be pyknotic.

Being unable to divide, an osteoclast is the result of fusion of cells rather than the product of repeated nuclear division. Recently studies confirmed the hemopoietic origin of osteoclasts from circulating monocytes. Some investigators have demonstrated that odontoclast precursors become fully differentiated and develop prominent ruffled borders only when they come in direct contact with mineralized dentin to be resorbed. They also observed that concomitant with the ruffled border formation, odontoclasts exhibit extensive synthesis and storage of acid phosphatase in many vacuoles and vesicles. Current information indicates that hard-tissue resorption occurs in two phases. The extracellular phase involves the initial breakdown of a small area of hard tissue into partially dissolved fragments. In the intracellular phase, the osteoclast appears to ingest and complete the dissolution of the breakdown products. Resorption of hard tissue occurs near the ruffled border of the osteoclast. The cell appears to surround the resorption site with a modified or clear zone of cytoplasm (Fig. 7–34B and D), which suggests that the seal increases the effectiveness of its hydrolytic enzymes. As the osteoclast attacks the hard-tissue matrix, the collagen meshwork is disrupted and crystals are released (Fig. 7–34C). The banding pattern characteristic of collagen fibrils at this stage can be seen with electron microscopy. Free crystals appear to be taken into cytoplasmic vacuoles of the osteoclast and are gradually digested within it (Fig. 7–35). The disrupted collagen fibrils are destroyed by *fibroblast-clasts*, cells in the periodontal ligament capable of both degradation and synthesis of collagen.

During the process of resorption, the pressure of the erupting permanent tooth is first directed to the bone separating the crypt of the permanent tooth from the alveolus of the primary tooth (Fig. 7–36). After this area is resorbed, the eruptive force is directed at the root of the primary tooth, which results in resorption of the cementum and dentin.

Resorption, like eruption, is not a continuous process; periods of activity alternate with periods of rest. During periods of rest, repair may take place by apposition of bone and cementum in limited areas of the root, which results in partial reattachment of the tooth. This explains why children experience periods when primary teeth alternate between looseness and fixation. Resorption usually proceeds faster than repair and ultimately results in the tooth being shed.

Resorption Pattern of Anterior Teeth

Resorption of the primary anterior teeth begins at about 4 to 5 years for the incisors and 6 to 8 years for the canines, depending on whether they are mandibular or maxillary canines. At these times, the crowns of the permanent successors are completed and situated in their own crypts lingual to the apical third of the roots of the corresponding primary teeth (Fig. 7–36).

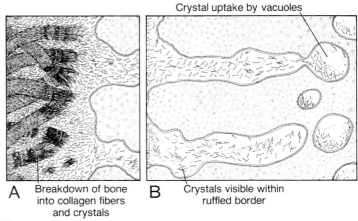

Figure 7–35. Uptake of mineral crystals in intracellular vacuoles. (A). Crystals appear within cytoplasmic extensions of the osteoclast. (B). Development of vacuoles in osteoclast cytoplasm.

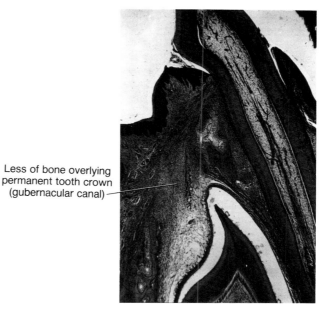

Figure 7–36. Histology of permanent incisor crown to primary tooth.

Clinical Application

In infants, tooth eruption may be accompanied by a slight rise in temperature, mild irritation of the gums, and general malaise. Any severe general symptoms, however, should not be associated with teething, although some systemic disturbance at the time of tooth eruption should be expected.

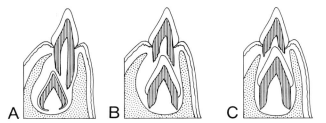

Figure 7–37. Relative position of a permanent anterior tooth to its primary predecessor during the process of shedding.

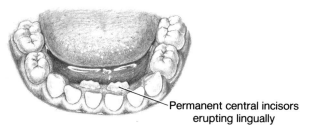

Permanent central incisors erupting lingually

Figure 7–38. Clinical view of eruption sites of permanent teeth lingual to primary crowns.

Plane of occlusion

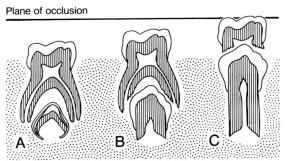

Progressive resorption and exfolation of primary tooth as permanent tooth develops

Figure 7–39. Relative position of a premolar to a primary molar during the process of shedding.

With the onset of eruptive movement of the permanent teeth, which proceeds in an incisal and labial direction, pressure is first directed at the bone separating the crypts of the permanent successors and the alveolus of the primary roots. With the loss of the separating bone, pressure is then directed at the primary roots (Fig. 7–37A). Thus, resorption of the primary anterior teeth first occurs along the lingual surface of the apical third of the root. It then proceeds labially until the crown of the erupting permanent tooth comes to lie directly apical to the primary tooth root (Fig. 7–37B). Resorption then proceeds horizontally in an incisal direction, causing the primary root to exfoliate and the permanent ones erupt in its place (Fig. 7–37C).

Sometimes, particularly in the region of the mandibular incisors, the labial movement of the permanent teeth does not cause complete loss of the primary roots. This may result in the primary incisors remaining in the jaw and attached to the labial alveolar bone. Then, when the crowns of the permanent incisors emerge through the gingiva, they appear lingual to the primary ones that are still in place (Fig. 7–38). Prompt removal of the primary crown and remaining root assists the permanent ones in correcting their positions.

In the maxillary jaw, however, if the permanent canines appear in a misplaced position, they usually do so labial to the existing primary canines. Again, prompt removal is beneficial. It is rare to see a maxillary permanent canine erupting lingual to a primary one, as the permanent canine could then become embedded in the heavy bone of the palate.

Resorption Pattern of Posterior Teeth

The growing premolar crowns are initially located between the roots of the primary molar teeth (Fig. 7–39A). The first signs of resorption around these crowns occur in the supporting interradicular bone. This is followed by resorption of the adjacent surfaces of the primary tooth roots (Fig. 7–39B). Meanwhile, the bony alveolar processes increase in height to compensate for the lengthening roots of the permanent teeth (premolars). As this occurs the primary molars emerge occlusally, which positions the premolar crowns more apical to the primary molar roots. The premolars continue to erupt as the primary molar roots further resorb, and these teeth then exfoliate (Fig. 7–39C). The premolars then erupt in place of the primary molars.

Abnormal Behavior of Primary Teeth
Retained Primary Teeth

The most common causes for retained primary teeth are *absence* or *impaction* of the permanent successor. The teeth most often affected are the upper lateral incisors; next affected are the lower second molars; the teeth least often affected are the lower central incisors. Retained primary teeth often remain functional for many years among the permanent teeth before they are lost through resorption of their roots. Their loss is believed to be contributed to by the heavy masticatory forces of adult life on the small roots and by the continued active eruption and progresssive elongation of the clinical crown of such teeth at the expense of root length.

Submerged Primary Teeth

Sometimes, primary teeth become *ankylosed*. Such teeth are prevented from active eruption and become submerged in the alveolar bone as a result of the continued eruption of adjacent teeth and the increase in height of the alveolar ridge (Fig. 7–40). Submerged primary teeth should be removed as soon as possible, particularly when their permanent successors are present. The major difference between retained and submerged primary teeth is that the latter are fused to the alveolar bone (ankylosed), whereas the former are not. Deeply submerged teeth suggest that the ankylosis occurred early during childhood.

Remnants of Primary Teeth

Remnants of primary teeth are parts of the roots of the primary teeth; these parts escaped resorption during the process of shedding. Such root remnants remain embedded in the jaw; are most frequently seen in ther interdental septa in the region of the lower second premolars; are usually asymptomatic; and, if observed on X-ray, should not be disturbed. Root remnants may exfoliate if they are near the surface of the jaws, or they may undergo resorption and become replaced by bone, thus disappearing completely.

Preprimary Teeth

In very rare cases, preprimary teeth appear in the oral cavity of newborn or neonatal infants. They are commonly found on the alveolar ridge of the mandible, in the incisor region, and usually number two or three. Because they possess no roots, they are not firmly attached. Frequently, they are shed during the first few weeks of life. They should be removed as soon as possible, however, to prevent discomfort to both the mother and the baby during suckling. Removal of the preprimary teeth does not affect the primary teeth. Sometimes, however, the teeth seen in the mouth of a newborn baby are premature primary teeth. Thus, they are not replaced after they fall out, and their place remains patent until the corresponding permanent teeth erupt.

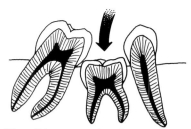

Figure 7–40. Diagram of submerged primary tooth.

Clinical Application

Ankylosis is a hard tissue union between bone and tooth. It probably occurs as a result of disturbance in the interaction between normal resorption and hard tissue repair during shedding. Primary molars are the teeth mostly affected, where ankylosis occurs mainly at the furcation area.

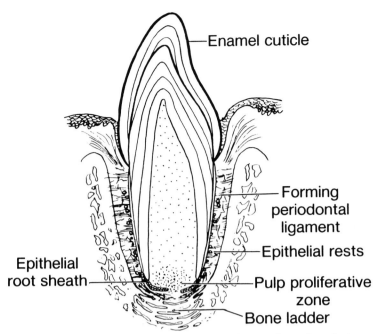

—Enamel cuticle

Forming
periodontal
ligament

Epithelial rests

Epithelial
root sheath

Pulp proliferative
zone

Bone ladder

Figure 7-41. Summary of changes in the tooth and periodontium with eruption-modification of alveolar bone and organization of ligament with root growth.

Summary

Eruption is the movement of the teeth through the bone of the jaws and the overlying mucosa, to appear and function in the oral cavity. These eruptive movements can be divided into three phases: preeruptive, prefunctional eruptive, and functional eruptive.

Active eruption is the result of occlusal movement of the tooth. After emergence of the tooth through the gingiva, active eruption is accompanied by gradual exposure of the clinical crown by separation of the attachment epithelium and the apical shift of the gingiva.

Clinical eruption begins with the appearance of the crown tip in the oral cavity and continues until the tooth comes into occlusion. During this period, the tooth moves faster than at any other time. Figure 7-41 indicates many of the changes occuring at this time. The periodontal fibers are organizing to stabilize the erupting tooth, the root sheath is growing, and root dentinogenesis follows as the bone in the fundic region organizes in response to the changes in root length.

Like most mammals, the human is a diphyodont creature—that is, possesses two sets of teeth: primary and permanent. The teeth of the primary set are small and fewer, to fit the small jaws of the infant. Because the teeth, once formed, cannot increase in size, the primary set of teeth must exfoliate and be replaced by the larger, more numerous teeth of the permanent set to accommodate the larger jaws of the adult.

Shedding of the primary teeth is the result of progressive resorption of their roots through the activity of the osteoclasts or odontoclasts. Hard-tissue resorption occurs in two phases: the extracellular, during which the matrix fragments and dissolution begins, and the intracellular, during which complete digestion of the products of resorption occurs. The process of resorption is not continuous; periods of activity alternate with periods of rest. Disturbance of the resorption process results in abnormal behavior of the primary teeth; some primary teeth may be retained because of the absence or impaction of their permanent successors; others may be ankylosed and submered.

In rare cases, teeth may appear in the oral cavity of newborn or neonatal infants, and are called preprimary teeth.

Self-Evaluation Review

1. What is the purpose of crown movements during the preeruptive phase of tooth eruption?
2. What are the characteristics of the intraosseus and supraosseus stages of the prefunctional phase of eruption?

3. What is the relation of the secretory phase of amelogenesis to the beginning of root formation?
4. Describe the characteristics of the functional stage of permanent tooth eruption.
5. What are three causes believed to be important in shedding of primary teeth?
6. What is the cause of periods of looseness and fixation during the eruption and shedding of the primary teeth?
7. Describe the two phases of bone resorption. Indicate which cells are believed responsible for each phase, and their function.
8. Explain the rule of "fours" for development of the permanent teeth.
9. Explain the "six/four" rule for emergence of the primary teeth.
10. What are some possible causes of tooth eruption?

Acknowledgments

The author wishes to recognize the contribution by David Johnson of Case Western University School of Dentistry of Figure 7–16. Dr. Roger Noonan, Program Director, Department of Pediatric Dentistry, Loyola University School of Dentistry, Maywood, Illinois, provided the clinical applications of the "Rule of fours" and "six fours." Dr. Sol Bernick (deceased) of the University of Southern California provided Figure 7–23.

Suggested Readings

Andreasen JO. External resorption: its implication in dental traumatology, paedodontics, periodontics, orthodontics, and endodontics. *Int. Endo. J.* 1986:67–70.

Berkowitz, BKB, Mohham BJ, Newman HN. The periodontal ligament and physiologic tooth movement. In BKB Berkowitz, BJ Moxham, HN Newman, eds. *The Periodontal Ligament in Health and Disease.* New York, NY: Pergamon Press; 1982:215–247.

Gorski JP, Marks SC Jr. Current concepts of the biology of tooth eruption. *Crit. Rev. Oral Biol. Med.* 1992;3:185–206.

Marks SC Jr, Gorski JP, Cahill DR, Wise GG. Tooth eruption, a synthesis of experimental observations. In: Davidovich Z, ed. *The Biological Mechanisms of Tooth Eruption and Root Resorption.* Birmingham, Ala: EBSCO Media; 1988:161–169.

Moxham BJ. The role of the periodontal vasculature in tooth eruption. In: Davidovich Z, ed. *The Biological Mechanism of Tooth Eruption and Root Resorption.* Birmingham, Ala: EBSCO Media; 1988: 207–233.

Proffit WR. The effect of intermittent forces on eruption. In: Davidovich Z, (ed). *The Biological Mechanisms of Tooth Eruption and Root Resorption.* Birmingham, Ala: EBSCO Media; 1988:187–191.

Steedle JR, Proffit WR. The pattern and control of the eruptive tooth movements. *Am. J. Orthodont.* 1985;87:56–66.

Thesleff I. Does epidermal growth factor control tooth eruption? *J. Dent. Child* 1987;84:321–329.

Topham RT, Chiego DJ Jr, Smith AJ, Huiton DA, Gattone VH II, Klein R. Effects of epidermal growth factor on tooth differentiation and eruption. In: Davidovich, Z, ed. *The Biological Mechanisms of Tooth Eruption and Root Resorption.* Birmingham, Ala: EBSCO Media; 1988:117–131.

Wise GE, Marks SC, Cahill DR. Ultrastructural features of the dental follicle associated with the eruption pathway in the dog. *J. Oral Path.* 1985;14:15–26.

Zajick G. Fibroblast cell kinetics in the periodontal ligament in the mouse. *Cell. Tissue Kinet.* 1974;7:479–492.

Agents Affecting Tooth and Bone Development

James K. Avery

Introduction

Certain vitamin and hormone deficiencies, if present during tooth formation will adversely affect formative cells and the matrix that they produce. Reduced organic matrix content results in production of hypoplastic tissue. Excessive levels of tetracycline or fluoride may become incorporated into mineralizing teeth and interfere with the mineralization process. Should both situations occur, a hypoplastic matrix that is also hypomineralized would result. The extent of the defect is dependent on the nature of the substance, the degree of excess or deficiency, and the developmental time frame. Vitamins A, C, and D, parathyroid hormone, tetracycline, and fluoride are discussed in terms of their relation to matrix development, and dentin and enamel mineralization in developing teeth. Most experiments have been conducted on the continuously developing rodent incisors, which adequately records developmental defects. Tooth development may be affected by many substances. The examples cited are those most frequently studied in animal and human research.

Objectives

After reading this chapter you should be able to describe in detail the effects of various vitamins, hormones, sodium fluoride, and tetracycline on developing teeth.

Vitamin A Deficiency

Although tissues of ectodermal origin—that is, the epidermis—are primarily affected in vitamin A deficiency, bones and teeth also record this deficiency. A vitaminosis A is evidenced by marked metaplasia of the enamel organ, which results in defective enamel and dentin formation (Fig. 8–1). Likewise, bone is laid down in abnormal locations, and its remodeling sequences seem to be affected. Both osteoclasts and osteoblasts have been shown to be affected by this disease process. Dentinal irregularities associated with vitamin A deficiency in developing teeth appear as areas characterized by either excessive osteodentin deposition (bonelike, with cell inclusions) or insufficient dentin depositions (Figs. 8–1 and 8–2). Alterations of the differentiated odontoblasts appear to be associated with these conditions. Some investigators, however, ascribe the primary effects of vitamin A deficiency to oral epithelial cells. This view originates from histological changes seen initially in the oral mucosa and extending to the degeneration of the epithelial-derived ameloblasts, which results in a hypoplastic enamel matrix. If the vitamin A deficiency is severe, ameloblast cells will become completely atrophied, which results in an absence of enamel formation. In less severe cases, the columnar ameloblasts apparently shorten, and adjacent enamel exhibits hypoplasia. An example may be seen in Figure 8–2. Several authors have described bone defects due to vitamin A deficiency. Most have noted that the defects are attributable to impaired endochondral ossification and faulty bone modeling. Figure 8–2 shows shortened ameloblasts and defective enamel and dentin formation. The normal appositional rhythm of dentin deposition may be altered. Vascular inclusions sometimes are seen in the dentin (Figs. 8–1 and 8–2). If the vitamin A deficiency is relieved during subsequent tooth development, normal dentin and enamel are produced, although defective tissue is not repaired (Fig. 8–2). Figure 8–3 illustrates enamel hypoplasia induced by vitamin A deficiency.

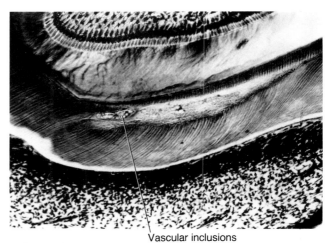
Vascular inclusions

Figure 8–1. Histology of vitamin A deficiency reveals enamel matrix deficiency and related defects in dentin at the dentinoenamel junction.

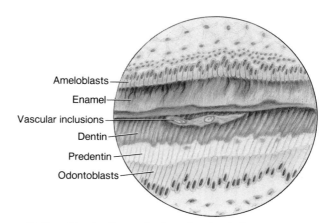

Ameloblasts
Enamel
Vascular inclusions
Dentin
Predentin
Odontoblasts

Figure 8–2. Illustration of vitamin A deficiency indicates shortened ameloblasts, enamel matrix deficiency, and vascular inclusions in dentin at the dentinoenamel junction.

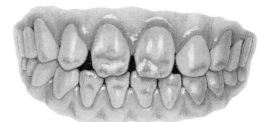

Figure 8–3. Illustration of clinical view of defective enamel resulting from vitamin A deficiency.

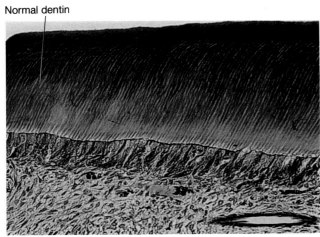

Figure 8–4. Normal-appearing dentin.

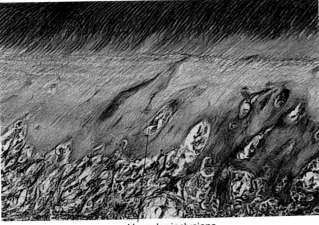

Figure 8–5. Appearance of defective dentin formation resulting from vitamin C deficiency, with vascular inclusions and degenerated odontoblasts.

Vitamin C Deficiency

Ascorbic acid deficiency has been described in guinea pigs, monkeys, and humans. Because none of these species synthesize vitamin C, they must depend on a dietary supply to maintain health. Scurvy, the disease resulting from vitamin C deficiency causes bone, dentin, and cementum deposition to cease and formative cells to atrophy, if severe. Vitamin C is required for collagen formation. It is necessary for the hydroxylation of the amino acids proline and lysine; an absence or deficiency of vitamin C during dentinogenesis results in defective dentinal tissue development. Dentinal tubules become irregular and reduced in number, vascular inclusions become apparent, and those odontoblasts present are short, with some taking on a spindle-shaped fibroblast-like appearance. Compare the appearance of normal dentin, in Figure 8–4 with that of dentin formed while vitamin C was deficient, in Figure 8–5. Figure 8–6 is an illustration of characteristics associated with vitamin C deficiency. Embryologically, vitamin C is essential for proper development of all mesenchymally derived structures, including bone, dentin, and cementum. Clinically, vitamin C deficiency is manifested by gingival bleeding and loosening of the teeth due to bone resorption. Weakness, anemia, and susceptibility to hemorrhage also may be evident. Administration of vitamin C results in rapid elimination of the symptoms associated with this deficiency.

Clinical Application

Clinically, vitamin C deficiency is manifested orally by gingival bleeding and loosening the teeth. Weakness, anemia, bone loss, and susceptability to hemorrhage may also be associated with this deficiency.

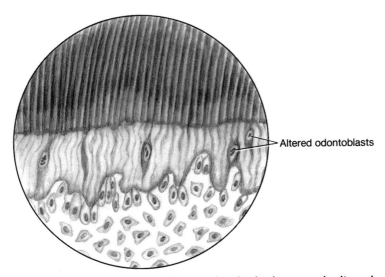

Figure 8–6. Illustration of vascular inclusions and altered odontoblasts resulting from vitamin C deficiency.

Vitamin D Deficiency

Vitamin D is essential for deposition of calcium and phosphorus in hard tissues. Its presence increases the absorption of dietary calcium and maintains proper levels of calcium and phosphorus in the blood. Primary deficiency of vitamin D results from insufficient exposure to the sun and insufficient dietary intake. Secondary deficiencies result from abnormal intestinal resorption. Secondary deficiencies may be overcome by alteration of dietary intake of calcium and phosphorus. A severe vitamin D deficiency in children results in rickets, a condition characterized by insufficient deposition of calcium salts in bony tissue. Hypoplasia of the enamel also may be evident. Although vitamin D deficiency is less common among adults, it is manifested by decreased mineralization of the bone matrix. Bones insufficiently mineralized, especially the weight-bearing long bones, are prone to bending and distortion.

In Figures 8–7 and 8–8, note the abnormally wide nonmineralized zone of predentin and the interglobular spaces in the dentin. Figure 8–8 also shows areas of enamel affected by hypoplasia and hypomineralization. Results of a study of children with rickets indicated that as many as 25% exhibited enamel hypoplasia. It has been reported that hypomineralized cementum is frequently found in these children. No other vitamin deficiencies have such notable effects on tooth formation as do vitamin A, C, and D deficiencies.

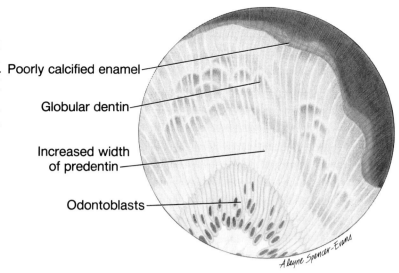

Poorly calcified enamel

Globular dentin

Increased width of predentin

Odontoblasts

Hypoplasia of enamel and dentin

Clinical appearance of "rickets" (a severe vitamin D deficiency)

Figure 8–7. Illustration of histology and clinical view of vitamin D deficiency.

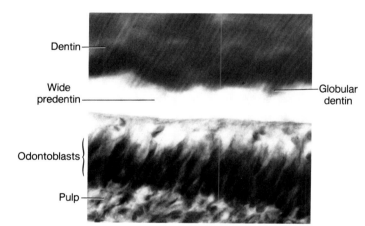

Dentin

Wide predentin

Globular dentin

Odontoblasts

Pulp

Figure 8–8. Histology of vitamin D deficiency. Globular dentin is indicated by irregular staining of matrix and by wide predentin.

Clinical Application

Osteoporosis results when calcium loss because of resorption is greater than calcium deposition. This may be evident orally with loss of alveolar bone and loosening of the teeth.

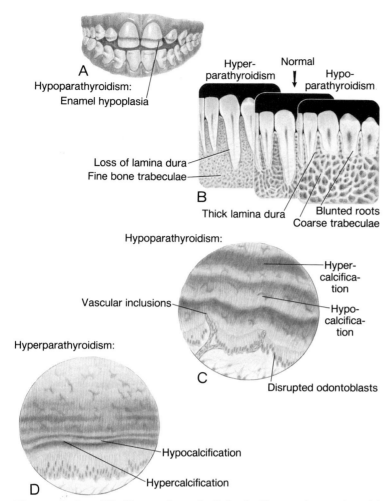

Figure 8–9. (A). Illustration of clinical effects of parathyroid hormone. (B). Diagrams of radiographs indicate altered supporting bone. (C) and (D) are the histological appearance of alternating bands of hypocalcified and hypercalcified dentin. These bands may demonstrate the clinical appearance of hypocalcified tooth and bone.

Parathyroid Hormone

The parathyroid glands regulae calcium balance in the body. An imbalance of parathyroid hormone (PTH), either deficiency or excess, may affect bone and tooth formation. Excess PTH (hyperparathyroidism) causes mobilization of calcium from the skeleton into the blood stream. Calcium ions may then be excreted in urine, feces, sweat, and milk. PTH may influence all of these mechanisms. Calcium excretion results in hypocalcemia or decreased levels of blood calcium, and the bone, in turn, mobilizes more calcium. When calcium resorption is greater than deposition, osteoporosis results. Osteoporosis may then, for example, weaken the supporting alveolar bone of the teeth. As shown in Figure 8–9, calcium mobilization in bone results in decreased bone density around the tooth, which is seen as a thinning of the lamina dura. Inactive parathyroids (hypoparathyroidism) results in low blood concentrations of ionized calcium, which causes an increase in gland activity. Bone density increases, which results in increased thickness of the lamina dura and an increased density of bone trabeculae (osteopetrosis). Calcium is not released from mature teeth as it is from bone; so the structure of teeth is not affected by hyperparathyroidism and hypoparathyroidism, except during development. Hyperparathyroidism will cause an initial hypocalcification of the forming dental tissue, followed by hypercalcification due to excessive blood calcium. Calcium excretion by the kidneys follows. The effect of hypoparathyroidism and hyperparathyroidism on teeth is illustrated in Figure 8–9. A section of defective dentin clearly shows the effects of both hypoparathyroidism and hyperparathyroidism (Fig. 8–10). The horizontally stained bands accentuate the hypocalcified and/or hypercalcified zones. A series of injections of parathyroid hormone into experimental animals were given to achieve this effect. Thus, both hyperparathyroidism and hypoparathyroidism produce calcium imbalance, which results in hypocalcified bands in the forming dentin. A loss of mineral in the supporting bone occurs with hyperparathyroidism, and increased deposition of mineral takes place with hypoparathyroidism.

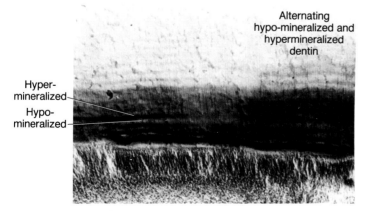

Figure 8–10. Alternating hypomineralized and hypermineralized dentin due to parathormone injections seen as bands of decreased and increased mineralization of the matrix.

Tetracycline and Fluoride

Tetracycline and fluoride, if available during the mineralization phases, may be incorporated in dentin, enamel, cementum, and bone. They are very different compounds. Fluoride is a binary compound of fluorine useful as an anticaries substance. Tetracycline, on the other hand, is used as an antibacterial agent. Both are deposited along with minerals in developing hard tissues. Tetracycline is derived from a yellow-gold fungus whose color is maintained in the purified antibiotic and transferred to the hard tissues in which it is incorporated. On prolonged exposure to light, tetracycline-stained dental tissue will change in color to a brown to gray (ie, these shades of discoloration are eventually seen in the teeth) (Fig. 8–11A). Other effects of tetracyclines include hypoplasia or absence of enamel. Staining is most notable in the dentin, especially in the first-formed dentin at the dentinoenamel junction. Notable staining of the crown is primarily from discolored dentin being seen through the translucent and relatively unaffected, enamel (Fig. 8–11B). Figure 8–12 is an example of a patient to whom tetracycline was given during early infancy. Staining is not visible in the central incisors, as the crowns were formed after cessation of treatment with tetracycline. The diffuse staining seen on the lateral incisors and cuspids indicates that they were undergoing development at the time. Tetracycline staining is more notable under ultraviolet (UV) light (Fig. 8–11B). The amount of damage is directly related to the magnitude and duration of the dosage; any defects caused by the tetracycline may be compounded by the effects of the illness itself. The precise mechanism of tetracycline incorporation into mineralizing tissue is not yet known, but it is believed that a chelate of calcium and tetracycline forms. At higher concentrations, cells may be altered, as is seen in Figure 8–11C. In both ameloblasts and odontoblasts, the cisternae of the endoplasmic reticulum become dilated, and protein synthesis is impaired. This, in turn, will result in hypoplasia of the enamel and dentin matrix.

Tetracycline and, to a limited extent, sodium fluoride cross the placental barrier and are available to the human fetus. If a pregnant female consumes fluoridated water during mineralization of the fetal teeth, the teeth will incorporate this compound. Such teeth exhibit higher resistance to dental caries. Compared with fluoride blood levels in the maternal circulation, fluoride blood levels in the fetus are relatively low. If, on the other hand, tetracycline antibiotics are administered to the mother during the period of tooth mineralization, the deciduous teeth may later be stained. Tetracycline staining of teeth is permanent; staining of bone is not permanent because bone is remodeled continuously.

The period marked by mineralization of crowns extends from approximately 5 months in utero to 12 years of age and includes the mineralization of both primary and permanent dentitions.

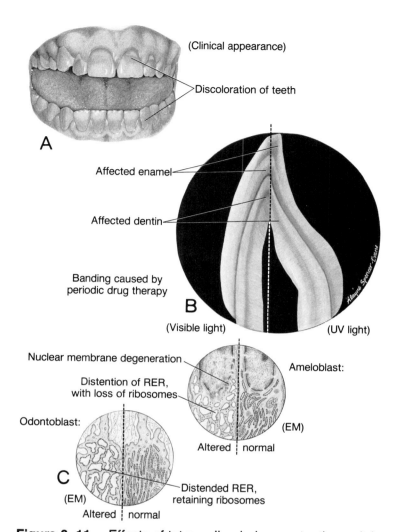

Figure 8–11. Effects of tetracycline in human teeth result in staining and hypoplastic enamel. Staining is evident in first-formed dentin. Both ameloblast and odontoblast endoplasmic reticula are altered.

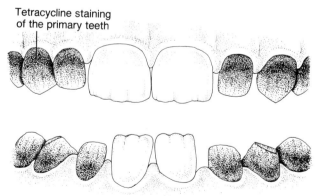

Figure 8–12. Illustration of tetracycline staining in teeth indicates that staining of those teeth developed when the injections were made.

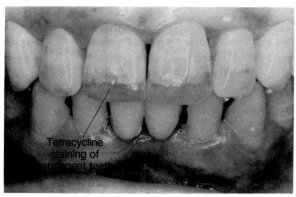

Figure 8–13. Clinical appearance of tetracycline staining.

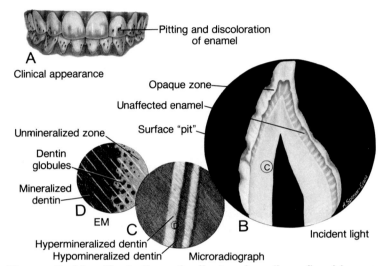

Figure 8–14. Illustration of effects of sodium fluoride on developing teeth. (A). The clinical picture reveals brown-stained hypoplastic pits. (B) illustrates the appearance of these pits in a ground section of the tooth seen in (A). (C) illustrates altered incremental lines of the encircled zone in (B). (D) illustrates the hypocalcified dentin of the encircled zone in (C), at higher magnification of the electron microscope.

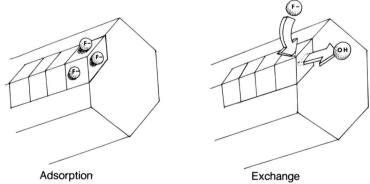

Figure 8–15. Diagram of two mechanisms of uptake of fluoride in enamel.

The teeth shown in Figure 8–13 exhibit brown staining of the incisal one third of the central incisors. This staining is due to tetracycline therapy that occurred during the initial phase of mineralization of these teeth; otherwise, the teeth would have been stained more cervically. Cervical staining is more characteristic of tetracycline because this agent deposits primarily in the dentin. The lateral permanent incisors, on the other hand, began mineralization after drug therapy and were not affected.

Figure 8–14A is a photograph of mottled enamel caused by sodium fluoride. Mottled enamel describes the scattered sites of pigmentation and hypoplasia (Fig. 8–14A). Sodium fluoride when taken into the body in concentrations of 5 ppm (which occurs in some naturally fluoridated areas in this country) is anticariogenic but often causes mottled enamel. The mottled areas may or may not be mineralized (Fig. 8–14C and D). The enamel rods follow an irregular course through these areas. Despite their unsightly appearance, these teeth are completely free of caries. Fluoride is most beneficial to the teeth in concentrations of approximately 0.5 to 1 ppm of water. Concentrations of 0.5 ppm may not prevent caries. Higher concentrations, such as 5 ppm, cause mottling and hypoplasia of the enamel and hypomineralized dentin, with increased interglobular spaces.

As hydroxyapatite crystals form, they may incorporate fluoride either by an *exchange* with the hydroxyl groups or by simple *adsorption*. The hydroxyl group exchange is slower and less reversible than adsorption. In the latter process, the fluoride may be adsorbed to the surface of hydroxyapatite crystals. This adsorptive process involves weak electrostatic bonding. Adsorption is believed to be rapid although reversible (Fig. 8–15).

> ### Clinical Application
>
> Effects of tetracyclines include staining of teeth, hypoplasia, and loss of enamel. Most of the staining is in the dentin, which is seen through the translucent enamel.

It is believed that fluoride found in inner enamel is taken up mainly during the secretory stage of amelogenesis and that fluoride found in the outer 30 to 50 μm of enamel occurs during the maturative stage. Because the latter stage lasts longer, there is time for more fluoride to be deposited in the outer enamel. The maturative stage lasts from 1 to 2 years in primary teeth and from 4 to 5 years in permanent teeth. This may be the reason for less fluoride being found in primary teeth than in permanent teeth.

When histological examination is conducted on teeth from areas of high fluoride concentration, the enamel is found to be altered more than is the dentin. Enamel rod formation is affected and zones of hypoplasia are commonly found. Figure 8–16, a photomicrograph, shows an area of hypoplasia and staining in the central fissure of a molar tooth; this area was caused by a high concentration of fluoride. Note that the inner enamel is stained less than the outer enamel. This is because the inner enamel is deposited prenatally, when less fluoride is available for incorporation.

Tetracycline was first discovered to be in human teeth and bones when traces were detected in bones being viewed under UV light. This observation provided a new method of marking bones and teeth for following their development. An example of this procedure is shown in Figure 8–17 in which the slab of dentin was photographed under UV light. The photograph shows that tetracycline had been incorporated into new dentin that was mineralizing. This created the vertical arched lines delimiting separate injections of the drug.

Tetracycline compound initially is deposited in the predentin as it mineralizes into dentin. Evidence of this marking is demonstrated in the increasing distance between new predentin formed and the area of fluorescent dentin. Because the therapeutic dosage level and visual tissue-labeling levels coincide, tetracycline has been widely used to visually record growth in experimental animals. The daily deposition rate of dentin can thus be recorded by measuring the width of dentin between each fluorescent line. In Figure 8–17, five discrete lines of tetracycline staining in dentin are seen. One is more widely spaced than the rest. In this instance, tetracycline injections were made on days 1, 6, 7, 9, and 11. Experimentally, if a second drug was administered on day 1, the effect of this compound could be measured on dentinogenesis by comparing the banding patterns in the dentin with those of a control-animal to which only tetracycline was administered. Some tetracycline is deposited in the dentinal tubules, which accounts for the near-horizontal fluorescent lines seen in Figure 8–17. Tetracycline may be used also to evaluate tooth movement by revealing bone and dentin formation (Fig. 8–18). This diagram shows two lines in the dentin of a crown, which indicates the time between injections. In this case, the crown was in the early stages of formation, prior to eruption. Observe that there is no line in the root dentin but that there are two vertical lines in the alveolar bone on the right of the roots and in the bifurcation zone. These lines were formed during a different time period,

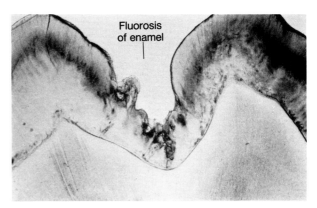

Figure 8–16. Histology of fluorosis of enamel indicates hypoplastic pits and altered brown-stained enamel.

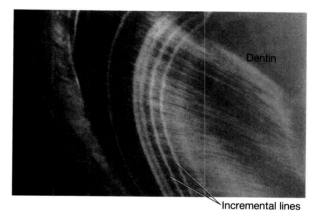

Figure 8–17. A series of lines of tetracycline staining in dentin mark the time of uptake. In enamel, there is less discrete staining. Photograph under UV light. E, enamel; D, dentin.

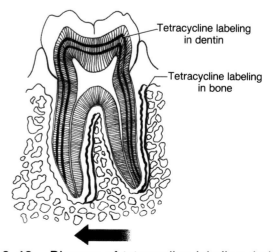

Figure 8–18. Diagram of tetracycline labeling during tooth development indicates lines in developing dentin and newly formed bone. Arrow indicates direction of tooth movement.

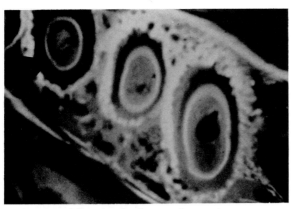

Figure 8–19. Histological section shows tetracycline fluorescence in roots and alveolar bone (cross section). Photographed under UV light.

before the roots were formed. The tooth moved to the left and the alveolar bone that formed behind the moving roots was clearly labeled by fluorescence.

In Figure 8–19, a UV photomicrograph of the tooth roots and the periodontium, there is heavy fluorescence in the roots and the alveolar bone. The tetracycline was taken up by both sites of hard-tissue deposition, which means that both the roots and the supporting bone were undergoing development at the time tetracycline was injected. As may be seen, tetracycline labeling is a valuable too for studying the development of teeth and bones.

Clinical Application

Brown staining or a defect in the enamel of the incisal third of crowns indicates the presence of a toxic substance in the body at the time of initial mineralization of the teeth. Location of the staining in the cervical area relates to introduction of a toxic substance at a time of final crown mineralization.

Summary

As noted on the left of Figure 8–20, the sectioned tooth exhibits normal appearing ameloblast, odontoblasts, enamel, dentin, and predentin. Compare this panel with the next, which illustrates the degenerative changes in the ameloblasts and affected enamel development associated with vitamin A deficiency. Note the altered appearance of the adjacent first-formed dentin.

In the next panel, vitamin C deficiency is seen to primarily affect connective tissue-forming cells, such as the odontoblasts, fibroblasts, and osteoblasts. As a result, the tissues for which they are responsible are also adversely affected.

Vitamin D deficiency which is indicated in the next panel is seen to affect mineralization of teeth. Increased areas of globular dentin result with corresponding interglobular spaces. There is also an increased width of predentin.

On the far right of Figure 8–20, parathormone deficiency is seen to have similar effects. Hyperparathyroidism results in hypomineralized dentin while hypoparathyroidism contributes to hypermineralized dentin.

Clinical Application

Fluoridation of water supplies throughout the United States is dentistry's most successful preventative program. When mottled enamel was first noted there was an association with the lack of dental caries. Sodium flouride was found to be the cause of this phenomenon when present in the water supply at a level of 5 parts per million parts water. Later, it was found that 0.5 ppm prevented caries and did not cause mottled enamel.

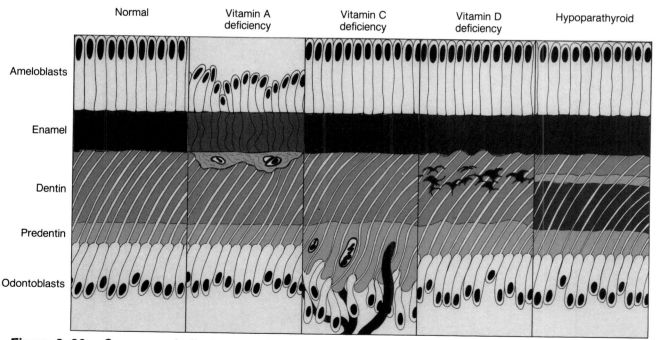

Figure 8–20. Summary of effects caused by vitamin A, C, and D deficiencies and hypoparathyroidism.

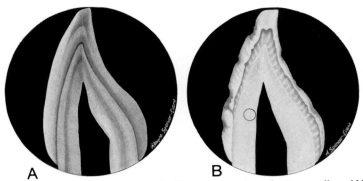

Figure 8–21. Summary of effect of uptake of tetracycline (A) and fluoride (B).

If replacement therapy is provided normal dentin deposition will resume in each of these thyroid deficiencies. Defective areas in the teeth are not restored, however, as occurs in bone that will be remodeled. All of the effects discussed are produced only during tooth development not in fully developed teeth.

Tetracycline and fluoride are absorbed during the mineralization phase of enamel and dentin formation, both can penetrate the maternal barrier in utero. Tetracycline can cause staining and hypoplasia of enamel, but with therapeutic doses, staining is usually most evident in the first-formed dentin. This antibiotic registers a mark on dentin and bone, which is only visible under UV light. Therefore, it is used for measuring mineralized tissue growth. Excessive fluoride causes brown staining and hypoplasia in enamel (Fig. 8–21A and B), but the enamel is caries resistant. The hypoplasia may appear as pits or be in broad areas of the crown. One part per million affords maximum caries protection and minimal hard-tissue alteration.

Self-Evaluation Review

1. Do tetracycline and/or fluoride cross the maternal barrier?
2. When, and in what form, are tetracycline and/or fluoride deposited in hard tissues?
3. Do clinical doses of tetracycline and high levels of fluoride produce an effect on human teeth? If so, what are the clinical symptoms.
4. List advantages of hard tissue labeling with tetracycline when one evaluates the effects of agents on tooth and bone development.
5. Compare differences between fluoride and tetracycline by contrasting the manner in which dentin and enamel are stained.
6. What tissues in the body are primarily affected by deficiencies of vitamins A, C, and D?
7. How is each of these deficiencies clinically characterized in the teeth?
8. Describe the effects of both parathormone deficiency and excess on tooth formation.
9. Why are these effects limited to developing teeth?
10. What are periodontal symptoms of vitamin C deficiency?

Suggested Readings

Cohlan SQ. Tetracycline staining of teeth. *Teratology* 1977;15:27.

Fejerskof O, Thylstrup A, Larsen MJ. Clinical and structural features and possible pathogenic mechanisms of dental fluorosis. *Scand. J. Dent. Res.* 1977;85:510.

Goodman, AG. *The Pharmacologic Basis of Therapeutics.* New York, NY: Macmillan; 1980.

Gregg JM, and Avery JK. Studies of alveolar bone growth and tooth eruption using tetracycline induced fluorescence. *J. Oral Therap. Pharmacol.* 1964;1:268.

Horowitz HS, Thylstrup A, Drisoll WS, Glenn FB. Perspectives on the use of prenatal fluorides: a symposium. *J. Dent. Child.* 1981;48:101.

Humerinta K, Thesleff I, Saxon L. In vitro inhibition of mouse odontoblast differentiation by vitamin A. *Arch. Oral Biol.* 1980;25:385.

Irving JT. A comparison of the influence of hormones, vitamins, and other dietary factors on the formation of bone, dentin and enamel. *Vitam. Horm.* 1957;15:291.

Kallenbach E. Microscopy of tetracycline induced lesion in rat incisor enamel organ, *Arch. oral Biol.* 1980;24:869.

Kawasaki K, and Fernhead RW. On the relationship between tetracycline and the incremental lines in dating. *J. Anat.* 1975;119:49.

Kruger BJ. Dose dependent ultrastructural changes induced by tetracycline in developing dental tissues of the rat. *J. Dent. Res.* 1975;54:822.

Moffert JM, Cooley RO, Olsen NH, Heffernew JJ. Prediction of tetracycline induced tooth discoloration *J. Am. Dent. Assoc.* 1974;88:547.

Pindborg JJ. *Pathology of the Dental Hard Tissues.* Philadelphia, Pa.: WB Saunders; 1970.

Shaw JH. *A Textbook of Oral Biology.* Philadelphia, Pa: WB Saunders; 1978.

Thylstrup A. Is there a biological rationale for prenatal fluoride administration? *J. Dent. Child.* 1981;48:103–108.

Thylstrup A. A distribution of dental fluorosis in the primary dentition. *Oral Epidemiol.* 1978;6:329.

Thylstrup A, Fejerskof O. Appearance of dental fluorosis in permanent teeth in relation to histologic changes. *Commun. Dent. Oral Epidemiol.* 1978;6:315.

Walton RE, Eisenman DR. Ultrastructural examination of dentin formation in rat incisors following multipole fluoride injections. *Arch. Oral Biol.* 1975;20:485.

Werstergaard J, Nylen NV. Dose and age dependent variations in effect of tetracycline on enamel formation in rat. *Scand. J. Dent. Res.* 1975;82:209.

Structure of the Periodontium and the Temporomandibular Joint

CHAPTERS 9–13

Histology of the Periodontium: Alveolar Bone, Cementum, and Periodontal Ligament

James K. Avery

Introduction

The periodontium includes the three supporting structures of the teeth: the bony alveolar process, the root-covered cementum, and the intervening periodontal ligament. The gingiva may also be considered part of the periodontium and is described in Chapter 19. The *alveolar process* is the bony extension of the mandible and maxilla that provides the necessary support for the teeth and serves a fibrous attachment for the periodontal ligament fibers. By resorption and deposition it also compensates for tooth movement. The *periodontal ligament* is also supportive, suspending the tooth in the socket, providing a cushion against various occlusal forces. Its nerve supply provides a delicate sense of touch and pressure to the tooth, and its blood vessels carry oxygen and nutrition to the ligament as well as to the periodontium and alveolar bone. *Cementum* covers the roots of the teeth and serves as an attachment for the periodontal ligament fibers. It provides compensation for occlusal wear by apical deposition and, at the same time, protection for the sensitive dentin (Fig. 9–1).

Objectives

After reading this chapter you should be able to describe the histological structures and function of the periodontal tissues, the root-covered cementum, the alveolar bone, and the intervening periodontal ligament.

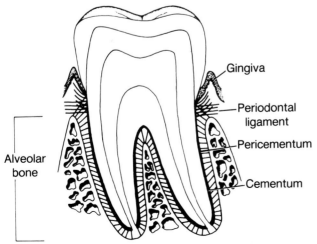

Figure 9–1. Diagram of periodontium.

Alveolar Process

The alveolar processes are those portions of the maxilla and mandible that support the roots of the teeth. They are composed of the *alveolar bone proper* and the *supporting bone.* The alveolar bone proper is the bone that lines the socket. In radiographic terms, it is referred to as the *lamina dura.* This process is the bony site of attachment of the periodontal ligament fibers. The supporting bone includes the remainder of the alveolar process, specifically the compact cortical plates on the outer surfaces of the alveolar processes and the spongy bone between the cortical plates and the alveolar bone proper (Fig. 9–2).

As discussed in Chapter 7, the alveolar process develops as a result of tooth root elongation and tooth eruption. Alveolar bone matures as the teeth gain functional occlusion; later, if the teeth are lost, the alveolar process disappears. Thus, the teeth are important in the development and maintenance of the alveolar bone. The alveolar bone proper is attached to the supporting cancellous and compact alveolar bone. Bone marrow containing blood vessels, nerves, and adipose tissue fills the space between the cortical plates and the alveolar bone proper (Fig. 9–3). The coronal border of the alveolar process is termed the alveolar crest (Fig. 9–2). It is located about 1 to 1.5 mm below the cementoenamel junction, and is rounded in the anterior region and nearly flat in the molar area. If the teeth are in buccal or lingual position, the alveolar process will be very thin or partially missing. The area of an apical root penetrating the bone is known as a *fenestration*, and its occurrence at the coronal root zone is termed *dehiscence* (Fig. 9–4).

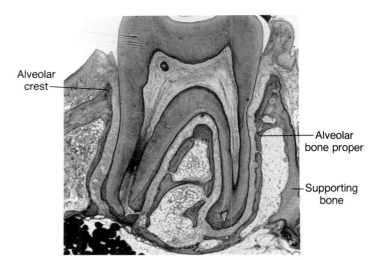

Figure 9–2. Histology of periodontium.

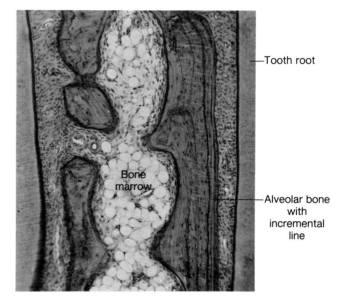

Figure 9–3. Histology of alveolar bone proper, with connective tissue communication between ligament and supporting bone shown.

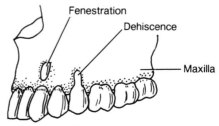

Figure 9–4. Diagram showing loss of alveolar bone adjacent to tooth. Bone loss near root apices is termed "fenestration," and bone loss in the region of the coronal root is termed "dehiscence."

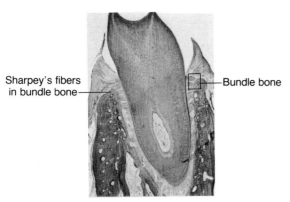

Figure 9–5. Alveolar bone proper. Silver stain illustrates the bundle bone. Outlined area is shown in Figure 9–6.

Sharpey's fibers in bundle bone

Bundle bone

Alveolar Bone Proper

On a histological basis, there are two types of bone: cancellous (spongy) and compact. Alveolar bone proper is a modification of compact bone, as it contains perforating fibers (Sharpey's) (Fig. 9–5). These collagen fibers pierce the alveolar bone proper at right angles or obliquely to the surface of the long axis of the tooth. This is the means of attachment for the periodontal ligament to the tooth. The fiber bundles originating from bone are much larger than the fiber bundles inserting in cementum. Perforating fibers occur elsewhere in the skeleton, wherever ligaments and tendons insert. Purely elastic perforating fibers are also found, but not in alveolar bone proper. Because the bone of the alveolar process is regularly penetrated by collagen bundles, it has been appropriately named *bundle bone* or alveolar bone proper (Figs. 9–5 and 9–6). When this bone is viewed radiographically, it is referred to as the *lamina dura* (Fig. 9–7). The lamina dura appears more dense than does the adjacent supportive bone, but this radiographic density may be due to the mineral orientation around the fiber bundles and the apparent lack of nutrient canals. Actually, there may be no difference in mineral content between the lamina dura and the supporting bone. The lamina dura is evaluated clinically for periapical or periodontal pathology.

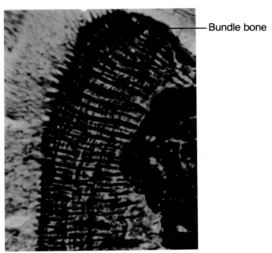

Bundle bone

Figure 9–6. Bundle bone with perforating fiber bundles.

Clinical Application

The lamina dura is an important diagnostic landmark in determining the health of the periapical tissues. Any loss of density in bone lining the socket usually indicates bone resorption, and can indicate a symptom of infection with inflammation of the periodontal tissues.

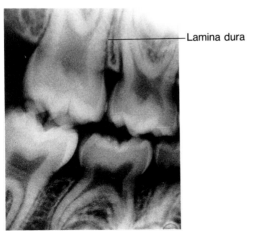

Lamina dura

Figure 9–7. Radiograph showing alveolar bone and density of lamina dura.

Tension created by occlusal forces is believed to be important in the maintenance of this bone. In physiological movement of teeth, this bone is readily resorbed in zones of compression and readily formed in zones of tension. Not all alveolar bone proper appears as bundle bone. At times, there are no apparent perforating fibers in the socket-lining bone (Fig. 9–8). Supporting bone constantly undergoes modification in adapting to minor tooth movements, and therefore fibers may be lost or replaced from time to time in some areas of root.

Compact Supporting Bone

The compact or dense bone of the alveolar process is like that found elsewhere in the human body. Compact bone in the alveolar process extends from the alveolar crest labially or bucally to the lower border of the sockets (Fig. 9–9). The cortical bone contains Haversian systems, radiating lamellae with lacunae, and canaliculi. The nutrient canals run in the direction of the long axis of the teeth and anastomose with "perforating canals" (Volkmann's canals) that pierce the bone at right or oblique angles. These canals establish a continuous system that houses the nerves and blood vessels of the bone. A sagittal view of the mandible demonstrates the vascular network in cortical bone (Fig. 9–9). Compact bone comprises the bulk of the interdental alveolar process; cancellous bone is located more apically between the alveolar process proper and the cortical bone (Fig. 9–10). Situated between osteons at the microscopic level are more irregular layers of bone, termed *interstitial lamellae* (Fig. 9–11). Bone cells (osteocytes) fill the oval lacunae situated in or between the lamellae. Minute *canaliculi* interconnect with adjacent lacunae; they contain processes of the osteocytes that contact other cells by a system of "gap" junctions.

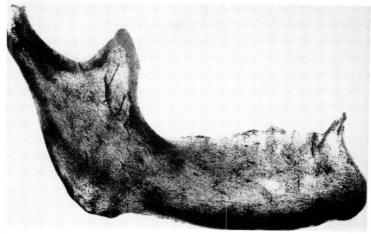

Figure 9–9. Blood vessels in cortical bone of the mandible, injected with India ink and cleaned to illustrate vascularity.

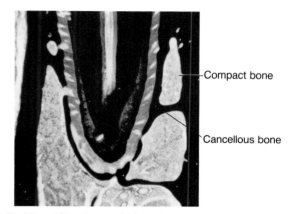

Figure 9–10. Histology of alveolar bone proper and supporting bone.

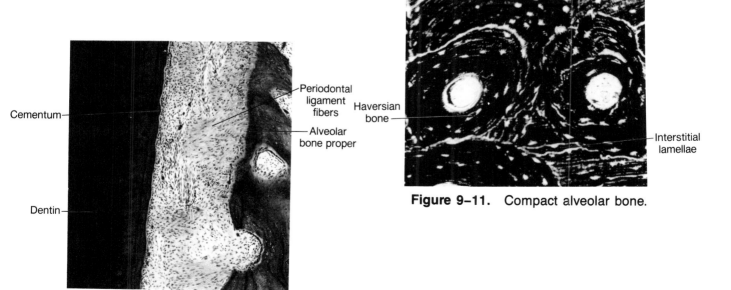

Figure 9–8. Organizing periodontal ligament.

Figure 9–11. Compact alveolar bone.

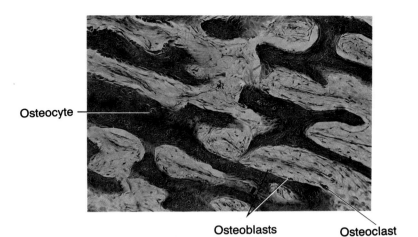

Osteocyte ——

Osteoblasts   Osteoclast

Figure 9–12. Cancellous supporting bone.

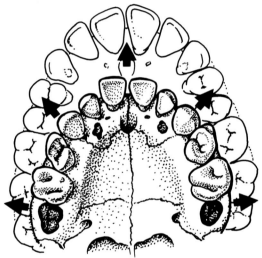

Figure 9–13. Migration of teeth and alveolar bone during growth of face.

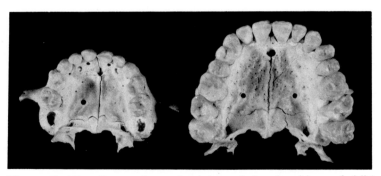

Figure 9–14. Comparison of palate and alveolar ridges of child (left) and adult (right).

Cancellous Supporting Bone

The cancellous or spongy bone of the alveolar process is generally composed of heavy trabeculae. The purpose of this supporting bone is to strengthen the alveolar bone proper with struts that pass to the cortical bone. Cancellous bone contains osteocytes in the interior and osteoblasts or osteoclasts on the surface of the trabeculae (Fig. 9–12). Between the bony struts that anastomose between the alveolar bone proper and the cortical bone are medullary cavities containing osteogenic cells, adipose tissue, and mature and immature blood cells. The maxillae are particularly rich in marrow tissue, such as megakaryocytes and immature white and red blood cells.

Physiological Tooth Movement

The preeruptive movements of both the primary and the permanent teeth have been discussed in Chapter 7. The eruptive process involves major remodeling of the alveolar processes to compensate for tooth growth and changes in position of the teeth. Repositioning of the teeth involves outward (facial and/or buccal) movement of the teeth as the face enlarges. Root growth results in growth in the height of the alveolar processes, which is compensatory for the increase in the length of the roots. Although the two growth processes—tooth eruption and an increase in facial size—have different origins, both relate to positioning of the teeth and to modifications of the fine structures of Haversian and cancellous bone of the alveolar processes. There are several causative factors of alveolar bone changes. First, the increase in the height of the alveolar process associated with root lengthening is "tooth controlled." In the absence of teeth, this change does not occur. Change is especially evident in an older person whose teeth may have been lost, which results in loss of the bone. Second, facial development involving condylar, maxillary, and mandibular growth also results in the movement of the teeth facially (Figs. 9–13 and 9–14).

Clinical Application

Physiological tooth movement can be monitored through radiographic examination noted at various angles of the changes in the alveolar bone. Monitoring changes in the appearance of the alveolar mucosa and gingiva is also important.

Because this process is not generated by the tooth, malformations of the face may result in tooth malalignment. Third, there will be further growth of the alveolar process unrelated to tooth eruption. This is part of the facial growth process. The teeth definitely control modifications of the alveolar process because, as a tooth moves, the alveolar bone responds with necessary compensatory changes. In this case, the resorption and deposition of bone around the teeth is a result, not the cause, of tooth movement. Thus, the alveolar process is guided in growth by tooth-related factors and extrinsic growth factors; the effects of these factors are difficult to separate as growth occurs (Fig. 9–15).

Aging of Alveolar Bone

A comparison of young and old alveolar bone reveals a shift with age from alveolar processes with smoothly lined sockets, and active bone formation with numerous viable cells, to alveolar sockets that appear jagged and uneven with fewer cells. The perforating fibers are inserted in an uneven pattern. Marrow appears to have a fatty infiltration, and osteoporosis indicates loss of some bony elements (Fig. 9–15).

Edentulous Jaws

The changes in the jaws resulting from tissue loading, compression, tissue conditioning, and denture retention coupled with the aging processes have not been clearly elucidated. It is apparent, however, that with age the alveolar process in edentulous jaws decreases in size (Fig. 9–16); loss of maxillary bone is accompanied by an increase in the size of the maxillary sinus. The internal trabecular arrangement is more open, which indicates bone loss. From a common radiographic viewpoint the location of various structures such as glands, fatty zones, muscle masses, and blood vessels varies little in the edentulous jaws.

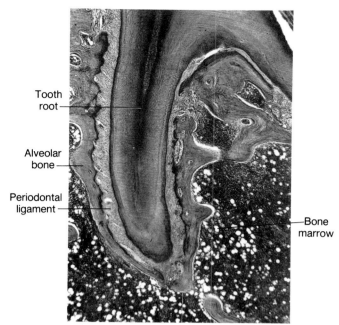

Figure 9–15. Aging alveolar bone illustrating scalloping of alveolar bone proper.

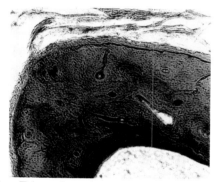

Figure 9–16. Edentulous jaw with loss of alveolar process. Remaining compact basal bone is seen.

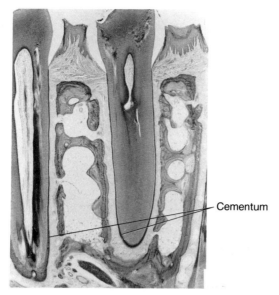

Figure 9-17. Relation of root to periodontium. Observe cementum on the root apex (right).

Table 9-1.
Comparison of Composition of Hard Tissues

	Cementum (%)	Bone (%)	Dentin (%)
Organic	50–55	30–35	30
Mineral	45–50	60–65	65.5

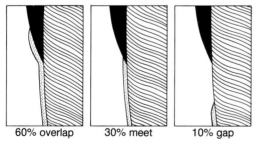

Figure 9-18. Relation of cementum to enamel at cementoenamel junction.

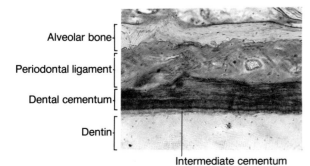

Figure 9-19. Histology of cementium on root surface.

Cementum

Cementum is the calcified tissue covering the roots of teeth (Fig. 9–17). It appears to be similar to bone and generally is of ectomesenchymal origin, although recent evidence indicates that the initial layer on the root surface is of epithelial cell origin. Cementum contains less mineral than does bone or dentin, as is seen in Table 9–1. Its histological appearances is similar to bone in that it contains cells within lacunae and exhibits incremental deposition lines. Unlike bone, cementum contains no Haversian canals and has neither blood vessels nor nerves in its matrix. Cementum is thinnest (20 to 50 μm) at the cementoenamel junction and gradually increases in thickness (150 to 200 μm) toward the root tip, where it surrounds the apical foramen. Generally, cementum is limited to the root surface, although in 60% of teeth it overlaps enamel for a short distance. In 30% of teeth, cementum meets enamel at a sharp point; and in 10% there is a short gap between the two (Fig. 9–18).

Intermediate Cementum

Recent investigations have confirmed an intermediate layer of cementum on the surface of the roots. Thus, it is situated between the granular layer of Tomes and the "dental cementum." This thin layer appears nearly identical to aprismatic enamel, that product of ameloblasts which is 10 nm thick and covers the mantle dentin in the crowns of teeth. It is best described as an amorphous layer of noncollagenous material containing no odontoblast processes or cementocytes. Because of the close similarity of this layer to the epithelial cell-originated aprismatic enamel, it has been suggested that intermediate cementum (Fig. 9–19) is formed by cells of the epithelial root sheath. If this process is accurate, deposition of this layer on the surface of the newly formed root dentin occurs shortly before these cells detach from the root surface and migrate into the periodontal ligament. The layer then mineralizes to an extent greater than that of either the adjacent dentin or the dental cementum. Intermediate cementum probably functions to seal the surface of the sensitive root dentin.

Cellular and Acellular Cementum

The initial layer of cementum deposited on the intermediate cementum is acellular. It is a thin layer, and subsequent increments usually alternate, with some containing cells and others not (Figs. 9–21 and 9–22). As a general rule, the thicker the cementum, the more lacunae are present. This rule is proven by the thick cementum at the root apex being highly cellular (Fig. 9–20). (Development of cementum is described in Chapter 6.) Cementum is incrementally deposited, with a new layer of cementoid being deposited as the preceding layer is calcified. Along the surface of the cementoid, numerous cementoblasts are observed (Fig. 9–21). The cementocytes found in the interior of the matrix appear polygonal (Fig. 9–24). As the cementoid calcifies, cementoblasts are incorporated into the cementum; these cells become cementocytes and are found in the lacunae. Near the surface they develop long processes that lie in canaliculi radiating from the cell body (Fig. 9–23). Their processes contact neighboring cell processes and may exhibit intercellular couplings by means of gap junctional complexes.

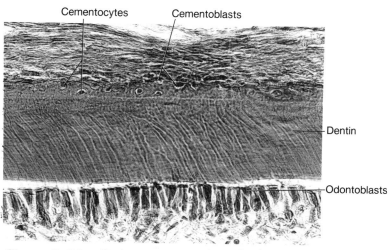

Figure 9–21. Early cementum deposited on root dentin.

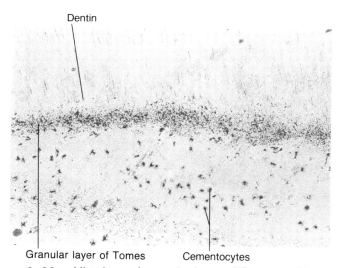

Figure 9–22. Histology of granular layer of Tomes and lacunae in cementum.

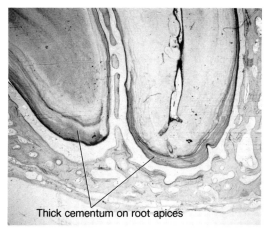

Figure 9–20. Thick cementum on root apices in an elderly person.

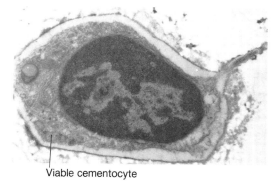

Figure 9–23. Ultrastructure of cementocyte near surface of cementum.

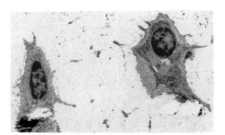

Figure 9–24. Ultrastructure of cementocytes deep in cementum.

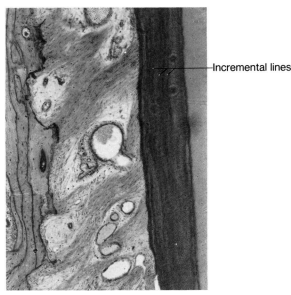

Incremental lines

Figure 9–25. Principal fibers arising from surface of cementum (right) and bone (left). Hematoxylin and eosin staining does not permit observation of penetrating fibers.

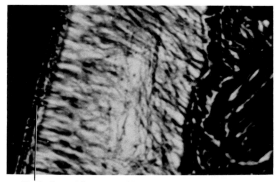

Periodontal ligament fibers penetrating cementum

Figure 9–26. Principal fibers arising from cementum and bone stained with silver to illustrate penetrating fibers.

In contrast, cementocytes in the deeper layers of cementum display few organelles and are in stages of degeneration (Fig. 9–24). The deepest layers of cementum may contain empty lacunae. Both cellular and acellular cementum are laid down incrementally, with these lines being more highly mineralized than are those in adjacent cementum. Incremental lines are best seen in decalcified sections (Fig. 9–25).

Cementum Surface Characteristics

Cementum attaches the periodontal ligament fibers to the tooth. Its surface thus has the appearance of numerous fiber bundles (Figs. 9–25 and 9–26). Basally, fiber bundles appear over the entire surface of the root, although some zones of cementum appear less active than others in fiber attachment. Some fiber bundles penetrate deeply, through a number of increments of cementum, whereas others are embedded more superficially. In general, the thinner the cementum, the more superficially the fibers penetrate the matrix. Perforating fiber bundles are smaller in cementum than in bone.

One characteristic of cementum is its resistance to resorption. This is clinically significant, as it allows orthodontic tooth movement with resultant remodeling of alveolar bone. Some investigators claim to have isolated an autoinvasive factor in cementum that may contribute to this resistance.

Clinical Application

Cementum is painless to scale and will repair itself by further deposition. Unlike bone, it is devoid of nerves, but like bone, it is a living tissue containing cells. Cementum serves to seal the ends of the dental tubules to prevent ingress of periodontally originated infections to the pulp.

The surface of cementum may reveal resorptive zones (Fig. 9–27). In some of these areas, cementum repair occurs and is an important feature of cementum. At the front, where resorption has ceased and repair by cementum has occurred, a *reversal line* is seen (Fig. 9–28). This line is so named because this is where the resorptive process has reversed. Periodontal fiber bundles attach to the newly formed cementum. One example of such an occurrence is an exfoliating tooth where, during root resorption, partial repair takes place. Because root loss is the eventual goal of physiological resorption, repair may provide some support to the tooth until the advancing exfoliation is complete (Fig. 9–29).

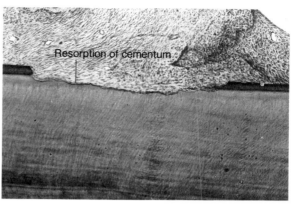

Figure 9–27. Cemental loss by resorption.

Clinical Application

Aging changes in the periodontium should be monitored. Changes in color, form, and density are signs of change. Gingival recession is seen along with changes in contour and stippling of the gingiva; this is why it is important to determine the normal appearance of the surface and its underlying structures.

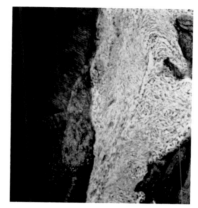

Figure 9–28. Reversal line in cementum (arrow): A healed root surface at an early stage.

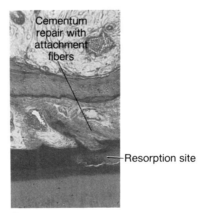

Figure 9–29. Cemental repair and fiber attachment. A healed root surface at a later stage.

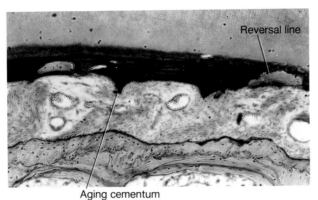

Figure 9-30. Aging cementum showing projection of spikes into ligament. Note the reversal lines (upper right).

Aging of Cementum

With aging, the surface of cementum becomes more irregular (Fig. 9-30). Generally, greater amounts of cementum may appear in the apical zone. An older root surface is less highly populated with fiber bundles than is a younger root surface. Seen microscopically, only the surface layer of cementocytes appears viable. All other lacunae appear empty.

Cementicles

Cementicles are calcified bodies appearing on or in the cementum and in the periodontal ligament. They usually are ovoid or round; their appearance is similar to that of the denticles; and they are classified as *free, attached,* or *embedded* (Figs. 9-31 and 9-32). Cementicles are a response to either local trauma or hyperactivity and appear in increasing numbers in the aging person.

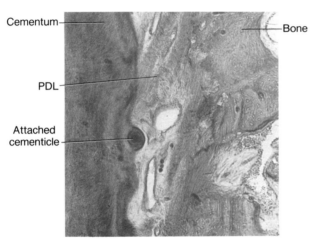

Figure 9-31. Attached or embedded cementicles. PDL, periodontal ligament.

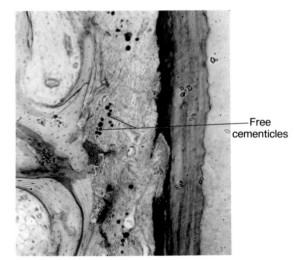

Figure 9-32. Appearance of free cementicles in periodontal ligament.

Periodontal Ligament

The periodontal ligament is the connective tissue located between the cementum and the alveolar bone proper (Fig. 9–33). Its functions are formative, supportive, protective, sensory, and nutritive. This ligament serves as a periosteum to the alveolar bone proper and as a pericementum to the cementum. The periodontium is also an extension of the gingival connective tissues. The periodontal ligament is fairly consistent in thickness, although it ranges from 0.15 to 0.38 mm. This thickness characteristically decreases slightly with age, measuring 0.21 mm in the young adult (11 to 16 years of age), 0.18 mm in the mature adult (32 to 52 years of age) and 0.15 mm in the older adult (51 to 67 years of age). The thinnest part of the ligament is located in the midroot zone. The periodontal ligament is composed of collagen fiber bundles connecting cementum and alveolar bone proper—hence, the name ligament. This ligament is highly cellular and contains a rich nerve and blood supply. The terms "periodontal ligament" and "periodontal membrane" are used interchangeably, although the former term more aptly describes this tissue.

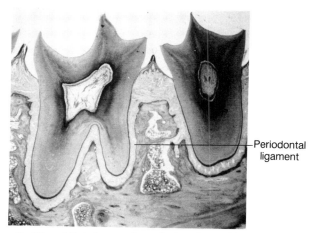

Figure 9–33. Histology of periodontium. Note the constant thickness of the periodontal ligament.

Principal Fibers

The fiber bundles that exit the cementum and alveolar bone proper to form the periodontal ligament are termed *principal fibers*. Groups of these fibers are named according to their location with respect to the tooth (Fig. 9–34). The *apical* fiber group is located at the apical area of the root, the *oblique* fibers are located immediately above them, the *horizontal* fibers appear in midroot, and the *alveolar crest* fibers are situated in the cervical region. The gingival group contains *circumferential, transseptal, free,* and *attached gingival fibers,* which are described below. Table 9–2 lists the function and the site of attachment for each of the principal fiber groups.

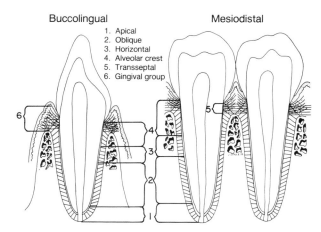

Figure 9–34. Principal fibers of periodontal ligament.

Table 9–2.
Principal Fibers

	Location of Attachment	Function
Dentoalveolar fiber group		
Apical	Apex of root to fundic proper	Resist vertical force
Oblique	Apical one third of root to adjacent alveolar bone proper	Resist vertical and intrusive force
Horizontal	Midroot to adjacent alveolar bone proper	Resist horizontal and tipping force
Alveolar crest	Cervical root to alveolar crest of alveolar bone proper	Resist vertical and intrusive force
Interradicular	Between roots to alveolar bone proper	Resist vertical and lateral movement
Gingival fiber group		
Transseptal	Cervical tooth to tooth; mesial or distal to it	Resist tooth separation; mesial distal
Attached gingival	Cervical tooth to attached gingiva	Resist gingival displacement
Free gingival	Cervical tooth to free gingiva	Resist gingival displacement
Circumferential	Continuous around neck of tooth	Resist gingival displacement

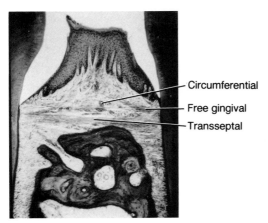

Figure 9-35. Gingival fiber group.

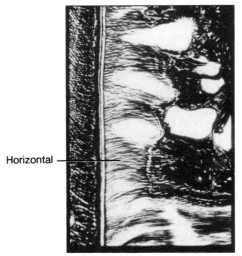

Figure 9-36. Horizontal fiber group in ligament.

Gingival Group

Histological identification of these fiber groups is not difficult. Although the groups appear similar, their origin and location in the gingiva are the best means of identification. In the gingiva, the transseptal fibers extend to adjacent teeth on their mesial and distal surfaces (Fig. 9–35). The free and attached gingival fibers arise from the cervical cementum and end freely in the lamina propria of the gingiva. The circumferential fibers circle the necks of the teeth and appear as dots in a longitudinal section (Fig. 9–35).

Dentoalveolar Group

The dentoalveolar group consists of *alveolar crest* fibers extending from the crest to the gingiva (Fig. 9–35) with *horizontal* fibers extending in a horizontal direction to the midroot alveolar bone proper (Fig. 9–36). *Oblique* fibers traverse above the apex and extend upward from the tooth to the bone (Fig. 9–37), *apical* fibers extend perpendicularly from the surface of the root to the fundic bone (Fig. 9–37), and *interradicular* fibers exend perpendicularly from the root surface to the interradicular alveolar bone proper in multirooted teeth (Fig. 9–38). In all Figures 9–35 to 9–38, the fiber bundles were prepared with silver stain to enhance viewing.

Vascular and Neural Supply

The principal fibers shown in Figures 9–35 to 9–38 were enhanced for viewing because of the spaces between fiber bundles termed *interstitial spaces*, which contain blood vessels, lymph channels, and myelinated and nonmyelinated nerves. With these structures, the periodontal ligament maintains the vitality of the periodontium. The blood vessels and nerves encircle the tooth and connect with others that extend vertically from the tooth apex to the gingiva. The

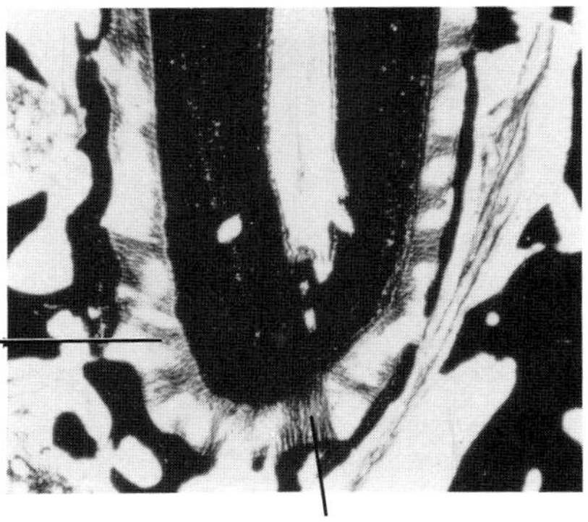

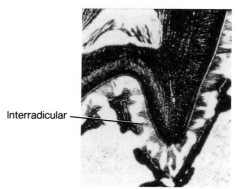

Figure 9-37. Oblique and apical fiber group in ligament.

Figure 9-38. Interradicular fiber group of periodontal ligament.

organization of these vessels can be seen in a cleared specimen after India ink injection (Fig. 9–39). On the left side in Figure 9–39 are vessels entering the ligament from the alveolar bone. Through the center a vascular plexus runs longitudinally in the ligament. On the right, this plexus is a clear zone, which is dentin. Further right are the blood vessels in the pulp. Figure 9–40 shows how the circular and longitudinal vessels of the ligament provide a network functioning in nutrition and "dampening" the change in the shape of the ligament that occurs when the teeth are occluded. In Figure 9–41, the interconnecting channels in the ligament are seen in a section longitudinal to the root surface. When a cross section of a tooth root is viewed, the regularity of the longitudinal vessels can be seen (Fig. 9–42). A longitudinal section through the periodontium illustrates the communicating branches of the longitudinal plexus (Fig. 9–43).

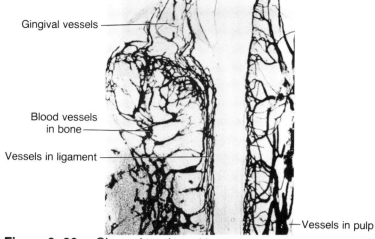

Figure 9–39. Cleared tooth and bone, with India ink injected blood vessels. Observe loops progressing from bone into periodontium and in tooth pulp (right).

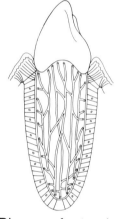

Figure 9–40. Diagram of network of blood vessels in periodontium. Dots indicate position between fiber bundles.

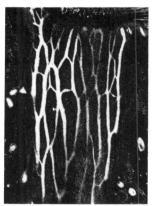

Figure 9–41. Histology of ligament in longitudinal section illustrating vascular and neural pathways.

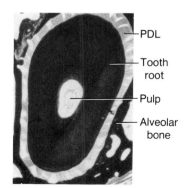

Figure 9–42. Histology of cross section of root, with interstitial spaces between fiber bundles shown. PDL, periodontal ligament.

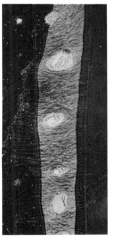

Figure 9–43. Histology of longitudinal section of periodontal ligament, with interstitial spaces shown.

Nerve trunks also travel in the interstitial spaces. The larger trunks traverse the ligament in the central zone, as is seen in a longitudinal view of the ligament in Figure 9–44. Higher magnification of this section reveals several arteries and veins, as well as a nerve, entering an interstitial space (Fig. 9–45). A clearer picture is seen under the electron microscope (Fig. 9–46). A few nerve endings, which appear to be Pacinian pressure receptors, may also be viewed (Fig. 9–47). In this figure the organized nerve ending is enclosed in a delicate connective tissue capsule.

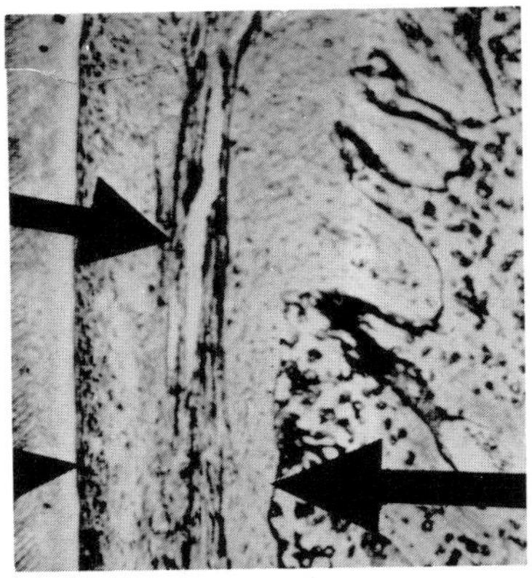

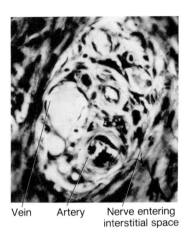

Vein   Artery   Nerve entering interstitial space

Figure 9–45. Interstitial space with vein, artery, and nerve.

Figure 9–44. Longitudinal section of nerve trunk in periodontal ligament. Top left arrow, nerve trunk; bottom left arrow, surface of root; bottom right arrow, surface of alveolar bone.

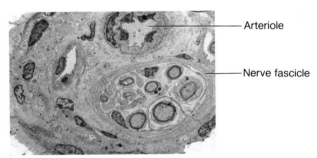

— Arteriole

— Nerve fascicle

Figure 9–46. Ultrastructure of interstitial space with nerve bundle (lower right) and arterioles (above).

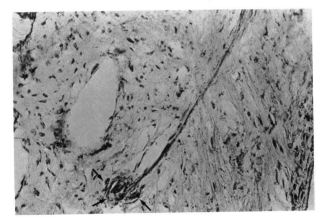

Figure 9–47. Nerve and nerve ending (arrows) in periodontal ligament (silver stain).

Organization of Periodontal Ligament

The principal fibers make up the bulk of the ligament and perform the important function of support. When the ultrastructure of the periodonal ligament is examined, it is found to be a dense, supportive network of collagen fibers. Some investigators believe a secondary network of fine fibers aids in supporting the primary principal fiber system. The supporting fiber system has been termed the *indifferent fiber plexus*. Transmission electron microscopic observations illustrate the presence of fine fibers supporting the principal fibers of the ligament (Fig. 9–48). The dense population of principal collagen fibers shows the presence of large numbers of fibroblasts. Throughout the ligament are additional fine fibers that appear elasticlike, termed *oxytalan fibers*. Their location appears to be around vessel walls, and they generally run parallel to the long axis of the tooth (Fig. 9–49). Oxytalan fibers can only be highlighted with special stains (aldehyde fuchsin with preoxidation); around each, there appears to be both a fibrillar and an amorphous zone. These fibers are in parallel arrangement and are about 150 Å in diameter. Although their function is unknown, oxytalan fibers may be part of the support system of the principal fibers. Figures 9–50 and 9–51 are electron micrographs of associated oxytalan and collagen fibers.

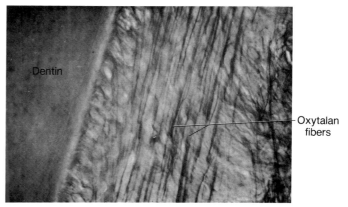

Figure 9–49. Histology of oxytalan fibers running longitudinally in ligament.

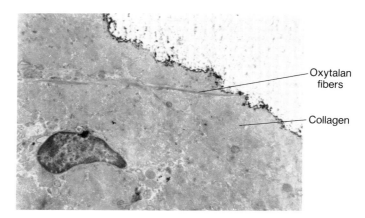

Figure 9–50. Ultrastructure of periodontal ligament, with relation of collagen and oxytalan fibers shown.

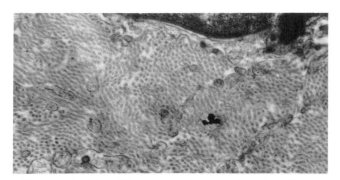

Figure 9–48. Electron micrograph of collagen fibers in ligament.

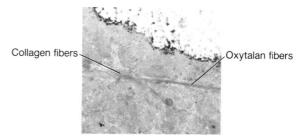

Figure 9–51. Ultrastructure of periodontal ligament, with relation of collagen and oxytalan fibers shown.

Ligament Cells

There are numerous cells in the ligament, as in most other tissues of the body. The most important is the fibroblast, because of the high density of collagen composing this tissue. Recent evidence that the ligament collagen "turns over" rapidly has added further importance to these cells. These cells are believed to function in resorption or destruction of the ligament collagen as well as in its formation. Moreover, there is evidence that a single cell, the *fibroblast/fibroclast*, can perform both functions (Fig. 9–52). One end of the cell is active in phagocytizing collagen and contains a lysosomal system; the other end of the same cell is active in assembling the procollagen chains. These will then form the superhelix of the collagen molecule (Fig. 9–52). With the aid of vitamin C, the hydroxylation of the amino acids proline and lysine occurs. The fibroblasts thus maintain a balance of collagen fibers in the ligament by balancing the rate of collagen formation and destruction.

Other cells in addition to blood vascular elements can be found in the ligament. Osteoblasts may exist along the alveolar bone proper, and cementoclasts may be seen. All may be called osteoclasts (Fig. 9–53) because they carry out the same function. These large multinucleated cells originate from circulating monocytes and are easily recognized by their size and the resorption lacunae. Cementoclasts, although similar in appearance to osteoclasts, are rare, being seen only during exfoliation of primary teeth, traumatic occlusion, or, possibly, tooth movement.

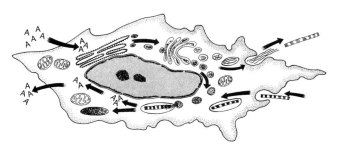

Figure 9–52. Diagram of fibroblast/fibroclast and, possibly, functional pathways.

Epithelial Rests

Epithelial rests are a normal constituent of the periodontal ligament throughout life and are discussed in Chapter 6. The epithelial cells that originated from the root sheath may appear as lacy strands, networks, or isolated nests of active or inactive cells. Epithelial cells are described as either proliferating, resting, or degenerating. An example of one of of these rests is seen in Figure 9–54.

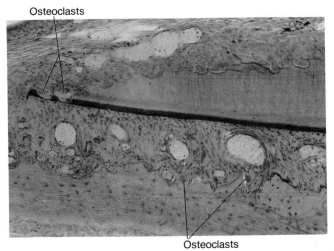

Figure 9–53. Periodontal ligament during period of resorption and repair.

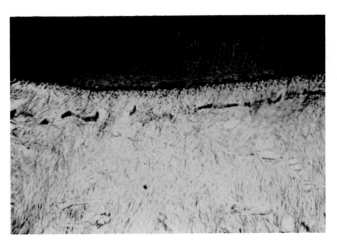

Figure 9–54. Epithelial rests in ligament near surface of root.

Summary
Alveolar Process

The alveolar process is the bone in the maxilla and mandible that supports the roots of the teeth. It is composed of the *alveolar bone proper*, which lines the sockets and attaches the ligament fibers to the bone. The remainder of the alveolar process is supporting bone, the compact cortical plate, and the cancellous bone situated between the cortical plate and the alveolar bone proper. The alveolar bone is constantly being modified, but its period of maximal change is during facial growth and tooth growth. The alveolar process is guided in growth by both extrinsic factors generated by the teeth and extrinsic factors generated by growth of the face. Finally, the alveolar process ages, as do other bones in the body, although in some cases tooth loss means bone loss.

Cementum

The calcified tissue covering the roots of the teeth is composed of epithelial root sheath-originated cementum, termed "intermediate cementum." Cementum can also be formed by cementoblasts. The latter is less highly calcified than is bone or dentin. Cementum is thinnest at the cervical region, and is thickest at the apical region. Cementoblasts incorporated into the cementum are termed "cementocytes." They appear in lacunae and are similar to bone cells. There are no Haversian systems in cementum, as in bone, because blood and nerves do not enter it. Cementum is resistant to resorption and, if resorbed, is likely to repair and form a reversal line. Cementum has free, attached, and embedded cementicles.

Periodontal Ligament

The periodontal ligament is the pliant tissue located between the root surface and the alveolar bone proper, and has a fairly constant thickness. It is composed of five groups of dentoalveolar fibers: apical, oblique, horizontal, alveolar crest, and interradicular. Free and attached gingival, circular, and transseptal fiber bundles comprise the dentogingival group. Each fiber group has a specific function. The periodontal ligament "turns over" collagen rapidly, and thus has an active population of fibroblasts that both form and destroy collagen. The periodontal ligament is highly vascularized by vessels in the interstitial spaces. Nerves transmit through these spaces, and several types of terminals respond to touch, pain, and the pressures of mastication. Fine fibers aid in the support of the ligament, and some of these are termed *oxytalan* fibers. They transverse the ligament in the long axis of the teeth.

Self-Evaluation Review

1. Name five functions of the periodontal ligament.
2. What type of bone composes most of the lamina dura?
3. The cortical plates of the jaws are classified as what type of bone? Why?
4. Name five cell types that may be found in the periodontal ligament in addition to blood cells. What are their functions?
5. What types of organized nerve endings have been found in the periodontal ligament? What is their function?
6. Describe the appearance of a "healed" root surface in early and late stages.
7. What forces would transseptal, free gingival, and circular fiber groups resist?
8. Describe the function of the attachment fibers of the periodontal ligament.
9. What is the name and function of the fibers found between molar roots?
10. What is the function of oxytalan fibers in the periodontium?

Suggested Readings

Alveolar Bone

Ash P, Loutit JF, Townsend KMS. Osteoclasts derived from hematopoietic stem cells. *Nature* 1980;283:669.

Bonucci E. New knowledge on the origin, function, and fate of osteoclasts. *Clin Orthop.* 1982;158:252.

Marks, BI. The microanatomy of the human edentulous maxillae. *Aust Dent J.* 1978;23:69.

Marks SC Jr. The origin of osteoclasts: evidence clinical applications and investigative challenges of an extraskeletal source. *J Oral Pathol.* 1983;12:226.

Quelch KJ, Melik RA, Bingham PJ, Mercuri SM. Chemical composition of human bone. *Arch Oral Biol.* 1983;665.

Severson JA, Moffett BC, Kokich V, Selipsky H. A histologic study of age changes in the adult human periodontal joint (ligament). *J Periodontol.* 1978;49:189.

TenCate AR, Mills C. The development of the periodontium: the origin of alveolar bone. *Anat Rec.* 1972;173:69.

Cementum

Boyde A, Jones SJ. Scanning electron microscopy of cementum and Sharpey fiber bone. *Z Zellforsch.* 1968;92:536.

Bravman D, Everhardt, D, Stohl S. Antigens found in cementum exposed to periodontal disease. *J Periodontol.* 1979;50:656.

Furseth R. The fine structure of the cellular cementum of young human teeth. *Arch Oral Biol.* 1969;14:1147.

Furseth R, Johansen E. The mineral phase of sound and carious human dental cementum studied by electron microscopy. *Acta Odontol Scand* 1970;28:305.

Held AJ. Cementogenesis and the normal and pathologic structure of cementum. *Oral Surg Oral Med Oral Pathol.* 1951;4:53.

Jande SS, Belanger LF. Fine structural study of rat molar cementum. *Anat. Rec.* 1970;167:439.

Jones SJ, Boyde A. A study of human root cementum surfaces as prepared for an exained in the scanning electron microscope. *Z Zellforsch.* 1972;130:318.

Lisodeskog S, Hammerstrom L. Evidence in human teeth of anti-invasive factor in cementum or perio ligament. *Scand J Dent Res.* 1980;88:161.

Listgarten MA, Kamin A. The development of a cementum layer over the enamel surface of rabbit molars—a light and electron microscopic study. *Arch Oral Biol.* 1969;14:961.

Selvig KA. An ultrastructural study of cementum formation. *Acta Odontol Scand.* 1964;22:105.

Selvig KA. 1965. The fine structure of human cementum. *Acta Odontol Scand.* 1965;23:423.

Schroeder HE. The gingival tissue. In: Cohen B, Kramer RH, eds. *Scientific Foundations in Dentistry.* London: Heinemann; 1976; chap 37.

Schroeder HE. Development and structure of the dental attachment apparatus. In: *Oral Struc Biol.* New York: Thieme Medical Publishers; 1991;187:290.

Periodontal Ligament

Berkowitz BKB, Moxham BJ Newman HN. The periodontal ligament and physiological tooth movements. In: Berkowitz BKB, Moxham BJ, Newman HN, eds. *The Periodontal Ligament in Health and Disease* Tarrytown, NY: Pergamon Press; 1982;215–247.

Bernick S, Levy BM, Dreize S, Grant, DA. The intra osseous orientation of the alveolar component of marmoset alveodental fibers. *J Dent Res.* 1977;56:1409.

Bhaskar SN, ed. *Orban's Oral Histology and Embryology,* 11th ed. St. Louis, Mo: CV Mosby; 1991.

Cho MI, Garnat PR. Mannose utilization by fibroblast of the periodontal ligament. *J Periodont Res.* 1987;21:64–72.

Edmunds RS, Simmons TA, Cox CF, Avery JK. Light and ultrastructural relationship between oxytalan fibers in the periodontal ligament of the guinea pig. *J Oral pathol.* 1979;8:109.

Fullmer HM, and Lillie RD. The oxytalan fiber: a previously undescribed connective tissue fiber. *J Histochem Cytochem.* 1958;6:426.

Garant PR. Collagen resorption by fibroblasts, a theory of fibroblastic maintenance of periodontal ligament. *J Periodontol.* 1976;47:380.

Griffin CJ, Harris R. 1968. Unmyelinated nerve endings in the periodontal membrane of human teeth. *Arch Oral Biol.* 1968;13:1207.

Levy BM, Bernick S. Studies on the biology of the periodontium of marmosets. II. Development and organization of the periodontal ligament of deciduous teeth in marmosets. *J Dent Res.* 1978;47:27.

Marchi F. Secretory granules in cells producing fibrillar collagen. In: Z. Davidovich, ed. *The Biological Mechanisms of Tooth Eruption and Root Resorption.* Birmingham, Ala: EBSCO Media; 1988;53–59.

Melcher AH, Bowen WH. *The Biology of the Periodontium.* New York, NY: Academic Press; 1969.

Nakamura, TK, Hanal H, Nakamura MT. Ultrastructure of encapsulated nerve terminals in hyman periodontal ligaments. *Jpn J Oral Biol.* 1982;24:126.

Ramfjord SP, Ash MM. *Periodontology and Periodontics.* Philadelphia, Pa: WB Saunders; 1979.

Simmons TA, Avery JK. Electron dense staining affinities of mouse oxytalan and elastic fibers. *J Oral Pathol.* 1980;9:183.

Slavkin HC. Towards a cellular and molecular understanding of peridontics. *J Periodontol.* 1976;47:249.

TenCate AR, Deporter DA. The role of the fibroblast in collagen turnover in the functioning periodontal ligament of the mouse. *Arch Oral Biol.* 1974;19:339.

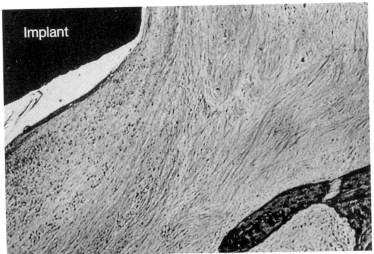

Figure 10–2. Light micrograph of fibrous tissue encapsulation around titanium blade implant in a human. The fibers run parallel to the implant surface rather than inserting into the titanium.

Bone-Implant Interfaces

In 1952, Branemark embarked on studies that resulted in the introduction of a treatment concept and implant design in the early 1980s after an extensive study of the cylindrical, threaded endosteal implants. A variety of implant models and surgical techniques have led to the development of our present concepts of fibro-osseous integration, osseointegration, and biointegration. Fibro-osseous integration is defined as the connective tissue-encapsulated implant within bone (Fig. 10–2). This type of integration was an early histological finding in implant development and resulted from early types of implant materials, possibly because of a lack of primary stability, premature loading of the implant, and/or a traumatic surgical procedure causing heat-induced bone necrosis. A long-term clinical study has demonstrated a success rate of approximately 50% over a 10-year period for this type of implant integration. Materials that stimulate this type of reaction are nonprecious metals, acrylates, polymers, and vitreous carbon. With the newer materials, fibro-osseous integration makes up a much smaller percentage of the interface to the implant, while osseointegration or biointegration comprise the majority of the interface (Figs. 10–3A through C).

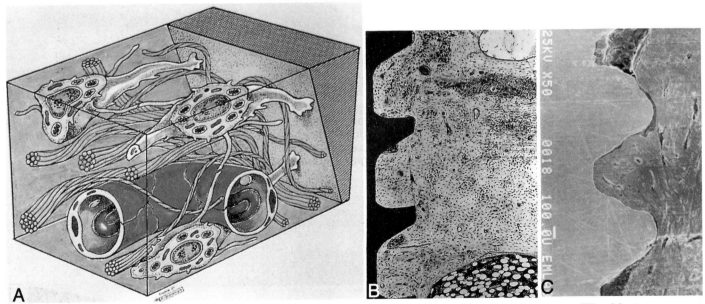

Figure 10–3. (A). High-resolution drawing of subgingival connective tissue at the boundary zone. Fibroblast processes are seen in immediate contact with the titanium oxide surface, but in reality are separated from it by a thin layer of proteoglycans. A network of collagen and blood vessels approaches the titanium surface and surrounds a normal blood vessel. (B). Implant threads of a titanium implant in contact with cortical bone in a rabbit tibia. (C). Scanning electron micrograph of combination cortical and cancellous bone contact on titanium surface.

Osseointegration was defined by Branemark as a direct structural and functional connection between ordered, living bone, and the surface of a load-carrying implant without soft tissue intervention at the light microscopic level. This type of integration has been shown to yield the most predictable success for long-term implant stability. Factors that enhance osseointegration include: (1) atraumatic surgical procedures with minimal heat generated, and (2) close fit of the implant fixture to the formed socket. Present implant surgical research indicates that the best result is achieved with a low drilling speed (under 800 rpm) and abundant irrigation with chilled saline, which minimizes bone tissue injury. Use of a precision drilling system increases the initial implant-bone contact. The implant materials, surface characteristics of the implant, and type of recipient bone are factors that help determine the final implant-tissue interface (Table 10–1). In addition, the appropriate timing of placing the implant in function supporting a prosthesis is an essential element in maintaining osseointegration.

Biointegration is a form of implant interface that is achieved with bioactive materials such as hydroxylapatite (HA) or bioglass that bond directly to bone, similar to ankylosis of natural teeth. The bone matrix is deposited on the HA layer as the result of a physiochemical interaction between the collagen of bone and HA crystals of the implant. HA-coated implants appear to develop bone contact faster than do non-coated implants. However, after a year, there seems to be little difference in bone contact between coated and non-coated implants. The HA-coated implants continue to be improved in their purity and manufacturing processes (Fig. 10–4A and B). Dental implants differ significantly from natural teeth in their interface with the alveolar bone and connective tissue fibers (Fig. 10–5). The junctional epithelium, however, appears to have the same interface characteristics with implants as with natural teeth. Because implants do not have a cemental surface for the insertion of the periodontal ligament and gingival connective tissue fibers, successful implants depend on direct contact with the alveolar bone and connective tissue adhesion coronal to the alveolar housing. A histologically successful implant would be defined as having 35 to 90% direct bone contact, a connective tissue adhesion above the bone, and an intact non-inflamed junctional epithelium. Clinically, the implant should be nonmobile and free of discomfort in function. An implant

Table 10–1.
Osseointegration Factors

Precision drilling system
Low-speed cutting
Chilled saline irrigation
Surface characterization of implant
Timing when placed in function

Clinical Application

HA-coated implants appear to achieve biointegration faster than other types of implant where there is minimal cortical bone available.

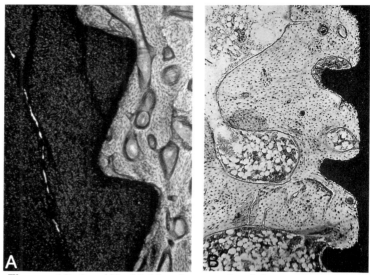

Figure 10–4. (A). Light micrograph of bone contact with aluminum oxide ceramic implant in a primate. (B). HA-coated implant in contact with cortical bone in a rabbit tibia.

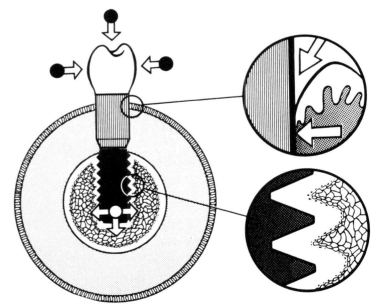

Figure 10–5. Diagrammatic summary of crucial problems in creating permanent tissue anchorage of an implant penetrating skin or oral mucous membrane. This penetration requires the establishment of a biologic barrier between the internal and external environments in the anchorage region. The connective tissue and bone interfaces to the implant are different compared with their interfaces with the natural tooth.

10: Histology of Endosseous Implants   **167**

could be considered successful if: (1) mucosal health is substantiated by clinical parameters such as a lack of redness, bleeding on probing, or suppuration. Soft tissue inflammation, when present, should be amenable to treatment; (2) there is no significant or progressive loss of supporting bone; (3) there is no persistent infection; (4) the implant functions in the absence of discomfort; (5) there is no increasing mobility of the implant when evaluated when the prosthesis is removed; and (6) the implant is prosthetically useful.

Bone is a specialized, calcified connective tissue. The alveolar bone is a combination of both cortical and cancellous bone. Both forms of bone have been shown to osseointegrate with the implant surface. In addition, blood vessels within the bone have been shown to proliferate in contact with the implant surface. To date, the implant materials that have demonstrated the most rapid ability for osseointegration are titanium (commercially pure, alloy, and plasma-sprayed), and the calcium phosphate ceramic material, HA. The biologically active surface on titanium is a dense protective oxide (T_1O_2) layer 15 to 50 μm thick. This layer forms quickly after processing and is relatively resistant to further corrosion by proteolytic enzymes or chemical attack. Titanium plasma-spraying of the implant increases the surface area for osseointegration almost six-fold. The HA-coated implants appear to osseointegrate more rapidly and have a higher percentage of bone contact than titanium. However, within a year's time, the difference does not appear to be clinically significant. The HA coating is used because it is manufactured with a commercially pure material that has proven to be nontoxic and has a resemblance to the inorganic phase of the human skeleton. The percentage of cortical bone in contact with implants appears to increase because of the remodeling of the bone associated with functional adaptation.

Epithelium Tissue Interface

The interface of epithelium to an implant is similar to that found with the natural tooth (Fig. 10–6). The sulcus and the junctional epithelium are both in contact with the implant. The healthy sulcus consists of a 5- to 15-cell layer of non-keratinized epithelium with wide intercellular spaces (Fig. 10–7). The junctional epithelium is approximately 2 mm in length and two to five cell layers thick, with basal and suprabasal cells in direct contact with the implant surface

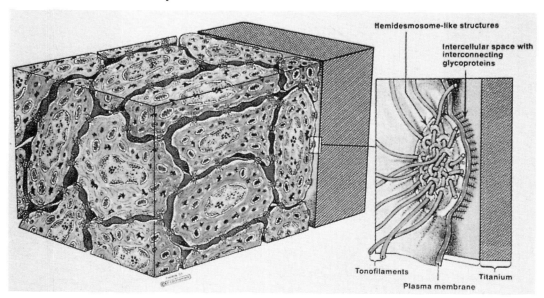

Figure 10–6. Enlarged schematic of gingiva-titanium oxide contact zone. Inset demonstrates a hemidesmosome-like structure anchoring the epithelial cells to the implant surface.

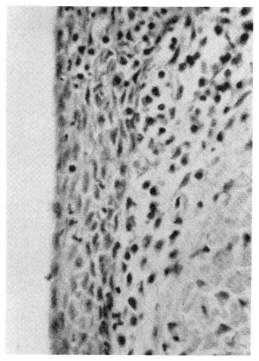

Figure 10–7. Light micrograph of the two- to five-cell-layer thickness of the junctional epithelium at the interface of a titanium screw in a miniature pig.

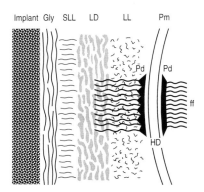

Figure 10–8. Schematic diagram of the hemidesmosome attachment to a dental implant. The attachment component of the gingival junctional epithelium to the implant surface is determined from interpolation of transmission electron microscope studies of this biologic seal. Pm, plasma membrane of the epithelial cell; HD, hemidesmosome; Pd, peripheral density; ff, fine filaments; LL, lamina lucida; LD, lamina densa; SLL, sublaminal lucida; Gly, glycocalyx; Im, implant.

(Fig. 10–8). These cells are attached to the implant surface by a basal lamina and hemidesmosomes (Fig. 10–9). The epithelial interface is similar to the natural tooth, whereas the connective tissue interface is significantly different.

Connective Tissue Interface

The initial success of dental implants is determined by the ability of the implant material to integrate with the alveolar bone (Fig. 10–10A and B). With the placement of the implant abutment through the oral mucosa, the long-term success is dependent on the "transmucosal seal" that forms

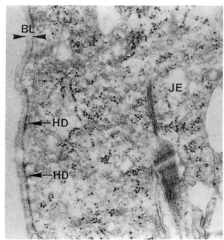

Figure 10–9. Transmission electron micrograph of hemidesmosomes at an epoxy resin implant in a monkey. BL, basal lamina; HD, hemidesmosomes; JE, junctional epithelium cell.

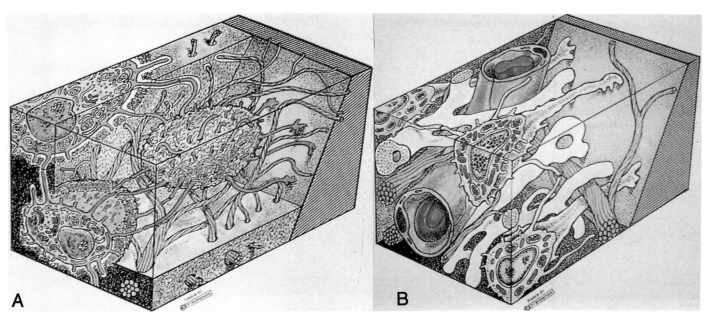

Figure 10–10. (A). Interface between cortical bone and titanium. An osteocyte with numerous processes in canaliculi approaches the titanium oxide surface. The calcified ground substance around the osteocyte is removed to show details. A meshwork of collagen surrounds the bone cell. There is an intimate contact between the ground substance of the Haversian bone and the titanium oxide. (B). Contact layer between cancellous bone and implant. Note fibroblast and osteoblast processes approaching the titanium surface. The bone trabeculae are seen in close relation to the implant surface and a blood vessel.

between the implant abutment's polished or machined surface and the mucosa's connective tissue and epithelium. In the peri-implant tissue, the vast majority of large collagen fiber bundles are attached to the marginal alveolar bone and insert into the marginal gingiva, not onto the titanium (Figs. 10–11, 10–12A and B, and 10–13A and B). These fiber bundles are highly organized and are oriented parallel to the surface of the machined titanium surface. The connective tissues adjacent to a tooth above the crestal bone are normally arranged into three different fiber groups: (1) dentogingival fibers extending from their insertion into cementum to the marginal connective tissue; (2) dentoperiosteal fibers extending from the cementum to the alveolar bone crest; and (3) circular fibers present in the connective tissue of the marginal gingiva and supra-alveolar connective tissue. All these fiber groups are functionally oriented (perpendicular) to the tooth. One research group has observed collagen fibers appearing to insert into the neck of a plasma-sprayed implant surface in monkeys. These collagen fibers were arranged in a perpendicular arrangement similar to the connective tissue fibers in cementum, as in a normal functioning tooth. The results of this research are not well understood.

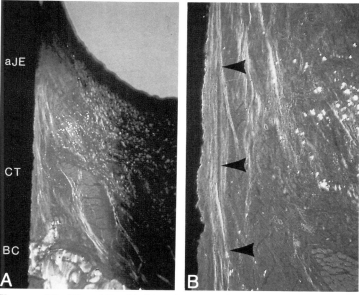

Figure 10–12. (A). Light microscopic view of an implant demonstrating the parallel arrangement of the connective tissue fibers. These fibers extend from the apical termination of the junctional epithelium to the marginal bone crest. (B). Higher magnification of (A) showing that the connective tissue fibers (arrows) run predominately parallel to the implant surface.

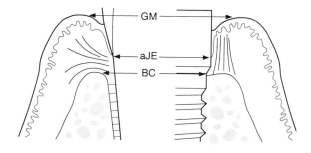

Tooth   Implant

Figure 10–11. Schematic drawing demonstrating the landmarks on the tooth and implant that separate the area of the sulcus and the junctional epithelium, the connective tissue, and the alveolar bone. The sulcus and junctional epithelium extend from the gingival margin (GM) to the apical termination of the junctional epithelium (aJE). The connective tissue interface extends from the (aJE) to the bone crest (BC).

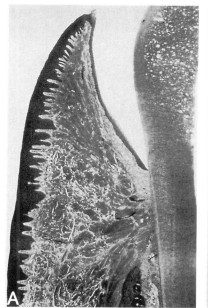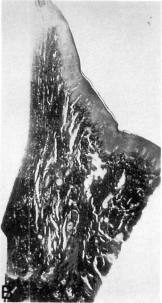

Figure 10–13. (A). Cross-section of the buccal dentogingival region in a dog, representing 2 months of plaque control. The junctional epithelium is thin and the distinct collagen fiber groups are well demarcated. (B). Cross-section of the buccal and coronal part of the peri-implant bone and mucosa interface in a dog, representing 2 months of plaque control.

The width of supracrestal connective tissue around the neck of a healthy implant is approximately 1 to 1.5 mm. This width may vary based on the initial thickness of the mucosa and the degree of adaptation of the mucosa at the time the transmucosal abutment is placed. If the direct bone implant contact is broken, connective tissue will fill the space between the alveolar crest and implant. These fiber bundles run parallel to the implant surface. Both the connective tissue and epithelial interfaces have proven to provide adequate resistance to oral function and marginal irritation.

Peri-implant Infections

Peri-implant health can normally be maintained for a long time with a supervised oral hygiene program. Although plaque accumulation and marginal inflammation are generally low, severe inflammation of the peri-implant tissue occurs in some cases. Clinical inflammatory reactions, as studied in animals, are histologically characterized by an increased number of inflammatory cells infiltrating the connective tissue. Microflora associated with implants in both healthy and slightly inflamed tissues are similar to those of teeth with healthy gingiva. The histological picture of early gingivitis is similar for both the tooth and the implant (Fig. 10–14). It consists of an inflammatory cell infiltrate in the connective tissue lateral to the junctional epithelium. With long-standing gingivitis, the inflammatory cell infiltrate around

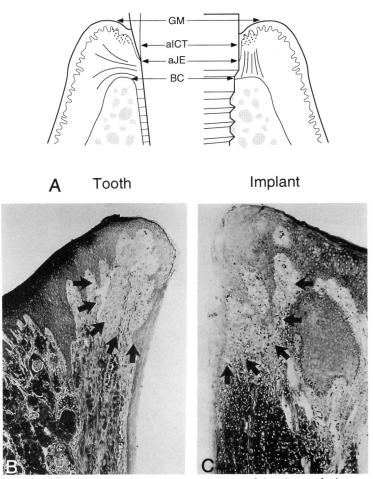

Figure 10–14. (A). Schematic drawing of 21 days of plaque formation, demonstrating the area of inflammatory connective tissue infiltrate that extends from the gingival margin (GM) to the apical termination of the connective tissue (a1CT). The area of the inflammation at 21 days is similar adjacent to both the tooth and the implant. GM, gingival margin; a1CT, apical termination of the connective tissue; aJE, the apical termination of the junctional epithelium; BC, bone crest. (B). Cross-section of the buccal and coronal part of the soft tissue adjacent to a tooth, representing 21 days of plaque formation. The infiltrate (arrows) is still above the base of the junctional epithelium. (C). Cross-section of the buccal and coronal part of the soft tissue adjacent to an implant, representing 21 days of plaque formation. The infiltrate (arrows) is still above the base of the junctional epithelium.

an implant has a more apical extension than a corresponding lesion in gingival tissue, and the junctional epithelium has the appearance of an ulcerated pocket epithelium (Fig. 10–15A through C).

The microbiota associated with implants and teeth affected by marginal bone loss are more complex and consists primarily of Gram-negative anaerobic rods. Histologically, bone loss around teeth occurs perivascularly. Despite this bone resorption, a layer of collagen-rich connective tissue usually separates the inflammatory cell-infiltrated connective tissue from the crestal bone adjacent to the tooth. Inflammatory cells are rarely seen in the periodontal ligament space. The inflammatory infiltrate causing resorption of bone around an implant is usually more pronounced than around a tooth, and the inflammatory zone extends directly to the

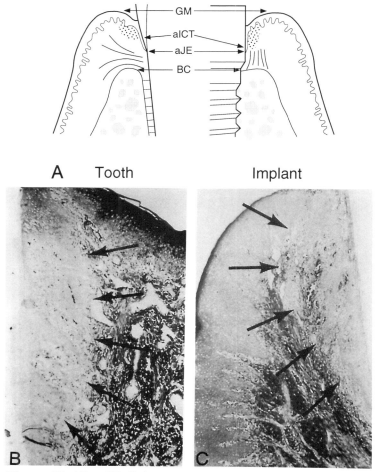

Figure 10–15. (A). Schematic drawing of 3 months of plaque formation, demonstrating the area of inflammatory connective tissue infiltrate that extends from the gingival margin to just short of the apical termination of the junctional epithelium with the tooth, and from the gingival margin to the apical termination of the junctional epithelium with the implant. GM, gingival margin; a1CT, apical termination of the connective tissue; aJE, the apical termination of the junctional epithelium; BC, bone crest. (B). Cross-section of the buccal and coronal part of the soft tissue adjacent to an implant, representing 3 months of plaque formation. The area illustrates the extension (arrows) of the inflamed connective tissue. (C). Cross-section of the buccal and coronal part of the soft tissue adjacent to a tooth, representing 3 months of plaque formation. The area illustrates the extension (arrows) of the inflamed connective tissue.

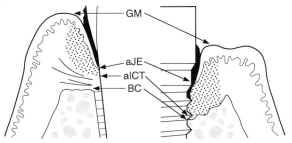

A   Tooth   Implant

crestal bone adjacent to the implant and even into the marrow spaces of the bone (Figs. 10–16A through C). This difference may be explained by the parallel orientation of the connective tissue adjacent to the implant, which is less resistant than collagen fibers, inserting at right angles into a cemental surface of a tooth. The parallel arrangement of connective tissue and the resulting pathway for bone resorption may help to explain the typical saucerization (circumferential cratering) defect associated with failing dental implants (Fig. 10–17).

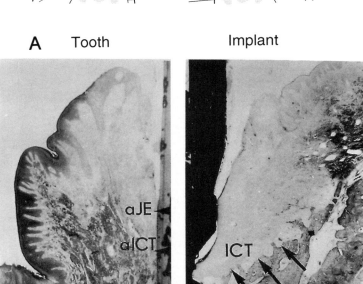

Figure 10–16. (A). Schematic drawing of destructive periodontitis demonstrating the area of inflammatory connective tissue infiltrate that extends from the gingival margin (GM) to just below the apical termination of the junctional epithelium (aJE) with the tooth, and from the gingival margin (GM) to the bone crest (BC) with the implant. (B). Cross-section of the dentogingival region adjacent to a tooth with destructive periodontitis. Arrows indicate the apical termination of the junctional epithelium (aJE), the apical termination of the inflamed connective tissue (a1CT) and the level of the bone crest (BC). Noninflamed connective tissue is present between the a1CT and the BC. (C). Cross-section of implant and peri-implant tissues with inflammation consistent with peri-implantitis. Arrows indicate the close relation between the inflamed connective tissue (ICT) and the bone. The bone margin is cupped out, demonstrating active bone resorption.

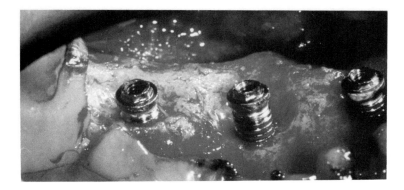

Figure 10–17. Implants with established peri-implantitis. With the soft tissues removed, the classic circumferential bone defect (saucerization) is apparent.

Surgical Correction of the Failing Implant

Successful regeneration of lost bone support around implants involves several clinical procedures. Regardless of the surgical technique, the most important step is decontamination of the implant surface. At present, most clinicians use either tetracycline or citric acid to remove the endotoxins that contaminate the implant surface. Some clinicians have also used air abrasive materials to clean the implant surface. The best method to decontaminate an implant surface has yet to be determined. The use of air abrasive material and citric acid along with guided tissue regeneration (GTR) principles (the exclusion of connective tissue and epithelium with an exclusive membrane material) allows 100% of bone height to be restored with 36% of this new height as new osseointegration (Fig. 10–18). As the techniques of decontamination and GTR are better understood, reosseointegration appears to be a predictable procedure for implants with bone loss.

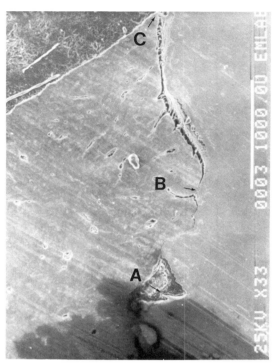

Figure 10–18. Scanning electron micrograph of bone contact to a titanium implant with connective tissue interface, which occurred in response to a regenerative procedure using guided tissue regeneration (GTR). new bone extends from (A), the most concave point below the second thread, to (B), the most coronal point of reosseointegration. (C) is the most coronal height of new bone (original magnification ×33).

Clinical Considerations

Osseointegration requires an implant composed of a biocompatible material. It must be placed in bone atraumatically and must be placed in function at the appropriate time. After an implant is integrated, the main condition for gingival health around implants is maintained by good oral hygiene. If oral hygiene is neglected, bacterial plaque forms, resulting in gingivitis, which can progress into periodontitis (Figs. 10–19). In the latter condition, bone resorption occurs and natural teeth or oral implants can be lost (Fig. 10–20). Because of the unique pattern (saucerization) of bone resorption around implants, every effort should be made in the design of the implant restoration

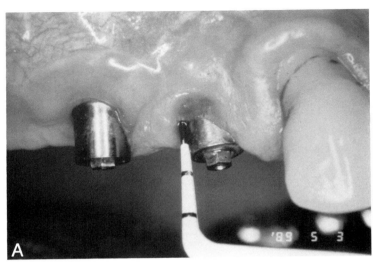

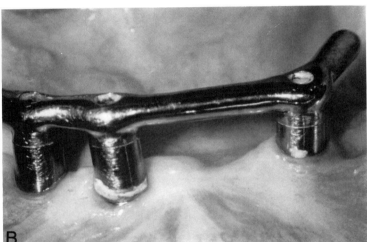

Figure 10–19. (A). Clinically, the tissue on the buccal of the implant is inflamed. Clinical probing should always be done with a plastic probe. This will prevent scratching of the implant surface. The inflammation can be reversed with improved oral hygiene. (B). Implants used to support a removable prosthesis. Although the patient maintains good plaque control, salivary calculus will form on the abutments. Removal of this calculus should always be performed with plastic instruments.

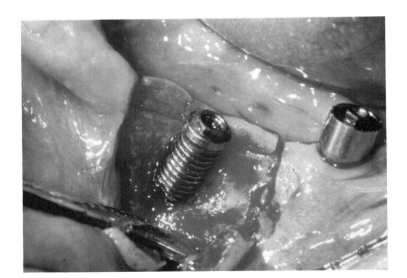

Figure 10–20. Severe bone loss around an implant that still has no mobility and clinically appears well integrated. The bone loss is secondary to heavy occlusal forces and marginal plaque accumulation.

to allow for optimal hygiene by the paitent (Fig. 10–21A and B). The shape and the texture of the implant surface that interfaces with the dentogingival complex is important. A geometrically simple, polished, conical, tooth-shaped design is ideal to minimize the deposition of bacterial plaque and calculus. The design of oral implants must consider the possibility of bone resorption and gingival recession, which would expose more of the implant to the oral cavity. Close professional supervision of the implant patient must include continual reassessment of the occlusal forces placed on the implant and the integrity of the prosthetic components. Clinical assessment of the peri-implant soft tissue interface and radiographic evaluation of the bone–implant interface must be carefully evaluated. Clinical parameters of mobility, tissue color and tone, probing and attachment levels, and bleeding upon probing must be recorded and compared over time. Standardized, reproducible radiographs must be compared to evaluate bone height and quality of osseointegration. Any deviation from normal should be corrected to ensure the long-term success of the dental implant.

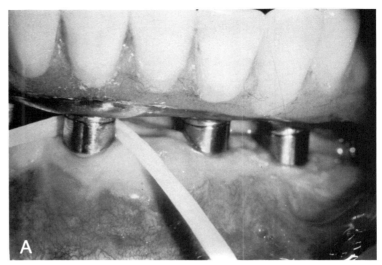

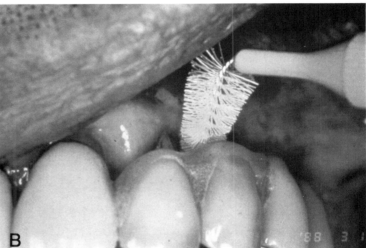

Figure 10–21. (A). To maintain a high level of plaque and calculus control, daily oral hygiene with dental floss or tape is imperative. (B). The use of an interproximal brush is an excellent method of personal oral hygiene, especially in areas difficult to reach with an ordinary toothbrush.

Clinical Application

Titanium implant abutments are easily marred and scratched by metallic instruments and abrasive oral cleaning materials.

Table 10-2.
Comparison of Natural Tooth and Implant

	Natural Tooth	Implant
Structure	PDL, cementum	No
Tissue interface	Junctional epithelium	Biologic seal
Fiber orientation	Perpendicular	Most parallel
Inflammation	Plaque induced	Plaque induced

Table 10-3.
Integration Quality

Fibro-osseous integration	Least successful
Bio-osseous integration	Good result
Osseointegration	Best result

Clinical Application

Implants and their prosthetic components must be designed so that adequate oral hygiene procedures may be performed.

Summary

The interfaces of oral tissues with an endosseous implant have been discussed and compared with the natural tooth (Table 10–2). Direct bone contact in the form of osseointegration or biointegration are the best choices of attachment (Table 10–3). The epithelial soft-tissue interface to endosseous oral implants is similar to the interface with natural teeth and is formed by a junctional epithelium and sulcus. The supracrestal collagen fibers run parallel to an implant's surface, whereas on natural teeth, they are functionally oriented (perpendicular) and insert into cementum. Oral implant necks should have a geometrically simple, polished, conical, toothshaped design to minimize plaque accumulation and facilitate oral hygiene procedures. The microbiota around dental implants and natural teeth are similar. Progression of inflammation directly from the connective tissue to the alveolar crest and into the marrow spaces is a unique pathway of inflammation seen around infected dental implants. This pattern of bone loss may be explained by the connective tissue interface to the dental implant. The interface appears to be protective as long as an adequate level of oral hygiene is maintained.

Self-Evaluation Review

1. Define an oral implant.
2. What are the three possible types of hard-tissue interfaces that can be formed between endosseous oral implants and alveolar bone?
3. What are the most preferred hard-tissue interfaces for endosseous oral implants?
4. What does the term "osseointegration" mean?
5. What materials can produce a bioactive chemical and mechanical interface with bone?
6. Why is a soft-tissue interface around an endosseous oral implant not desirable by most implantologists?
7. What is "saucerization"?
8. What is the most important condition for healthy tissue around endosseous oral implants?
9. What is the difference between the interface of connective tissue to a tooth and an implant?
10. Adherence to what five factors will ensure the greatest probability of achieving osseointegration of implants?

Acknowledgments

We thank Dr. M.A. Listgarten of Philadelphia, Pennsylvania for use of Figure 10–9; Drs. B.E. Gysi and J.R. Strub of Freiburg, Germany, for use of Figures 10–2 and 10–7; Dr. P.I. Branemark and Dr. T. Albrektsson of Göteborg, Sweden, and the Quintessence Publishing Co., Inc., Chicago, Illinois, for use of Figures 10–1, 10–3A, 10–5, 10–6, and 10–10A and B; Dr. B. Gottlander and Dr. T. Albrektsson of Göteborg, Sweden, and Munksgaard International Publishers, Ltd. for use of Figures 10–3B and 10–4B; Dr. M.A. Listgarten and Munksgaard International Publishers, Ltd. for use of Figure 10–12A and B; Dr. T. Berglundh and Munksgaard International Publishers, Ltd. for use of Figures 10–13A and B, and 10–14B and C; Dr. I. Ericsson and Munksgaard International Publishers, Ltd. for use of Figures 10–15A through C; Dr. J. Lindhe and Munksgaard International Publishers, Ltd. for use of Figure 10–16A through C; and Drs. R.V. McKinney and R.A. James and Mosby-Year Book, Inc., for use of Figures 10–5 and 10–8.

Suggested Readings

Adell R, Lekholm U, Rockler B, Branemark PI. Marginal tissue reactions at osseointegrated titanium fixtures *Int J Oral Maxillofac Surg.* 1986;15:39–52.

Berglundh T, Lindhe J, Ericsson I, Marinello CP, Liljenberg B, Thompson P. The soft tissue barrier at implants and teeth. *Clin Oral Imp Res.* 1991;2:81–90.

Berglundh T, Lindhe J, Ericsson I, Marinello CP, Liljenberg B, Thompson P. Soft tissue reaction to de novo plaque formation on implants and teeth. *Clin Oral Imp Res.* 1992;3:1–8.

Buser D, Warrer K, Karring T. Formation of a periodontal ligament around titanium implants. *J Periodontol.* 1990;61:597–601.

Hickey JS, O'Neal RB, Scheidt MJ, Strong SL, Turgeon D, Van Dyke TE. Microbiologic characterization of ligature-induced peri-implantitis in the microswine model. *J Periodontol.* 1991;62:548–553.

Listgarten MA, Buser D, Steinemann SG, Donath K, Lang NP, Webber HP. Light and transmission electron microscopy of the intact interfaces between non-submergd titantium-coated epoxy resin implants and bone or gingiva. *J Dent Res.* 1992;71:364–371.

Listgarten MA, Lang NP, Schroeder HE, Schroeder A. Periodontal tissues and their counterparts around endoosseous implants. *Clin Oral Impl Res.* 1991;2:1–19.

McCollum J, O'Neal RB, Brennan WA, Van Dyke TE, Horner JA. The effect of titanium implant surface roughness on plaque accumulation. *J Periodontol.* 1992;63:802–805.

McKinney RV, Steflik DE, Koth DL. The epithelium-dental implant interface. *J. Oral Implant.* 1988;13:622–641.

Ten Cate AR. The gingival junction. In: Branemark PI, Zarb GA, Albrektsson T, eds. *Tissue Integrated Prostheses.* Chicago, Ill: Quintessence; 1985:145–153.

Thomsen P, Ericson LE. Light and transmission electron microscopy used to study the tissue morphology close to implants. *Biomaterials.* 1985;6:421–424.

11

Histologic Changes during Tooth Movement

Carla A. Evans and James K. Avery

Introduction

Adjustments in tooth position are possible throughout life because the components of the periodontium (periodontal ligament, alveolar bone, cementum, and gingiva) remodel continually. Some tooth movements occur spontaneously. Tooth buds may change position within the jaw before beginning to erupt. After active eruption to the occlusal level, teeth continue to erupt passively and migrate as they compensate for late growth changes and tooth wear.

Tooth movement also may occur in response to the sustained mechanical forces emanating from orthodontic appliances or other stimuli. This chapter focuses on the histological features of mechanically induced tooth movement. The tissues used as examples in this chapter are from a rhesus monkey because it is not possible to obtain equivalent samples from human patients.

In most instances, the periodontal structures respond well to movement induced by the clinician because the alveolar bone and gingiva show a remarkable ability to be modified (Figs. 11–1 and 11–2). Mechanical loads activate cells, and tissues remodel to resist stresses and strains. The sequence and timing of the remodeling process are known, but the biologic basis for orthodontic tooth movement is not well understood.

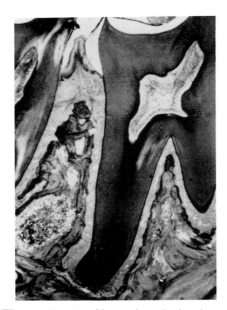

Figure 11–1. Normal periodontium.

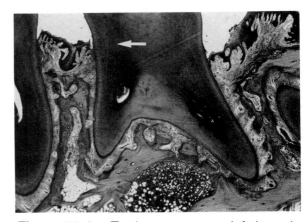

Figure 11–2. Tooth movement to left (arrow).

Objectives

After reading this chapter, you should be able to describe typical histological changes in the periodontium that result from tipping, bodily movement, and intrusive, extrusive, and rotational forces on the tooth root during clinical treatment. Also, you should be able to describe potential adverse changes resulting from orthodontic tooth movement.

Fundamentals of Tooth Movement

Clinical tooth movement requires a periodontal ligament. Forces applied to teeth are mediated through the periodontal ligament and result in remodeling of the periodontal tissues (Figs. 11–1 and 11–2).

When an appliance is attached to a tooth and the tooth is moved as shown in Figure 11–2, the entire surface of the socket is affected. The pressure side of the tooth root compresses the periodontal ligament and alveolar bone, which results in bone resorption. On the opposite surface of the root, the movement stretches the ligament fibers, which causes tension to occur. This situation is, of course, similar in the case of a single or multirooted tooth, although it is more complex in the latter (Fig. 11–2). Forces had only recently been applied to the tooth in Figure 11–2; consequently, the ligament is narrower on the compression side than on the tension side.

Sites of Remodeling

On the compression side of the ligament, collagen fiber bundles initially are disorganized and compacted. Vascular flow decreases and cell death may occur (Fig. 11–3). On the tension side of the ligament, the collagen fibers are stretched. The fibroblasts become more spindle-shaped and appear oriented with their long axis in the direction of the fiber bundles (Fig. 11–4). A two-rooted tooth, as shown in Figures 11–2 and 11–5), has two or more zones of compression as well as two or more zones of tension. Note that the bifurcation zone has a region of tension toward the left root and a region of compression toward the right root. The

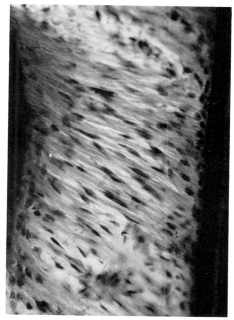

Figure 11–4. Tension zone (early).

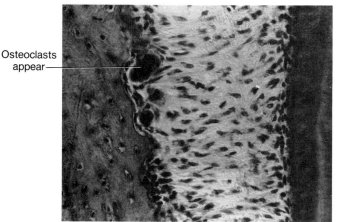

Osteoclasts appear

Figure 11–3. Compression zone (early).

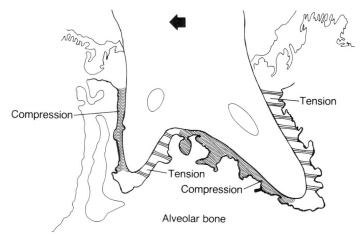

Compression

Tension

Tension

Compression

Alveolar bone

Figure 11–5. Zones of compression and tension in tooth movement.

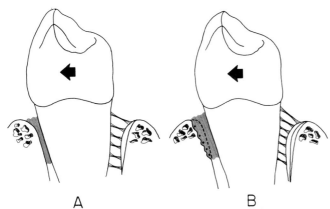

Clinical Application

Clinically applicable advances related to tooth movement have come primarily from improvements in orthodontic materials and statistical observations on growth and development. Basic biologic research on the remodeling process and mechanisms of tooth movement is desirable to produce faster and more stable tooth movement.

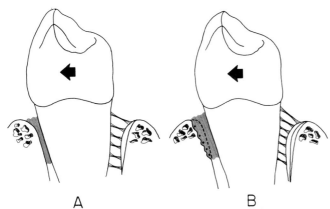

Figure 11–6. Results of tipping type of tooth movement. (A). Early. (B). Late.

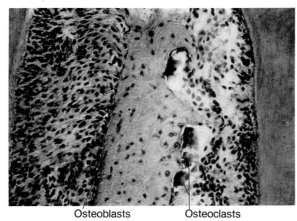

Osteoblasts   Osteoclasts

Figure 11–7. Osteoblasts and osteoclasts in bifurcation zone. Left, tension zone; right, compression zone.

apical areas demonstrate transition from tension to compression and are vulnerable locations during tooth movement because too much pressure could cause death of the pulp tissue by interfering with the tooth's vascular supply.

The initial response to physical force is displacement of the tooth; permanent structural changes follow. The histological features accompanying the changes include changes in cell type and number, vascular changes, and changes in the extracellular matrix.

Transduction

The mechanism of *transduction*—that is, the conversion of physical force into biologic response—is not known, but numerous hypotheses have been introduced. Some of the mechanical and chemical signals proposed as initiators of metabolic changes are: altered blood and lymphatic flow; pressure and volume changes within the periodontal space; distortion of matrix molecules, cell membranes and cell cytoskeleton; stress-generated bioelectric effects from alveolar bone bending; hormonal influences; and inflammatory phenomena and other nervous and immune cellular events. The explanations propose ways for local and systemic factors to influence alveolar bone, periodontal and gingival fiber bundles, cells (mesenchymal, vascular, neural, gingival epithelial), and tissue fluids. However, more investigation is needed to elucidate the cascade of changes involved in remodeling of the periodontium during tooth movement.

Force Variables

Time is an important variable in the response of alveolar bone to tooth movement. As might be expected, the histology of the compression and tension zones will change with time. Alveolar bone resorption allows for the gradual movement of the tooth into the space provided and begins on the compression front. On the tension side, bone formation compensates for tooth movement away from the bone under tension, shown in Figure 11–6A and B. Figure 11–6A illustrates a tooth tipping to the left; on the left is seen a compression zone whereas on the right is seen a tension zone. Later (Fig. 11–6B), the zone of direct osteoclastic resorption is seen on the left, with bony deposition occurring in the tension zone on the right. Direct or frontal resorption is a desirable clinical goal because it is not a destructive process.

Osteoclasts appear a few hours after tooth movement begins as they are recruited from monocytes arising from blood vessels. Both osteoclasts and osteoblasts stain with oxidative enzymes. Figure 11–7 illustrates both osteoblasts (left) and osteoclasts (right) in the interradicular bone between the roots of a molar tooth. Compare the resorption sites that have large, multinucleated, black-stained osteoclasts (right) with the highly cellular and fibrous zone (left). The tooth is therefore moving in which direction? Fibroblasts proliferate and synthesize new matrix in tension sites and participate in the degradation of necrotic periodontal ligament in areas of compression along with osteoclasts and macrophages.

Histologic Changes

The tissue response to mechanical forces in tooth movement will vary with force *magnitude* (light, heavy), *duration* (continuous, intermittent), *direction*, and *point of application*. Should the force be too great in magnitude or the movement too rapid, *hyalinization* of the periodontal ligament may occur. Hyalinization results in the loss of cell activity and vascularity in the pressure zone of the ligament. This zone of the ligament may appear glasslike; hence, the origin of the term. A hyalinized ligament is shown in Figure 11–8A, where the tooth is in close apposition to bone. Viewed at higher magnification (Fig. 11–8B), a loss of the fibrillar nature of the collagen fibers can be seen. Loss of cells interrupts bone resorption and tooth movement stops temporarily.

Another feature of hyalinization is its association with *undermining resorption*. Because resorption cannot occur on the compressed surface of the alveolar bone, osteoclasts are activated in the marrow spaces opposite the compressed alveolar bone surface. When the osteoclasts finish removing the intervening bone, the tooth will move again. Note the osteoclasts in Figure 11–8B that are destroying the bone adjacent to the hyalinized zone. Some of the cells in the zone of compression do not recover. As they are destroyed and resorption relieves the compression, new cells from adjacent tissues rebuild the destroyed zone. It is not yet known why compression of the ligament and alveolar bone results in undermining resorption, but lack of blood supply and cell death in the hyalinized zone may contribute. Also, changes in bioelectric potential may signal the onset of resorption.

In addition to delaying orthodontic treatment, *undermining resorption* of alveolar bone is potentially more damaging to the alveolar process than is *direct resorption*, as it may result in extensive bone loss and root resorption. What protects the root surface from damage during routine tooth movement is not known. Undermining resorption is not easily controlled and the extent of damage is unpredictable.

Forces applied to the teeth can also produce cause distant changes, such as those in periosteum, endosteum, sutures, and possibly even mandibular condyles. A complete explanation of tooth movement must include mechanisms for bone remodeling in alveolar bone marrow spaces, alteration of the gingiva, and transmission of forces to distant sites.

Intermittent force and continuous force cause different histological appearances. When the tissues are temporarily relieved of stress, circulation is partially restored, cell activity is restored, and repair takes place. Tooth mobility may be increased, however, which can become a problem.

A lower level of cellularity in the periodontal ligament is found in older individuals and may be related to an initial slower rate of response during tooth movement. Increased age, however, does not reduce the prospect of a successful clinical outcome.

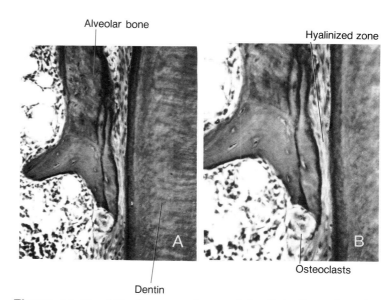

Figure 11–8. (A). Compression and hyalinization of periodontal ligament caused by excessive tooth movement. (B). Higher magnification of (A) shows undermining resorption adjacent to the hyalinized zone.

Clinical Application

The clinician must choose a force level and an appliance that are effective, efficient, and safe. Regular monitoring of the progress of treatment is extremely important so that forces and appliances can be altered as required.

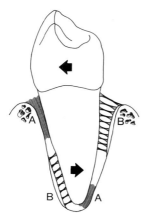

Figure 11–9. Tipping of tooth, causing crown movement to the left and root movement to the right. Observe the zones of compression and tension.

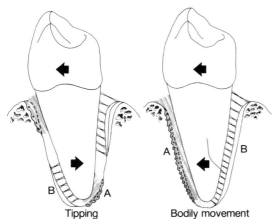

Tipping   Bodily movement

Figure 11–10. Tipping movement compared with bodily movement. In the latter, changes occur over the entire periodontium of the root surface.

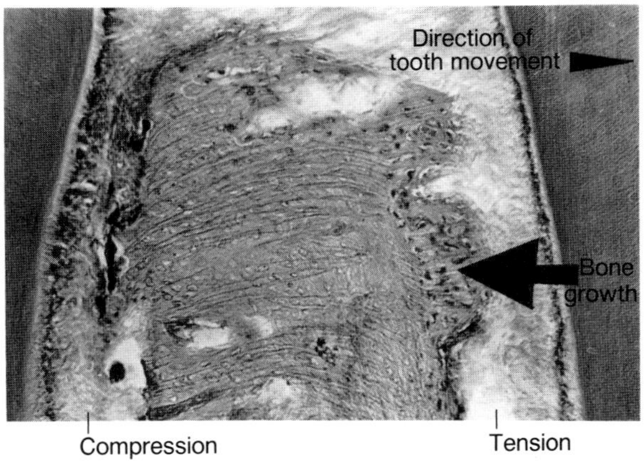

Tipping and Bodily Movement

Tipping of a tooth (Fig. 11–9) results in nonuniform alteration of the sockets, whereas bodily movement affects the entire socket in a more constant fashion, as is illustrate in Figure 11–10. Compression, and possibly hyalinization, occur at *points A* whereas tension and bone deposition occur at *points B*. When the crown tips to the left, the root apex moves to the right producing zones of compression and tension on opposite sides of the tooth apex relative to the cervical region. Likewise, both bone resorption and deposition occur on the same side of a tooth as it is tipped (Fig. 11–10).

Figure 11–11 shows a histological section of the bifurcation zone of a molar tooth during the process of being tipped to the right. Direction of force is indicated by the small arrow in the upper right-hand corner. At the point of the large arrow, on the tension side of the tooth, new alveolar bone is being formed. The active bone-forming osteoblasts as well as osteocytes are seen stained black by a histochemical stain, which indicates vital functioning cells. Along the dentin (right), the cementoblasts are also stained, which indicates the formation of new cementum in response to tension on the perforating fibers. Resorption of bone and degenerative changes are occurring in the compression zone on the left of the alveolar bone. This is indicated by inactivity of the bone front. Most of the lacunae are unstained, which indicates the absence of vital cells. Spaces where bone loss has occurred indicate resorptive activity.

In Figure 11–12, the small circle on the roots indicate the *center of resistance*, or the fulcrum of rotation of each tooth. In the case of a short, incompletely developed root (Figure 11–12A), tipping causes resorption at two sites and tension at the opposite two sites. The root apex of a young, completely formed tooth, as shown in Figure 11–12B, tips in a direction opposite to the crown. In the adult, as shown in Figure 11–12C, tipping is complicated by strong apical fibers that resist movement and a narrow ligament space. In this case, tipping causes less movement at the root apex, but causes resorption along most of the length of bone on the compressed side.

Compression   Tension

Figure 11–11. Bifurcation zone during late tooth movement. Left, active resorption; right, bone formation.

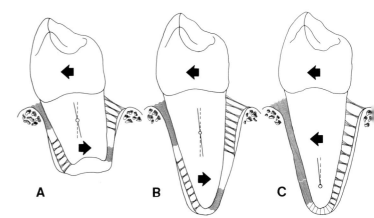

A   B   C

Figure 11–12. Change in point of rotation of tooth in young forming root (A), completed root (B), and mature periodontium (C).

A micrograph of the cemental surface reveals the activity of oxidative enzymes during tooth movement in the cementoblasts adjacent to the cementum (Fig. 11–13, center). Observe the bundles of collagen fibers projecting from the cementum. The stain indicates that the cementocytes, probably newly differentiated, have high functional activity. This is also true for the osteoblasts in the adjacent alveolar bone. New cementum will be deposited, and attachment fiber bundles will be formed in response to the tension.

Both the cementum and the alveolar bone may undergo resorption (Fig. 11–14). If compression is great and over a long period, both opposing surfaces will be affected. Note the osteoclasts along the bone and cementum (Fig. 11–14).

Extrusive and Intrusive Movement

Figure 11–15A illustrates the orientation of principal fibers when *extrusive forces* are applied to the tooth. Note the direction of the arrows. This type of movement causes tension in all the ligament fibers with resultant bone deposition along the lamina dura, especially in the alveolar crest and fundic regions. Light extrusive forces are most effective at producing compensatory bone growth.

Intrusive forces cause relaxation of the free and attached gingival fibers, as well as bone loss at the alveolar crest and over the entire socket (Fig. 11–15B). Good results are less easily obtained with intrusive movements than with tipping. This mode of movement requires a light, persistent force proceeding at a slow rate.

The tooth shown in Figure 11–16 is in the process of being intruded. The applied forces, depicted by the arrow on the left of this micrograph on the pulpal side of the root dentin, cause the principal fibers to appear oblique except at the gingival area at the top of the field, where they are collapsed. The bone in this area has been partially resorbed and will undergo further resorption, as will the compressed alveolar bone in the apical zone.

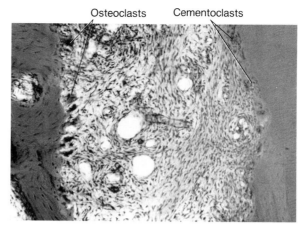

Figure 11–14. Activity in compression zone (late). Observe the osteoclasts on bone and the resorption of the root surface.

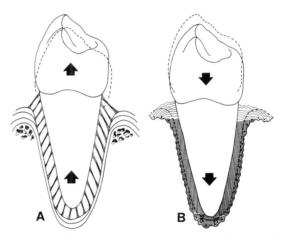

Figure 11–15. (A). Extrusion of tooth, causing tension over entire socket. (B). Intrusion of tooth, causing resorption over entire surface of alveolar bone proper.

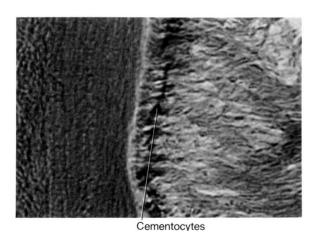

Figure 11–13. Activation of cementocytes along surface of root.

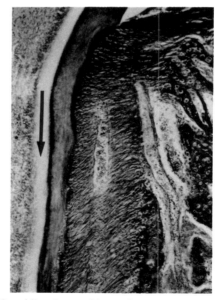

Figure 11–16. Histology of intrusive movement. Note the loss of bone and cementum.

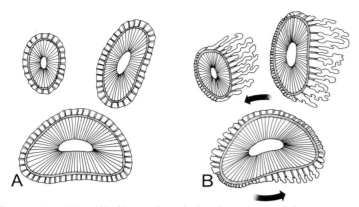

Figure 11-17. (A). Normal periodontium around three-rooted tooth. (B). Rotation of three-rooted tooth, causing bone loss and deposition of new bone.

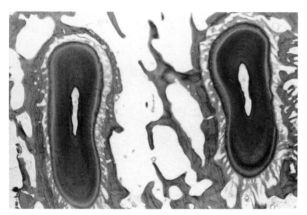

Figure 11-18. Histology of rotation of roots. Observe the direction of periodontal fiber bundles.

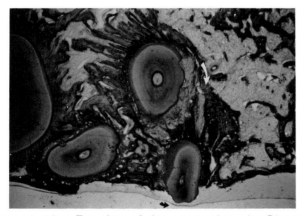

Figure 11-19. Rotation of three-rooted tooth. Observe the bone formation along the tension surfaces of the bone. White upper arrow, direction of rotation; black lower arrow, perforation of cortical bone by root.

Rotation and Bodily Movement

Figure 11-17 illustrates the consequence of rotational forces on a three-root molar tooth. At the left in these diagrams is the direction of the principal fibers before treatment. As the tooth is rotated, deposition will occur along the tension surface. The result after 4 months is shown in Figure 11-17B. Observe the distance each root has moved. Not all roots may move the same distance; for example, one root rotates in place whereas the others are moved around this axis. Restructuring of the socket in the alveolar bone during rotation thus occurs by development of zones of tension and compression as shown in Figure 11-17B. The oval shape of the root also complicates resorptive patterns.

Figure 11-18 shows two teeth in the early stages of clockwise rotation illustrated by the direction of the collagen fiber bundles of the periodontal ligament. Bone resorption and bone formation are minimal at this early time, although resorption of bone on the inferior aspect of the root on the right and some cemental loss along the root surface on the right are seen.

Figure 11-19 illustrates the clockwise rotation of a three-rooted molar in the monkey after 4 months. In this micrograph, the root on the left has rotated in position, which demonstrates the characteristic changes in socket shape that result from movement of an oval root. These are the same changes shown in Figure 11-17. The other two roots also show evidence of clockwise movement and more extensive remodeling of the socket. The pattern of bone deposition, stimulated by tension placed on the periodontal ligament fibers, can be seen on the left of the uppermost root. Observe that bone formation has occurred along the direction of the periodontal ligament fibers. This deposition pattern indicates the path of root movement. Excessive application of rotational force in the tooth of this laboratory animal has resulted in the undesired perforation of the cortical bone plate by the buccal root, which can be seen at the lower right of the micrograph (Fig. 11–19, arrow). In Figure 11–20, the long horizontal trabeculae of bone can be seen deposited behind the moving tooth root. Incremental deposits of cementum also can be seen along the tension side of the root (Fig. 11–20) Cementum, like bone, will resorb or form in areas of pressure and tension. This figure demonstrates an extreme case of socket remodeling and shows the alveolar bone's potential for remodeling.

Figure 11–21 demonstrates an extreme case of intrusion of a tooth in a socket. The molar tooth in this monkey is in contact with the underlying bone. Observe the extent of bone loss on the left and the right. Bony change is indicated by the darkly-stained bone surrounding the root. Resorption has caused a thinning of the bone on the left of the root.

Remodeling of the bony tooth socket and alteration of the periodontal ligament fibers are not the only considerations in tooth movement. As shown in Figure 11–22, black-stained neural elements pass from the periodontal ligament (right) into the alveolar bone (left). These neural elements must adjust to positional changes of the tooth and bone. The vascular network within the periodontal ligament will be modified according to any changes caused by tooth movement and will adapt to maintain a normal vascular supply (Fig. 11–23). Lack of vascular supply to this area results in hyalinization, possibly with resultant undermining and surface resorption.

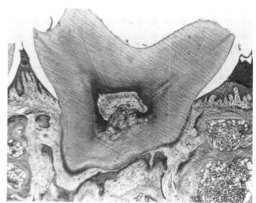

Figure 11–21. Intrusion of tooth (early). Observe the contact of the tooth and aleolar bone.

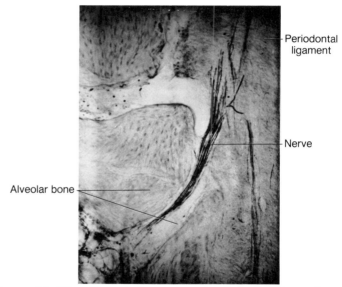

Periodontal ligament

Nerve

Alveolar bone

Figure 11–22. Neural elements enter ligament from alveolar bone.

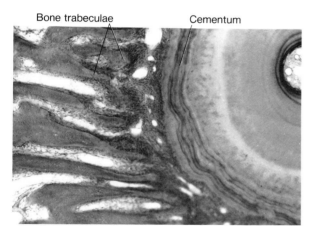

Bone trabeculae

Cementum

Figure 11–20. Bone trabeculae and cementum on tension side of root. This tooth is undergoing rotation.

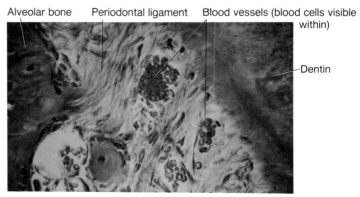

Alveolar bone   Periodontal ligament   Blood vessels (blood cells visible within)

Dentin

Figure 11–23. Normal vascularity of periodontal ligament.

Root resorption is a potential complication of orthodontic tooth movement. Figure 11–24A and B shows an unusual case of generalized extreme root resorption that occurred during orthodontic treatment.

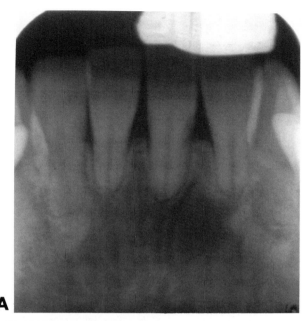

A

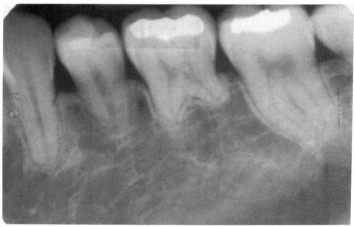

B

Figure 11–24. (A) and (B). A rare case of generalized extreme root resorption.

Clinical Application

Although commonly associated with excessive force or long duration of treatment, root resorption may also arise surprisingly quickly during use of light forces; however, this is very rare.

Stability and Relapse

Teeth remain in position on a day-to-day basis because the forces acting on them from the tongue and cheeks and from chewing and swallowing are in equilibrium. Even in severe malocclusions (Fig. 11–25), the alignment of the teeth is stable. The clinician faces two challenges: first, to move the teeth and second, to find a second position of equilibrium so that the results of tooth movement with orthodontic appliances will be stable. Figure 11–26 shows relapse of dental crowding after completion of comprehensive treatment, which included extraction of premolars, fixed orthodontic appliances, and a long period of retention with removable retainers.

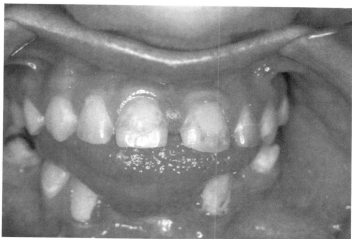

Figure 11–25. Tooth position is stable in this anterior open bite malocclusion associated with a lymphatic malformation.

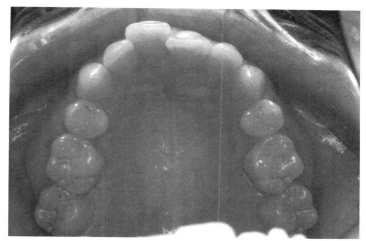

Figure 11–26. Orthodontic relapse.

Clinical Application

Stability of the orthodontic outcome depends on attaining equilibrium of forces and total remodeling of the periodontium. Gingival fibers in particular remodel very slowly and will cause rotations and spacing anomalies to recur. Gingival fiber resection and permanent fixed retention may be required to maintain the correction.

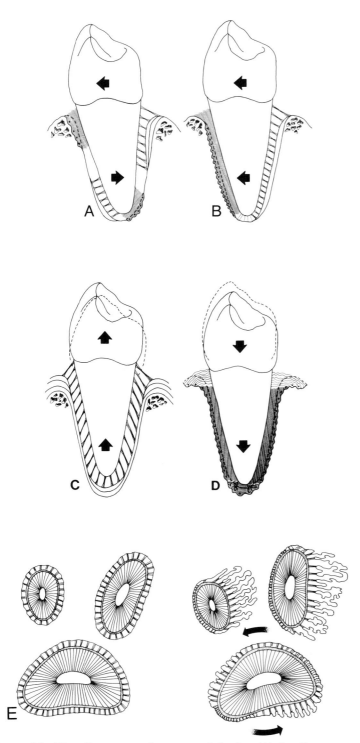

Summary

Changes in the periodontal structures during tooth movement depend on the magnitude, duration, direction, and point of application of the force, as well as health and age of the tissues. Changes on the tension side of tooth movement are characterized by an initial increase in periodontal ligament width with stretching of the periodontal ligament fibers. Later, bone deposition follows in the form of plates or spurs. On the compression side of the tooth, either direct bone resorption or hyalinization with undermining resorption ensues. Variations of these changes are demonstrated in Figure 11–27, which illustrates forces causing tipping (A), bodily movement (B), extrusive force (C), intrusive force (D), and rotational force (E). Determination of the center of resistance of the tooth is an important factor in planning treatment mechanics.

Most routine clinical tooth movement produces a successful, stable, nondestructive result. In some unusual instances, however, substantial permanent loss of bone or root structure may occur. Remodeling of the periodontium after tooth movement is necessary to maintain the correction. In contrast to the rapid reorganization seen in alveolar bone, gingival fibers require a prolonged period of retention and may never fully remodel.

Figure 11–27. Summary diagrams of tipping (A), bodily movement (B), extrusion (C), intrusion (D), and rotation (E).

Self-Evaluation Review

1. What differences would you expect in the periodontium of a young versus a mature tooth from tipping?
2. What changes are noted along the cemental surface at a tension site?
3. Describe hyalinization of the periodontal ligament. From what may it result?
4. What complications may arise from hyalinization of the periodontal ligament?
5. What adverse results would you expect when a tooth is moved too rapidly?
6. Compare the effects of intrusive and extrusive forces.
7. Describe undermining resorption. What complications may arise?
8. What role would vascularity play in bone resorption?
9. Which tissue resorbs more rapidly, tooth or alveolar bone? Why?
10. Compare rotation with rotation plus bodily movement of a tooth.

Suggested Readings

Atherton JD. The gingival response to orthodontic tooth movement. *Am J Orthod.* 1970;58:179.

Azuma M. Study on histologic changes of periodontal membrane incident to experimental tooth movement. *Bull Tokyo Med Dent Univ.* 1970;17:149.

Baumrind S, Buck DL. Rate changes in cell replication and protein synthesis in the periodontal ligament incident to tooth movement. *Am J Orthod.* 1970;57:109.

Beertsen W, Everts V, Hoeben K, Niehof A. Microtubules in periodontal ligament cells in relation to tooth eruption and collagen degradation. *J Periodont Res.* 1984;19:489–500.

Davidovitch Z. Tooth movement. *Crit Rev Oral Biol Med.* 1991; 2:411–450.

Davidovitch Z, Montgomery PC, Eckerdal O, Gustafson GT. Cellular localization of cyclic AMP in periodontal tissues during experimental tooth movement in cats. *Calcif Tissue Res.* 1976;19:317.

Edwards JG. A study of the periodontium during orthodontic rotation of teeth. *Am J Orthod.* 1968;54:441–459.

Kuam E. Organic tissue characteristics on the pressure side of human premolars following tooth movement. *Angle Orthod.* 1973;43:18–23.

Proffit WR. The biologic basis of orthodontic therapy. In: *Contemporary Orthodontics.* St. Louis, Mo: CV Mosby Co; 1993:266–288.

Roberts WE, Goodwin WC Jr, Heiner SR. Cellular response to orthodontic force. *Dent Clin North Am.* 1981;25:3–17.

Rygh P. Orthodontic root resorption studied by electron microscopy. *Angle Orthod.* 1977;47:1–16.

Rygh P. Ultrastructural changes in pressure zones of human periodontium incident to orthodontic tooth movement. *Acta Odontol Scand.* 1973;31:109–122.

Stenvik A, Mjor IA. Pulp and dentine reactions to experimental tooth intrusion. *Am J Orthod.* 1970;47:370–385.

Ten Cate AR, Deported DA, Freeman E. The role of fibroblasts in the remodeling of periodontal ligament during physiologic tooth movement. *Am J Orthod.* 1976;69:155.

Thilander B, Lindhe J, Okamoto H. The effect of orthodontic tilting movements on the periodontal tissues of infected and non-infected dentitions in dogs. *J Clin Periodontol.* 1977;14:231.

12

Wound Healing

Francisco Rivera-Hidalgó

Introduction

Healing is the process by which tissues are restored to an anatomic and a physiological arrangement after they have been injured. Figure 12–1 illustrates the normal arrangement of the gingival mucosa and Figure 12–2 diagrams an incision through this tissue. Whether injury results unintentionally from accidental trauma, or intentionally from the blade of the surgeon or from the removal of a tooth, events are triggered that will eventually restore it to its normal state. *Injury* is cell and intercellular matrix damage that may result in cell death, damage to capillaries with disruption of their blood flow, and alteration of the normal structure and function of the area. When injury occurs, blood or plasma leak into the injured area, bringing cells and chemical substances that start a complex series of events. These events are: clotting, inflammation, mobilization of cells, formation of granulation tissue, repair, and remodeling. In this chapter we will review these events as they relate to an incisional wound of the gingival tissues. Our incision cuts through and damages epithelium, connective tissue matrix, and capillaries of the area.

Objectives

After reading this chapter, you should be able to present the events that follow injury and the histologic changes associated with the repair process; to present fundamental knowledge of wound healing and some of the biochemical and immunologic events associated with it; and to understand the special healing cases associated in the healing adjacent to a tooth surface, in guided tissue regeneration, and in the extraction wound.

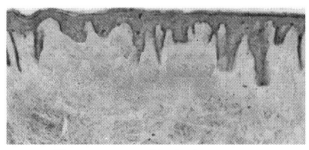

Figure 12–1. Gingival mucosa.

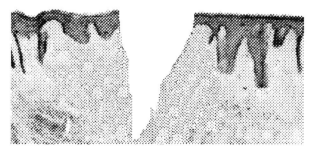

Figure 12–2. Incisional wound.

Early Events Leading to Clotting and Inflammation

The first changes resulting from injury are believed to occur at the vascular level. A transient episode of vasoconstriction (lasting a few minutes) is followed by a prolonged vasodilation, which results in increased vascular permeability. Albumin and other blood constitutents are spilled into the wound space, which changes hydrostatic pressure and leads to fluid accumulation (*edema*) and swelling. The resultant increase in extravascular pressure is sufficient to collapse adjacent capillaries and veins, and in that way to contribute to controlling the bleeding.

Extravasation of blood spills cells, platelets, and other blood substances into the wound site (Fig. 12–3). Prothrombin, plasma fibronectin, fibrinogen, plasminogen, kininogens, clotting factors, complement, and immunoglobulins are among the blood substances spilled.

Platelets reach the wound as a result of the hemorrhage from damage to capillaries. Platelets become activated by the exposed collagen from injured capillaries (collagen types IV and V are found in association with small blood vessels). Activated platelets become sticky and change their shape, projecting pseudopods to aid in the aggregation of other platelets. Platelets attach themselves to the exposed collagen through a *glycoprotein receptor* (GIb) on their surface that in turn attaches to a protein (known as the *von Willebrand factor*) released by platelets and endothelial cells in response to the injury (Fig. 12–4). The platelets reshape themselves to achieve broad contact with the exposed subendothelial structures, then release their granules, which contain important mediators (including adenosine diphosphate [ADP], fibronectin, platelet-derived growth factor [PDGF], platelet-activating factor [PAF], serotonin (5-hydroxytryptamine [5HT]), clotting factor V, insulinlike growth factor 1 (IGF-1, and synthesize thromboxane (TX), a potent mediator of inflammation).

Most platelets aggregate through the action of calcium ions, ADP, and TX. This platelet aggregation and plug formation occurs within 3 min after injury (Fig. 12–5). The platelet plug that forms aids in the temporary sealing of the damaged blood vessels. TX activates the blood-clotting cascade that leads to the formation of fibrin. Clotting factor V binds to the activated platelets and, together with clotting factor X, activates thrombin, which in turn leads to platelet activation and fibrin formation.

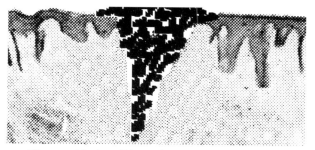

Figure 12–3. Blood fills the wound gap.

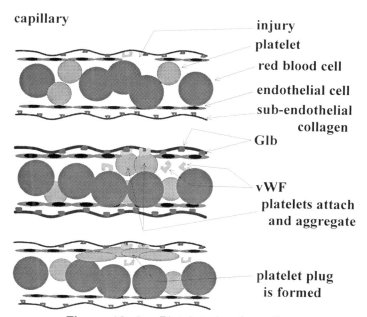

Figure 12–4. Platelet plug formation.

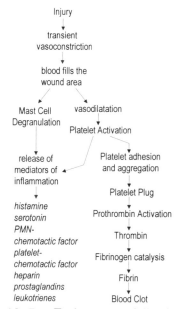

Figure 12–5. Early events following injury.

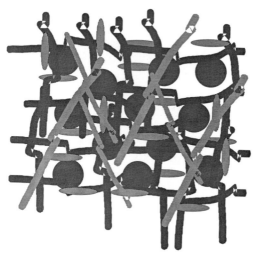

Figure 12–6. The clot is formed by a meshwork of fibers, red blood cells, and platelets.

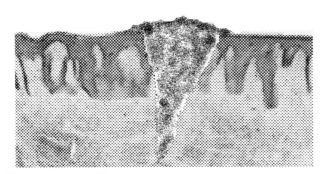

Figure 12–7. The blood clot fills the wound space.

Clotting proceeds in the area of the platelet plug. *Hemostasis*, the process of clot formation, proceeds via intrinsic and extrinsic pathways that cascade to form a clot. Prothrombin is first converted to thrombin. In the presence of thrombin, fibrinogen is converted to fibrin monomer, which polymerizes, forming fibrin strands. Cross linkage is established between the fibrin strands, and a dense, tight clot is formed within 5 to 10 min after injury (Fig. 12–6). A matrix of fibrin, blood constitutents, and cellular debris fills the wound defect and provides protection (Fig. 12–7). In skin, the surface of the clot dehydrates, forming a scab. In the oral cavity, the scab is soft and appears white because pigment has been washed away.

Plasma fibronectin is abundant in the wound. Found in plasma and in tissue matrix, fibronectin comprises a group of glycoproteins that are secreted by fibroblasts, platelets, and endothelial and epithelial cells. In the wound, fibronectin accumulates to help in the removal of bacteria and to help in cell adhesion to the extracellular matrix.

As a result of injury, mast cells synthesize mediators and degranulate to release many bioactive substances, which include lysosomal enzymes, hyaluronic acid, heparin, prostaglandins, chemotactic mediators for leukocytes, PAF, and histamine (Fig. 12–8). *Histamine*, a vasoactive amine, is responsible for vasodilation and increased vascular permeability during the first few minutes after wounding.

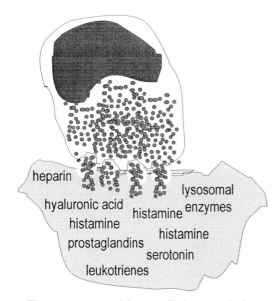

Figure 12–8. Mast cell degranulation.

Damage to the cell membrane activates *phospholipase A2*, an enzyme that cleaves phospholipids normally found with cholesterol and triglycerides in the cell membrane. This enzyme will break down arachidonic acid, producing mediators known as eicosanoids (Fig. 12–9). *Eicosanoids* are compounds that have a cyclopentane ring, contain 20 carbon atoms, and consist of prostanoids and leukotrienes (Table 12–1). *Prostanoids* are converted via the cyclooxygenase pathway into *thromboxane A2* (vasoconstrictor), *prostacyclin* (vasodilator), *prostaglandin E2* (vasodilator), and *prostaglandin F2α* (vasoconstrictor and chemotactic). The *leukotrienes* are converted via the lipoxygenase pathway into *leukotriene B4* (chemotactic) and *leukotriene C4*, known as *slow-reacting substance* (SRS), which induces smooth muscle contraction.

The *Hageman factor*, or *clotting factor XII* is one of several blood clotting factors spilled as a result of injury. This factor is activated by exposed collagen of damaged tissue and blood vessels. Its activation results in the establishment and amplification of an inflammatory response. Once activated, the Hageman factor activates directly or indirectly four important systems: (1) the clotting system, (2) the anticlotting (plasmin) system, (3) the kinin system, and (4) the complement system (Fig. 12–10).

Plasminogen, bound to tissues and present in blood, is activated by the Hageman factor and converted into plasmin, which activates the anticlotting system. *Plasmin* prevents the clotting process from spreading throughout the blood vessels (intravascular coagulation) and helps in the eventual dissolution of the fibrin clot.

Kininogens are the product of the interaction between kallikrein and Hageman factor. Kininogens are subsequently transformed into kinins, which exhibit potent biologic effects similar to those of histamine (Table 12–1). The *kinins* cause contraction of visceral smooth muscle and dilation of vascular smooth muscle. They increase capillary permeability, attract white blood cells, and are responsible for inducing pain. Once released, the kinins and the prostaglandins remain active longer than histamine (which is just a few minutes), and in that way lengthen the vasoactive changes. The kinins are considered to be responsible for prolonging the inflammatory state.

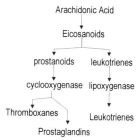

Figure 12–9. Inflammatory mediators from arachidonic acid.

Table 12–1.
Mediators of Inflammation

Histamine/serotonin	Vasodilation
	Increased vascular permeability
	Smooth muscle contraction
Kinins	Vasodilation
	Increased vascular permeability
	Smooth muscle contraction
	Pain
Prostaglandins	Vasodilation
	Increased vascular permeability
	Pain
Leukotrienes	Vasodilation
	Increased vascular permeability
	Smooth muscle contraction
	PMN chemotaxis
Complement products	Vasodilation
	Increased vascular permeability
	Smooth muscle contraction
	PMN chemotaxis
	MΦ chemotaxis
	Mast cell degranulation

PMN, polymorphonuclear neutrophils; MΦ, macrophage.

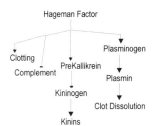

Figure 12–10. The Hageman factor activates four systems.

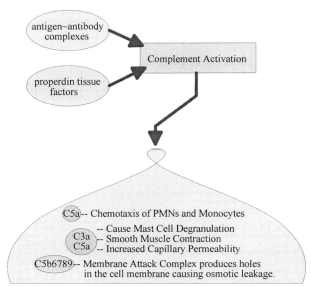

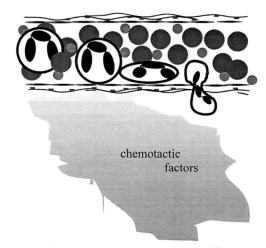

Figure 12–11. Complement activation and products.

Figure 12–12. Polymorphonuclear neutrophils start to adhere to the endothelial cells in postcapillary venules (pavementing) and migrate through gaps between endothelial cells (diapedesis) following a chemotactic gradient.

Complement is a group of 20 or more proteins that, when activated, generate mediators of the acute inflammatory response and damage or kill foreign cells (Table 12–1). These products of the activation induce the release of histamine from mast cells and platelets; attract granulocytic leukocytes; help in the elimination of foreign substance (*antigen;* Ag) such as bacteria, viruses, and their products; and help in the mediation of the inflammatory process. Complement is classically activated by *antibody-antigen complexes* (Fig. 12–11). Activation of the complement cascade via an alternative pathway that bypasses the need for antibody is possible. This alternative pathway, dependent on the presence of thrombin, plasmin, and other factors present in tissue, may play an important role in defending the body against invaders during the initial phase of the inflammatory response, when antibody to a particular antigen may not be available.

Cellular Events and Establishment of Acute Inflammation

The *granulocytes (polymorphonuclear neutrophils* [PMNs], *basophils,* and *eosinophils*) are important to the defense of wound areas. Blood flow in the capillaries and arterioles of the wound area is slowed in responding to the action of chemical mediators. Changes in the cells surface are responsible for the PMN accumulation (adhesion) next to the area of injury followed by a flattening or pavementing against the endothelial cells within a postcapillary venule (Fig. 12–12). This process is controlled by cell-adhesion molecules. *Lymphocyte functional antigen* (LFA-1) is an adhesion molecule found on the surface of the PMN that attaches to another adhesion molecule, *intracellular adhesion molecule* (ICAM-1), on the endothelial cell. As PMNs begin to pass between endothelial cells, they release some of their granules containing enzymes that may aid in this passage. The migration of PMNs through gaps between endothelial cells is called *diapedesis.* Their subsequent directional movement toward the injury site is guided by chemical substances such as complement product C5a. This movement toward higher concentration of the mediator is known as *chemotaxis.*

During the first day the number of PMNs in the wound increases rapidly and their accumulation at the wound site is considered to be a histological sign of acute inflammation. Clinical signs of inflammation, known as the classic signs of inflammation, are: pain (dolor), heat (calor), redness (rubor), swelling (tumor), and loss of function (functio laesa). These are signs of changes that allow increased blood flow to the area (heat and redness), release of mediators such as kinins (pain), and accumulation of fluid resulting in edema (swelling and loss of function).

Polymorphonuclear neutrophils function by engulfing (phagocytosis) and digesting foreign material and wound debris (Fig. 12–13). PMNs carry on their cell surface *complement receptor one* (CR$_1$), a receptor for *antibody fragment c* (Fc) and nonspecific receptors for bacterial carbohydrate. *Opsonization* is when bacteria and debris are coated with antibody or complement products, facilitating their uptake by phagocytes (Fig. 12–14). The PMN binds to particles through these receptors, extends pseudopodia around the particles, and internalizes them into a phagocytic vacuole. The lysosomes merge with it (forming a phagolysosomal vacuole) and the PMN killing mechanisms are activated (Table 12–2). Eventually, the vacuole is opened to the cell exterior and the breakdown products of particles are engulfed and active or unused enzymes are released. The enzymes released can digest debris or normal tissue that comes in contact with them. These unused enzymes can aid in the wound-cleansing process or may damage normal tissue.

Polymorphonuclear neutrophils constitute the first line of defense and are the first phagocytic cell to arrive at the wound site. Their numbers reach a maximum during the first day and start to decrease during the third day after wounding, partially because their life span is limited to 2 days. PMNs release their enzymes toward the end of their life cycle or sometimes right after phagocytosis uses up all of their energy reserve (glycogen). The wound fluid that contains dead PMNs, wound debris and other factors is known as *pus*.

Basophils and eosinophils are the other two granulocytes besides the PMNs. Basophils are found in blood vessels and are similar to mast cells in tissues. They can migrate into the tissue and function like a mast cell. Basophils are long-lived and can multiply in tissues.

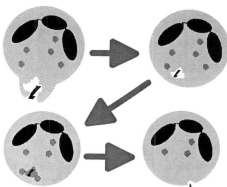

Figure 12–13. Steps involved in phagocytosis: engulfing, phagosome, phagolysosome digestion, and excretion.

Table 12–2.
Phagocyte-Killing Mechanisms

Oxygen-dependent killing within the phagosome oxygen is converted into superoxide, which becomes singlet oxygen, hydrogen peroxide, and hydroxyl radicals. These reactive oxygen intermediates (ROI) can kill bacteria. Lysosomal granules contain enzymes such as myeloperoxidase, lysozyme, and lactoferrin that can kill bacteria.

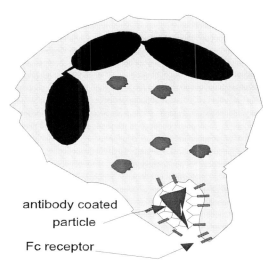

antibody coated particle

Fc receptor

Figure 12–14. An opsonized particle or Ag is engulfed by a PMN.

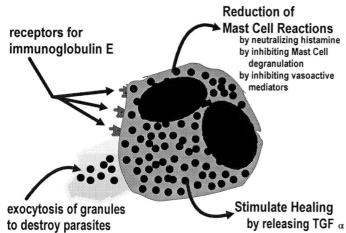

receptors for immunoglobulin E

Reduction of Mast Cell Reactions
by neutralizing histamine
by inhibiting Mast Cell degranulation
by inhibiting vasoactive mediators

exocytosis of granules to destroy parasites

Stimulate Healing
by releasing TGF α

Figure 12–15. Eosinophils contribute to the enhancement of inflammation, and later, to the healing process.

Clinical Application

Continuous stimulation of macrophage leading to overproduction of IL-1 can lead to an exaggerated destruction of bone. IL-1 induces the osteoclastic resorption typical of periodontal disease.

Table 12–3.
MΦ Substances with Activities

Collagenase: collagen breakdown.

Arachidonic acid metabolites: influence inflammatory response.

IL-1: causes fever; releases vasodilators from endothelium; increases endothelial adhesiveness to PMNs, monocytes, and lymphocytes; causes endothelial release of PAF; induces degradation of cartilage and bone resorption; enhances fibroblast proliferation, activates T-lymphocytes; and co-regulates B-cell antibody production.

TNF (or cachectin): same activities as IL-1 plus induction of production of IL-1 by MΦ and endothelial cells.

IL-6 (or IFN-β_2): same activities as IL-1.

PDGF: chemotactic for fibroblasts and PMNs.

TGF-α: promote epithelial growth, keratinization, and angiogenesis.

TGF-β: chemoattractant for monocytes, stimulates fibroblast production of collagen and fibronectin, promotes formation of granulation tissue.

CSF: promotes the development of leukocytes and PMN activity.

IL-1, interleukin-1; PMN, polymorphonuclear neurophils; PAF, platelet-activating factor; TNF, tumor necrosis factor; MΦ, macrophage; IFN-β_2, interferon-β_2; PDGF, platelet-derived growth factor; TGF, transforming growth factor; CSF, colony-stimulating factor.

Eosinophils are phagocytic cells with a bilobed nucleus and eosinophilic granules. They respond to chemotactic factors, especially those released by the mast cells. They have receptors for antibodies of the E class (*IgE*) and play a role in protection against parasitic infection. They release their granules by exocytosis to kill parasites too large to engulf. They may play a role in modulating the reactions mediated by mast cells. Later in the healing process, eosinophils produce an important growth factor known as *transforming growth factor* (TGF-α) (Fig. 12–15).

Growth factors are proteins or peptides that induce cells to initiate DNA synthesis and to divide. Some growth factors can also be chemotactic. PAF, TGF-α, TGF-β, tumor necrosis factor (TNF-α or TNF-β), and platelet-derived growth factor (PDGF) are some of the factors involved in wound healing. Some of these factors are also considered cytokines.

Cytokines are a group of nonantibody molecules produced by white blood cells and tissue cells and that influence or signal other cells. They are involved in regulating the activity of cells. Lymphokines are cytokines produced by lymphocytes whereas monokines are cytokines produced by monocytes. Cytokines include four main groups: colony-stimulating factors (CSF), interferons (IFN), interleukins (IL), and tumor necrosis factors (TNF). Another cytokine produced by keratinocytes is nitric oxide (NO). NO, a short-lived mediator of inflammation, is a gas that functions as a biologic messenger and induces vasodilation.

Monocytes in circulation are mobilized at the same time as PMNs. They are attracted into the area by chemotaxis induced by C5a and preferentially by TGF-β (probably from platelets), to which they are especially sensitive. As monocytes migrate into the wound site, they are activated by high concentrations of TGF-β or bacterial products and are transformed into tissue macrophages (MΦ). The phagocytic function of the macrophage is similar to the function of the PMN, but MΦs have a longer lifespan than PMNs and have the ability to synthesize enzymes at the wound site. The phagocytic role of the PMN as a barrier to bacterial infection is different from the role of the MΦ, which is one of cleaning up the wound site in preparation for repair.

Macrophages release prostaglandins and leukotrienes to influence the inflammatory response, collagenase, which is required to degrade the collagen in the connective tissue, interleukin-1 (IL-1), interleukin-6 (IL-6), TNF, PDGF, CSF, TGF, adhesion molecules, and other mediators of inflammation. Growth and chemotactic factors leading up to the proliferation and migration into the wound of fibroblasts and endothelium are released by the MΦ (Table 12–3).

In the wound, MΦ numbers reach a maximum during the second day and decrease after the fourth day. The presence of MΦs at the wound site is histologically associated with late acute inflammation or with chronic inflammation.

Macrophages aid the specific immune response by preparing antigens for lymphocyte recognition and by producing soluble mediators required for *T-lymphocyte* activation. A somewhat similar role has been attributed to the *Langerhans epithelial cells*. Both of these cells function as immunologic accessory cells. Cells that support the activities of other cells are called *accessory cells*; those that carry out those activities are called *effector cells*. An immunologic accessory cell is a lymphoid cell capable of presenting antigens to B- and T-lymphocytes. Accessory cells are also called *antigen presenting cells* (APCs). MΦs can function as APCs (Fig. 12–16).

Lymphocytes are not normally associated with acute inflammation, but they are found at the wound site. Their role is mediation of the specific immune response. Accessory cells help T-lymphocytes (helper) in the recognition of antigen. These activated cells in turn induce effector T-lymphocytes to produce lymphokines that mediate delayed hypersensitivity (cell-mediated) reactions. After antigen recognition and help from helper T-lymphocytes, B-lymphocytes are transformed into plasma cells. These cells produce and release specific antibodies (Fig. 12–16). These antibodies react with available antigens to form the complexes that activate complement through the classic pathway. These antibodies will opsonize antigens and prepare them for phagocytosis.

As the inflammatory response continues, the acidity of the wound site increases, in some cases reaching a pH of 6.8. Complement activation produces more chemotactic factors for attracting PMNs and monocytes. These cells phagocytize wound debris and release their enzymes, enhancing the inflammatory state (Fig. 12–17). Fluid continues to accumulate

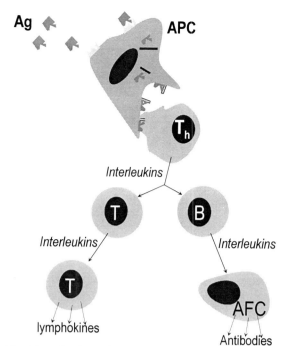

Figure 12–16. Antigen is endocytosed and processed by an APC and subsequently presented to a T$_h$ cell. In turn, the T$_h$ presents the antigen to a B-lymphocyte and releases interleukins that influence other T- and B-lymphocytes ultimately to produce antibodies and lymphokines.

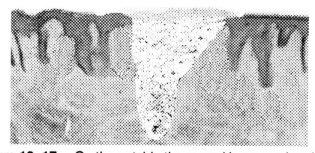

Figure 12–17. On the outside the wound is covered and protected by the blood clot, whereas on the inside the inflammatory mechanisms are actively establishing an acute inflammation.

Clinical Application

Some anti-inflammatory agents such as corticosteroids act by reducing the production of collagenase from macrophage and other phagocytes.

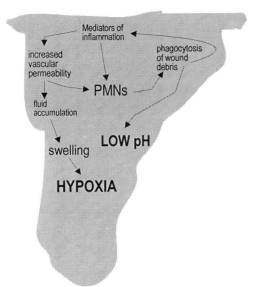

Figure 12–18. Inflammation induces changes that lead to low pH and hypoxia of the wound.

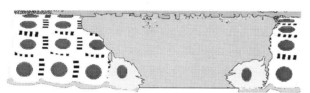

Figure 12–19. Dedifferentiation of cells at the wound edges leads to motile and phagocytic activity.

Figure 12–20. Cells migrate over the clot's dense fibrillar matrix digesting debris and, at the same time, re-form a new basement membrane.

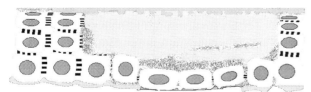

Figure 12–21. When contact between cells is established (contact inhibition) cells differentiate, become more mature, increase the production of keratins, and eventually form the original epithelial architecture.

as a result of the combined effects of increased blood vessel permeability, the action of enzymes, and increased protein concentration in the extravascular space. As the inflammatory events peak, the degree of hypoxia (low oxygen content) in the wound microenvironment increases (Fig. 12–18).

The lymphatic circulation contributes an important role in the inflammatory process. The lymphatic endothelial cells and vessels next to the wound contract rhythmically moving fluids, cells, large molecules, and debris along the lymphatic vessels and away from the wound toward regional lymph nodes. This activity aids in resolution of the inflammatory state. Antigens, debris, and particulate are brought to the regional lymph nodes, where cells remove them by phagocytosis and where they are processed by APCs. In the nodes, APCs and lymphocytes interact and mount an immunologic response.

The inflammatory response is an essential step that prepares the wound site for the repair that follows.

Events Leading to Repair of the Wound

Once acute inflammation peaks, numerous other activities begin to shift the wound environment from one where inflammation is being constantly amplified and enhanced to one where reparative processes are amplified and enhanced. At a cellular level, the shift is a decrease in inflammatory mediators coupled with an increase in growth mediators. The wound microenvironment itself may trigger some of these changes.

Epithelial-related Events

In their normal state the epithelial cells (ECs) at the basal layer are occupied with the production of keratin as their principal activity, and thus are called *keratinocytes*. Keratin is a family of 20 proteins that constitute the intermediate filaments, also known as tonofilaments of the EC. Some of these filaments are connected to the hemidesmosomes and the desmosomes that attach the ECs to each other. ECs express different keratins at different layers, mainly expressing keratin 5 and 14 at the basal layer and 1 and 10 at the upper layers.

Upon wounding, the basal cells at the wound margin undergo significant changes. During the initial 12 hours after injury, ECs at the margin of the wound undergo a *dedifferentiation* process (become more primitive) (Fig. 12–19). Dedifferentiation of these cells results in a number of cellular modifications: cells acquire the potential for ameboid movement, that undergo organelle reduction, their membranes exhibit ruffled borders, they have fewer cell junctions (desmosomes), they have a higher metabolic rate, their surface expresses receptors that interact with the wound environment, and they become phagocytic. The modified ECs increase the number of gap junctions (for better cell-to-cell communication), flatten out toward the wound, and use the clot as a scaffold for ameboid movement into the wound phagocytizing fibrin and debris as they dissect their way (with the help of collagenase and plasminogen activator) as a one- or two-cell-thick layer between the clot and the base of the wound (Figs 12–20 and 12–21).

As they move, the cells rest on a dense fibrillar matrix principally composed of fibrin and fibronectin. Fibronectin promotes keratinocyte motility and phagocytosis. TGF-β promotes motility and secretion of fibronectin by the EC (Fig. 12–22). The movement of ECs along fibrin has been termed *contact guidance*. A cell receptor that attaches the cell to fibronectin (known as the *fibronectin receptor*) mediates this attachment. This receptor is probably an integrin transmembrane link protein that constitutes a family of cell surface molecules. Hyaluronic acid, a component of the extracellular matrix, interacts with fibrin and aids in the establishment of a scaffold for EC migration.

As they move, the ECs have to reform the missing *basement membrane* (BM). ECs produce fibronectin, collagens type IV and V, and laminin to form an immature BM. The BM (a structure seen with light microscopy) attaches the basal epithelial cells to the underlying connective tissue matrix. Ultrastructurally, the BM consists of an electron-lucent layer (lamina lucida) made of laminin (glycoprotein) and heparan sulfate (polysaccharide), followed by an electron-dense layer (basal lamina) or lamina densa containing type IV collagen, and an electron-lucent layer, the fibroreticular lamina that contains anchoring fibrils (type VII collagen) exending from the basal lamina into the connective tissue matrix (Fig. 12–23). The fibroreticular lamina merges with the extracellular matrix.

In cases where the BM remains intact after wounding, the movement of EC is facilitated, resulting in faster repair of the wound.

It is mostly accepted that the EC at the wound margin moves toward the wound while the cell next to it divides to fill the space. This sequence is repeated until the wound is covered. However, there is some evidence to suggest that once the marginal EC has moved it stays put, and the cell immediately behind "leapfrogs" to become the leading cell.

Epithelial-cell movement as a layer stops when cellular contact is re-established (contact inhibition) (Fig. 12–21). When contact is re-established, these cells differentiate (become more specialized) and begin to multiply, eventually returning to their usual stratified arrangement (Fig. 12–24). Internal rearrangement of the cell occurs again to produce keratins as the main activity. Recent studies suggest that epithelial growth and differentiation is enhanced by the release of TGF-α by the eosinophils in the wound area. The chemical structure of TGF-α is partially similar to *epidermal growth factor* (EGF), a factor produced by the salivary glands that promotes epithelial growth and differentiation.

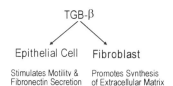

Figure 12–22. Cell activities induced by TGF-β.

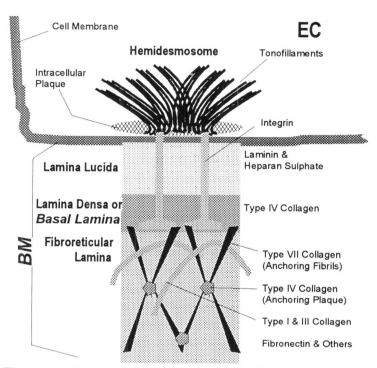

Figure 12–23. Basement membrane (BM) is formed as the EC migrates across the wound.

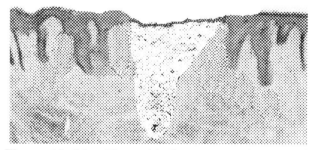

Figure 12–24. The epithelium covers the wound.

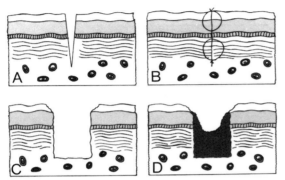

Figure 12–28. Primary and secondary intention healing is a function of the width of the wound.

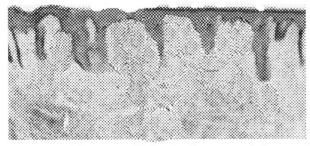

Figure 12–29. The wound is healed but remodeling continues for several months. It may take 6 months or more for the tissue to achieve its usual tensile strength.

Normal gingival tissue contains type I and type III collagens at a ratio of 5:1, which account for 99% of the collagen; type IV, which is associated with the basal lamina and produced by the EC, accounts for 1%. In granulation tissue, type III collagen predominates initially and, as it matures, decreases gradually to approximately 20% of the total collagen. The ratio of type V to type I collagen is increased at extraction sites in the early healing stages and gradually diminishes to usual levels, as does the ratio of type III to type I. The increase is probably related to angiogenesis, in which type V collagen may facilitate the migration of endothelial cells. The tensile strength of the wound augments as the content of type I collagen increases. Through the healing process collagen is formed, broken down, and re-formed.

The assembly of collagen type I and III occurs extracellularly within the tissue matrix. This matrix has a high content of water (70% in the periodontal ligament).

Maturation of the Wound

As healing progresses, vascularization diminishes as granulation tissue is replaced by young new connective tissue. This tissue is different from normal connective tissue in that it is more cellular and has many immature collagen fibers. Early in the maturation process wound contraction begins. Wound contraction results from the contraction of connective tissue, which starts around the fourth day and continues for several weeks. It involves the movement of the wound edge, both the epithelium and the connective tissue, as a whole.

Interspersed throughout the wound, *myofibroblasts*, highly differentiated fibroblasts that have contractile microfilaments and properties associated with smooth muscle cells, are found. Their intracellular proteins (vinculin and actin) join extracellular material composed of fibronectin and collagen types I and III, to interconnect to other myofibroblasts. These connected myofibroblasts apply the forces necessary to achieve contraction. It appears that the force is generated uniformly throughout the wound. These cells increase early in the repair process and diminish gradually, eventually disappearing from the site. In wounds where the edges are far apart and large volumes of tissue are to be replaced more contraction occurs. When the wound edges are closely approximated the amount of contraction is less.

The width of the clot formed between the edges of a wound determines whether the wound will heal by *primary intention* (narrow clot) or by *secondary intention* (wide defect) (Fig. 12–28). The net result of contraction is a scar area that is significantly smaller than the wound. A scar is a mark left in the tissue after a wound heals. Histologically, a scar represents an area that has a slightly higher than normal ratio of collagen fibers to cells. In an incision made to reflect a mucosal flap (mucosa that has been partially detached), the wound edges are closely approximated (coapted), which makes the intervening clot and area to be repaired very narrow; thus, the resultant scar is small (Fig. 12–29). The gingival tissues will heal with practically no scar formation whereas the alveolar mucosa will form scar tissue. Contraction is observed in the alveolar mucosa but practically not observed in the attached gingiva; the reason for this is not clearly understood.

Remodeling is a process that results in the rearrangement of the collagen fibers and proteoglycans. It starts around the third week and continues for several months. There is always a certain level of remodeling that occurs as part of the maintenance of normal tissue. Remodeling is the result of the breaking down of collagen that was deposited in excess, increasing collagen cross linking and decreasing the proteoglycan content. Once formed, collagen fibers continue to undergo chemical changes that decrease their solubility and increase their tensile strength for several months. Because of its capacity to simultaneously degrade and synthesize collagen, the FIB plays an important role in this process.

Wounds Associated with Teeth

Tissue–Tooth Interphase

How a wound edge heals against a tooth represents a special case of healing that will be explored in this section. The *normal tissue–tooth interphase* (NTTI) (Fig. 12–30) is a complex structure that includes a multitude of tissues: junctional epithelium (JE), connective tissue matrix (CT), periodontal ligament (PL), cementum, and bone (AB) (Fig. 12–30). Whenever a surgical separation occurs, most of these tissues are involved in the healing process that follows. When this interphase has been *modified* (MTTI), as with periodontal disease and treatment, the local morphology may dictate how the healing will occur.

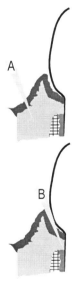

Figure 12–30. Normal tissue–tooth interphase. (A). Simple incision. (B). Intrasulcular incision.

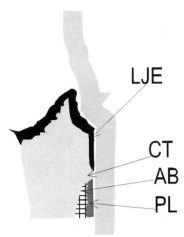

Figure 12–31. Healing with an LJE is an MTTI, the result of repair.

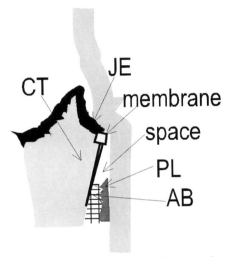

Figure 12–32. Guided tissue regeneration membrane in place to allow cells from bone, PL, and cementum to repopulate the space.

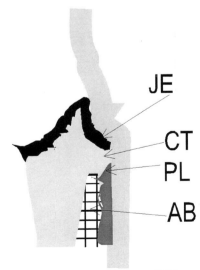

Figure 12–33. Regeneration after GTR and removal of membrane.

In the case of a simple incision through the soft tissue the previous description of how an incisional wound heals applies (Fig. 12–30A). In other cases, as with an intrasulcular incision, additinal activity must occur to reestablish the tooth–tissue interphase (Fig. 12–30B). This activity will result in either regeneration (healing by re-establishing lost tissues and normal architecture) or repair (healing that does not re-establish lost tissues or normal architecture). Regeneration is the most desired result of surgical interventions of this area. However, the result obtained most frequently is repair.

In many instances when the tooth surface has been exposed to the oral environments as the result of periodontal disease, repair by an *abnormally long junctional epithelium* (LJE) is obtained. This MTTI may occur as a result of the different rates at which tissues can fill the wound (Fig. 12–31).

Guided Tissue Regeneration

The rate at which the ECs can move exceeds the rate at which other tissues in the wound can move to fill the wound. The migration rate for epithelium is between 0.1 and 1 mm/day. Epithelium will migrate down a root surface until it encounters CT. At that point an epithelial attachment to the tooth will be established. A CT zone follows immediately apical. This zone of 1 to 2 mm of attachment to the root is always present. Apical to this zone AB, PL, and cementum are re-formed. When the root surface is exposed by periodontal disease-induced changes in the attachment, the most commonly observed healing is by an LJE (Fig. 12–31).

If the epithelial movement down the root could be slowed or prevented, a virtual empty space would be created to allow the growth of slower moving tissues, and there would be an opportunity for regeneration (Fig. 12–32). This is the principle behind *guided tissue regeneration* (GTR). In GTR an inert membrane is placed in the wound to satisfy these requirements.

In GTR the membrane is a two-part semipermeable structure of polytetrafluoroethylene (Teflon). The part that forms the collar of the membrane is a multilayer structure that when implanted looks to the ECs like CT. The main portion of the membrane has a cell-occlusive structure. The membrane is placed on top of the AB and the collar is tightly sutured to the tooth to prevent apical migration of the ECs and to exclude the CT. After being implanted for 4 to 6 weeks the membrane has to be surgically removed. The tissue that forms under the membrane will eventually mature to become normal tissue (Fig. 12–33).

These membranes are also used in conjunction with endosseous implants. Other membranes are being developed, most notably some that are resorbable.

The Extraction Wound

After the removal of a tooth the wound that remains represents a special case of healing. An extraction wound, with injury extending to the alveolar bone, heals by secondary intention.

At the precise instant of extraction, the tooth socket can be visualized as an area in which JE, gingival fibers, PL fibers, blood vessels, and nerve fibers have been torn or severed, and AB may have been fractured.

Figure 12–34 is the clinical picture of a site immediately after an extraction. No blood clot can be seen in this photograph. In Figure 12–35, however, bleeding has occurred and a clot can be seen forming.

The lining bone of a socket after a wound would be covered by PL fibers that anchor in the AB and by blood vessels that pierce its surface as they traverse into the supporting bone (Fig. 12–36). The lining bone, being somewhat more dense than spongy bone but less dense than cortical bone, is recognized radiographically as a radiopaque line that parallels the root (the lamina dura, Fig. 12–37). The dynamic events secondary to tooth extraction lead to the formation of a clot that fills the socket (Fig. 12–35). During the first 3 days, basal and peripheral changes occur in the clot as FIBs migrate up toward the converging ECs.

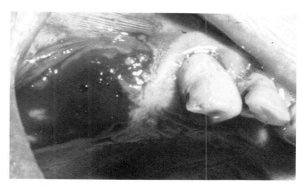

Figure 12–35. Bleeding shortly after extraction, clot forming.

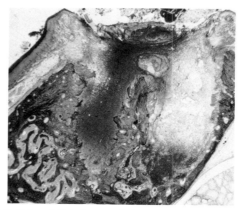

Figure 12–36. Histology of the extraction site at 24 h.

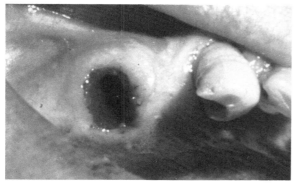

Figure 12–34. Tooth socket immediately after extraction.

Lamina Dura

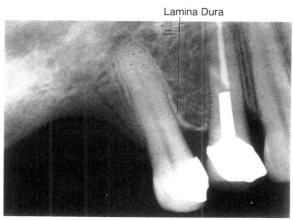

Figure 12–37. The lamina dura is a radiographic structure depicting the bone that lines the socket.

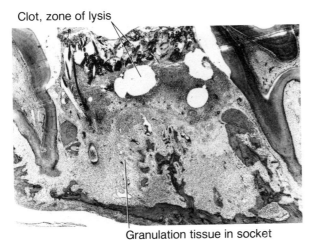

Clot, zone of lysis

Granulation tissue in socket

Figure 12-38. Histology of extraction site at 4 days.

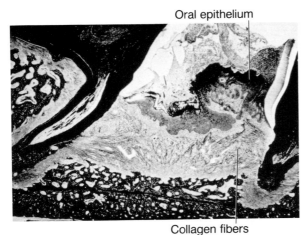

Oral epithelium

Collagen fibers

Figure 12-39. Histology of extraction site at 14 days.

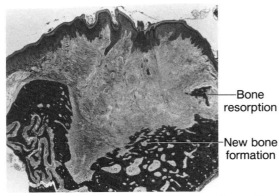

Bone resorption

New bone formation

Figure 12-40. Histology of extraction site at 3 weeks.

At 4 days a vascular network within the clot is evident (Fig. 12-38). Bone resorption begins to take place at the adjacent areas of the socket, at the alveolar crest, and in the interradicular area. Figure 12-38 shows FIBs migrating into the clot and the PL area being remodeled. Thus, at the end of the first week, the clot has become organized into granulation tissue, and bone formation has begun.

During the second week, collagen bundles can be seen running through the area (Fig. 12-39). The oral epithelium grows in an attempt to cover the surface of the wound. The area appears to be well vascularized, and bone formation is continuing.

By the third week, the epithelim has migrated under the remaining clot that covers the granulation tissue, and new bone is evident at the base of the socket (Fig. 12-40). The granulation tissue is maturing into CT.

The fourth week is characterized by the presence of collagen bundles and new bone. This new bone fills a large portion of the socket (Fig. 12-41).

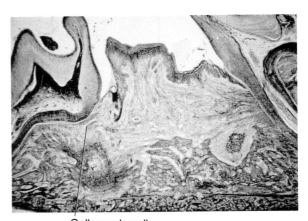

Collagen bundles

Figure 12-41. Histology of extraction site at 4 weeks.

By the eighth week, the keratinized oral mucosa overlying the socket is well differentiated, as is the lamina propria (CT, blood vessels, and other components). The base of the socket has been filled with AB to a new height below the previous level (Fig. 12–41). The height of the lingual plate is usually higher than the height of the buccal plate. During this period, the bone is remodeled by alternating events of resorption and deposition. The process of remodeling continues throughout the life of the individual.

After 12 weeks, the extraction site cannot be distinguished from the normal adjacent tissues (Fig. 12–42). Approximately 85% of individuals who have undergone extractions exhibit a residual ridge whose density is greater than that of the trabecular bone forming the inner portion of the alveolar bone, but is less than that of the cortical bone of the buccal and lingual plates.

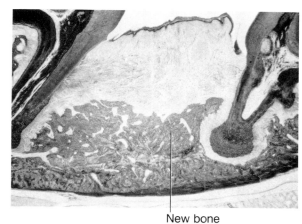
New bone

Figure 12–42. Histology of extraction site at 12 weeks.

Clinical Application

A common complication associated with tooth extraction is a "dry socket" the clinical diagnosis when the blood clot is missing from the socket and there is a localized infection (sometimes called focal osteitis).

Table 12–6.
Healing Phases with Approximate Start and Duration

0–2 d
    Establishment of inflammation
2 d to 1 wk
    Clean-up of the wound
1–2 wk
    Proliferation and production
        Epithelial migration starts 12 h
        Collagen synthesis starts 2–3 d
        GAGs synthesis starts 4–5 d
    Orientation and organization
        Functional changes in collagen
        Fiber orientation
        Wound contraction
1–6 mo
    Maturation and Remodeling
        Increase in tensile strength

Summary

Although the events reviewed in this chapter are depicted as independent events, wound healing is a continuous process. Many of these events occur concurrently, and their activities may overlap each other. In a large wound many microenvironments may exist with variations in the duration of healing events. Based on estimated duration of events from animal and human studies, the healing process could be divided into five phases, as summarized in Table 12–6.

Factors not directly associated to the wound may affect the healing process and the length of healing. Some of these factors are associated to the location of the wound, the circulation of the area, the nutritional or hormonal status of the patient, and the existence of infection at the site. Wounds that are located in an area where trauma can reinjure the wound, or in cases where infection occurs, will heal more slowly. In areas where the blood supply is compromised either by the wound trauma itself or secondary to another factor such as radiation therapy, the capacity of the tissues to heal properly will be affected. Healing in malnourished individuals is altered or defective. Hormonal problems such as those in diabetes may lead to an impaired inflammatory response, which in turn could lead to diminished formation of connective tissue elements.

Children and younger individuals will heal faster than older individuals. How aging affects healing is not completely understood. Overall, the available information suggests that in older individuals the start of the healing process is slightly delayed whereas changes that add strength to the wound stop earlier than in a younger individual.

Smoking can also affect healing. Several clinical studies have implicated smoking as a factor leading to the postsurgical loss of bone or implants. Other clinical studies have found the development of postextraction pain to be associated to smoking immediately after tooth extraction. Smoking can induce vasoconstriction and affect the oxygenation of the tissues.

Table 12–7 is a summary of the major events of the wound-healing process. Without the capacity to heal we could not survive.

Table 12–7.
Important Events in Healing

Injury
↓
Formation of platelet plug
Activation of clotting system
Release of chemoattractants
Release of inflammation mediators
↓
Blood clot
↓
Mast cell degranulation
Production of eicosanoids
Activation of plasmin, kinin, and complement systems
Infiltration by granulocytes, especially PMNs
↓
Inflammation
↓
Opsonization and phagocytosis
Production of cytokincs
Infiltration by macrophages
Production of growth factors
Angiogenesis
Infiltration by fibroblasts
Epithelial cell migration
Formation of basement membrane
Epithelial differentiation
↓
Granulation tissue
↓
Production of proteoglycans
Production of collagens
organization of cell products
Establishment of young connective tissue
Maturation of new tissues
Maturation of matrix components
Increase in myofibroblast activity
↓
Wound contraction
↓
Rearrangement of collagen
Rearrangement of proteoglycans
Formation of scar
Increased wound strength
Increased collagen strength
Decreased collagen solubility
Decreased vascularity
↓
Remodeling

Self-Evaluation Review

1. Describe the events that lead to the formation of a blood clot.
2. Describe the contribution of PMNs to the establishment of acute inflammation.
3. Describe the role of the Hageman factor in inflammation.
4. Describe the role of the eosinophils in inflammation and healing.
5. Why is the monocyte-macrophage cell considered to play such an important role in wound healing?
6. Describe the composition of the basement membrane.
7. What is the role of hypoxia and lactate in the healing of the wound?
8. What is granulation tissue?
9. Describe the major components of connective tissue.
10. Define long junctional epithelium, guided tissue regeneration, and lamina dura.

Acknowledgments

Leo Korchin, DDS, MS, and Sol Bernick, PhD contributed some of the histological material.

Suggested Readings

Gutmann JL, and Harrison JW. Surgical wound healing. In: *Surgical Endodontics*. Boston, Blackwell Scientific Publications Inc; 1991;300–337.

Hill MW. The influence of aging on skin and oral mucosa. *Gerodontal.* 1984;3:35–45.

Janeway CA. How the immune system recognizes invaders. *Sci Am.* 1993;269:73–79.

Jones JK, Triplett RG. The relationship of cigarette smoking to impared intraoral wound healing: a review of evidence and implications for patient care. *J Oral Maxillofac Surg.* 1992;50:237–239.

Keene DR, Sakai LY, Lunstrum GP, Morris NP, Burgeson RE. Type VII collagen forms an extended network of anchoring fibrils. *J Cell Biol.* 1987;104:611–621.

Pelissier A, Ouhayoun, JP, Sawaf MH, Forest N. Changes in cytokeratin expression during the development of the human oral mucosa. *J Periodont Res.* 1992; 27:588–598.

Ross R. Wound healing. *Sci Am.* 1969;220:40–50.

Rothe MJ, Nowak M, Kerdel, FA. The mast cell in health and disease. *J Am Acad Dermatol.* 1990;23:615–624.

Todd R, Donoff BR, Chiang, T, Chou MY, Elovic A, Gallager GT, Wong DT. The eosinophil as a cellular source of transforming growth factor alpha in healing cutaneous wounds. *Am J Pathol.* 1991;138:1307–1313.

Whalen GF, Zetter BR. Angiogenesis. In: Cohen IK, Diegelmann RF, and Lindblad WJ. *Wound Healing: Biochemical and Clinical Aspects*. Philadelphia Pa: WB Saunders, 1992:77–95.

Structure and Function of the Temporomandibular Joint

James K. Avery and Sol Bernick

Introduction

The temporomandibular joint (TMJ), the mandibular articulation, is a bilateral diarthrosis between the condyles of the mandible and the articular eminences of the temporal bone, arteriorly, and the mandibular fossae, posteriorly. The temporomandibular joint allows the mandible to move as a unit in both a hinge and a gliding movement.

The temporomandibular joint consists of (1) the condylar head of the mandible, (2) the articulating surfaces of the temporal bone, (3) the articulating disc, and (4) the articulating capsule. The disc separates the head of the condyles from the temporal bone. Therefore, the disc divides the joint into two portions, an upper and a lower compartment. The disc is an oval plate of fibrous tissues whose periphery blends into the articulating capsule. In front, the disc is anchored to the tendon of the lateral pterygoid muscle. It is lightly attached to the condyle, so that it follows the jaw in sliding movements. There are two synovial membranes in the joint: one lines the capsule above the disc, and the other lines the capsule below the disc.

A loose articular capsule is attached to the articular tubercles, the squamotympanic fissure, and the margins of the mandibular fossa between these two attachments. Below, it is attached to the neck of the mandible, so that posteriorly a portion of the mandible is intracapsular (Fig. 13–1).

The lateral (temporomandibular) ligament is intimately related to the fibrous capsule. Above, it is attached to the zygoma, and below, it is attached to the lateral surfaces and posterior border of the neck of the mandible.

In addition, there are two accessory ligaments associated with the temporomandibular joint. The sylomandibular ligament attaches to the styloid process and to the posterior border of the ramus; the sphenomandibular ligament extends between the spine of the sphenoid bone and the lingula of the mandible (Fig. 13–1C).

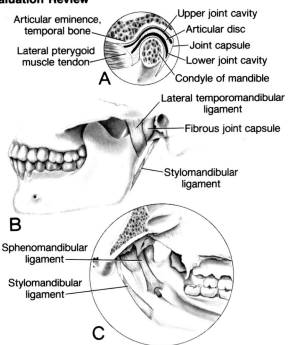

Articular eminence, temporal bone
Lateral pterygoid muscle tendon
Upper joint cavity
Articular disc
Joint capsule
Lower joint cavity
Condyle of mandible
A

Lateral temporomandibular ligament
Fibrous joint capsule
Stylomandibular ligament
B

Sphenomandibular ligament
Stylomandibular ligament
C

Figure 13–1. (A). Diagram of TMJ compartments. (B). Diagram of lateral and posterior ligaments of TMJ. (C). Diagram of medial ligaments of TMJ.

Objectives

After reading this chapter you should be able to describe the structure of the condyles, the temporal fossae, and the articulating disc and capsule. You should also be able to discuss the function of this joint and the relation of the muscles of mastication to its actions.

Histological Structure

The microscopic structure of the TMJ reveals a fibrous capsule enclosing the joint, which is attached anteriorly to the articulating tubercle of the temporal bone above, and the neck of the condyle below (Fig. 13–2). Posteriorly, the capsule is attached to the temporal bone anterior to the external auditory canal above and the posterior aspects of the condyle below (Fig. 13–2). Suspended from the internal walls of the capsule between the condyles and the fossae is the fibrous disc, which is composed of collagen fibers (Fig. 13–3). This disc is seen to separate the superior and inferior joint cavities. In this diagram, the cartilage is in the condyle head underlying the fibrous periochondrium. Therefore, the condition indicates that the mandible has not completed its growth, as cartilage has not been entirely replaced by bone. Growth occurs at two sites, one in formation of new cells underlying the periochondrium of condyle surface and the other at the site of the transformation of cartilage to bone in the neck of the condyles. As long as there is cartilage in the condyle head, growth may occur. Observe (Fig. 13–2) the inclined plane of the anterior articulating surface of the condyle, the thin area of the articulating disc anteriorly and the thick zone posteriorly. On the extreme posterior, a number of blood vessels appear, known as the *vascular triangle* (Fig. 13–3). Above the vascular triangle the elastic fibers of the disc emanates from the borders of the petrotynysanic fissure, as seen in Figure 13–3. The articulating disc is composed of collagen fibers, as seen in Figure 13–4. Because the condylar head slides along the articular plane during function, the capsule is described as loose, and is a supported by a medial ligament (sphenomandibular), a lateral ligament, a lateral (temporomandibular), and a posterior one, (stylomandibular). These relative positions are seen in Figure 13–1B and C.

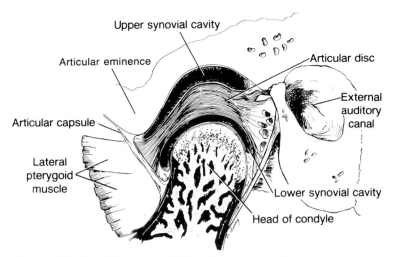

Figure 13–2. Diagram of TMJ. with articular disc, capsule, and relations to lateral pterygoid muscle and external auditory canal illustrated.

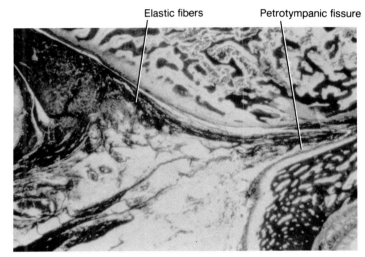

Figure 13–3. Light micrograph of posterior region of the glenoid fossa shows location of elastic fibers attached to the petrotympanic fissure.

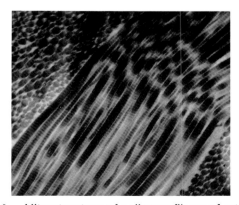

Figure 13–4. Ultrastructure of collagen fibers of articular disc.

13: Structure and Function of the Temporomandibular Joint　　**215**

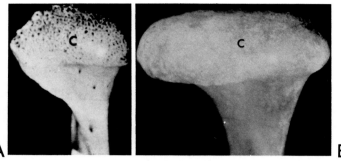

Figure 13–5. Comparison of 6-year-old condyle (A) and adult condyle (B), respectively. Note the increase in the lateral dimension.

Condyles

Condyles are ovoid in shape mediolaterally and consist of a smooth bony surface covered with a fibrous connective tissue (Fig. 13–5B). The condyles grow laterally during development, gaining the oval shape as they reach maturity at 6 years of age. For example, the porous appearance of the cartilage-covered condyle is apparent in Figure 13–5A. Histology of the condyle confirms this as the 6-year-old exhibits a wide band of cartilage whereas in an early-teenaged individual the condyle has thinned considerably, with further thinning occurring as the age of the individual nears 20 (Fig. 13–6). The head of the condyle and that of long bones differ in that long bones form secondary ossification sites (Fig. 13–7). These secondary ossification sites produce epiphyseal lines where lengthening of the long bones occurs.

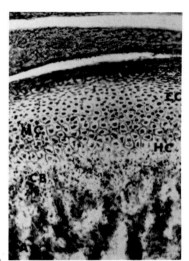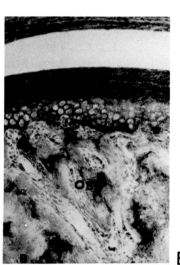

Figure 13–6. (A). Histology of young postnatal condyle and disc. (EC) Reserve cartilage zone, (MC) multiplication of cells, cartilage zone, (HC) hypertrophy zone (CB) calcifying zone. (B). Thin cartilage zone at later postnatal time, (OB) bone formation.

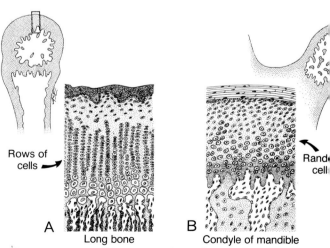

Clinical Application

The heads of the condyles provide bilateral growth sites during their long period of pre- and postnatal development. From 20 weeks in utero to 25 years of life, this joint enlarges, modifies, and functions as cartilage covering the heads of the condyles is remodeled and bone is formed. It keeps pace with the growth of the face and functions during the entire developmental time.

Figure 13–7. Diagrams of cartilage of long bone (A) and condyle (B). Observe the lack of palisading and the thick perichondrium in the condyle.

The heads of condyles accomplish growth like that of a long bone by development of new chrondoblasts, with growth of new cartilage matrix and replacement by bone. In long bones, however, the cartilage cells appear to be arranged in long rows adjacent to the cartilage bone junctions. In the mandibular joint cartilage the cells appear scattered, as seen in Figures 13–6 and 13–7.

Temporomandibular Fossa (Glenoid Fossa)

The TM fossae is composed of an anterior zone in the form of an eminence (articular) and a posterior part, which is a depression or cavity on the inferior aspect of the temporal bone. This fossa is located at the posterior medial end of the zygomatic arch (Fig. 13–8). To compensate for the increase in lateral dimension of one condylar head, the glenoid fossa extends laterally as well (Fig. 13–8). By maturity, the articular eminence becomes prominent. The articular eminences are smooth with rounded ridges on whose posterior slope the condyles slide during articulation. On the posterior wall of the fossa, the petrotympanic fissure separates the anterior squamosas and the more posterior petrous parts of the temporal bone (Figs. 13–3 and 13–8). It is the only location in the disc in which elastic fibers are found. Because of their location, these fibers may be a remnant of the anterior ligament of the malleus.

Synovial Membrane

A synovial membrane (stratum synovial) lines the entire articular capsule of the joint, both the upper and the lower compartments. The synovial cells appear to be a continuous layer, but usually are intermingled with connective tissue fibers and fat cells. Thus, the synovium is not a true membrane (Fig. 13–9). In this posterior region of the joint, synovial folds may be found on the free surfaces of the joint. Within these folds the cells may be piled up and may project into the cavity. Some folds may be nonvascular; others have associated connective tissue, and others contain adipose cells (Fig. 13–10). Ultrastructurally, it has been shown that there are two types of synovial cells, types A and B (light and dark cells). It has been suggested that type A secretes

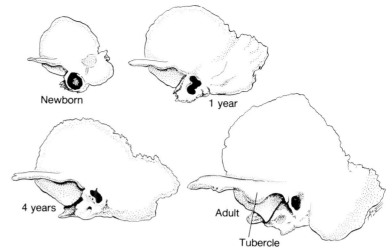

Figure 13-8. Development of the glenoid (temporomandibular) fossa from birth to maturity.

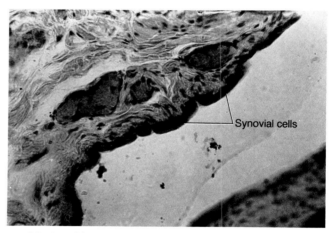

Figure 13-9. Light micrograph of synovial cells lining TMJ.

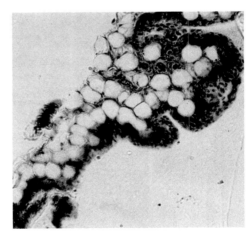

Figure 13-10. Light micrograph of synovial and fat cells in TMJ.

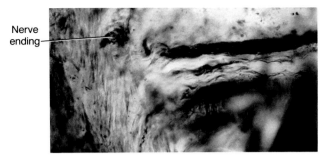

Figure 13–17. Nerve ending in disc.

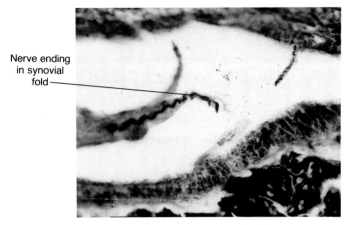

Figure 13–18. Nerve ending in synovial fold.

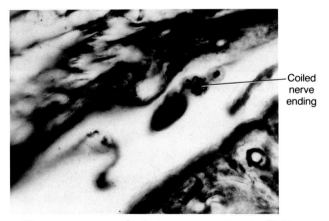

Figure 13–19. Coiled nerve ending in TMJ.

pressure, are found in, and pass from, the joint into the peripheral region of the articular disc and synovial folds (Figs. 13–17 and 13–18). Only free nerve endings, probably for pain, have been found in the peripheral region of the disc (Fig. 13–17). The thin central portion of the disc is free of nerves. both myelinated and nonmyelinated nerves are found in the connective tissue core of the synovial folds (Fig. 13–18). Those nerves that terminated in various encapsulated structures appear to be coiled or glomerular in nature, and are embedded in the connective tissue of the articular disc or capsule (Fig. 13–19). In the condylar region, myelinated nerves are traced passing through the muscle to enter the capsular connective tissue. These nerves may end as nonmyelinated free nerve endings or specialized coiled endings, which are similar to a Ruffini ending (Fig. 13–20).

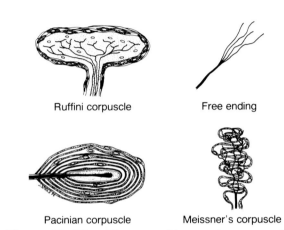

Figure 13–20. Diagram of types of nerve endings in joint capsule and disc.

Muscles of Mastication

There are eight powerful muscles of mastication, four on each side. Each has a different location; therefore, the direction of fiber contraction results in a different functional relation. Three of the muscles on each side—the medial pterygoid, the masseter, and the temporalis—exert vertical forces in closing of the jaws whereas the lateral pterygoid muscles function to protract the mandible and stabilize the joint. These muscles do not function alone, but work as a group with the muscles of the tongue and the superhyoid muscles. *Free movements* of the mandible relate to the interplay of masticatory muscles and the morphology of the teeth without food whereas *masticatory movement* is the synergistic action of the three groups of muscles—the elevators, depressors, and protractors that function together and at different times during mastication of food.

The *medial pterygoid* muscle arises from the medial surface of the lateral pterygoid plate and inserts in the inferior surface of the ramus and angle of the mandible. A blood supply is from the maxillary artery with a nerve supply from the mandibular division of the trigeminal. It functions to protract and elevate the mandible (Fig. 13–21). From this inferior view, the medial part is seen to run down and backward, below and behind the angle of the mandible to meet the externally located masseter in a tendinous raphe, and forms the pterygomasseteric sling (Figs. 13–21 and 13–22).

The *lateral pterygoid* muscle has two heads: the upper arising from the greater wing of the sphenoid and the lower from the lateral pterygoid plate. They insert into the front of the neck of the condyle and the capsule (Fig. 13–22). The blood supply is from the maxillary artery and the nerve supply is from the pterygoid branch of the mandibular nerve. Both heads of this muscle function to protrude the mandible and pull the articular disc forward (Figs. 13–21 and 13–22).

Clinical Application

Myofacial pain dysfunction is usually a result of masticatory muscle spasms, and the major etiologic agent is psychological stress. There are four cardinal symptoms: preauricular pain, muscle tenderness, limitation of mouth opening, and clicking.

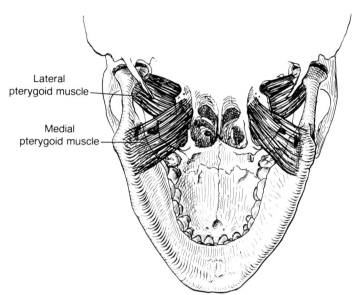

Figure 13–21. Inferior view of lateral and medial pterygoid muscles of mastication.

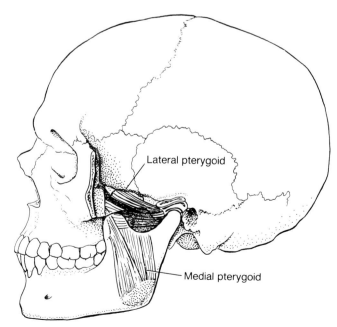

Figure 13–22. Lateral view of lateral and medial pterygoid muscles of mastication.

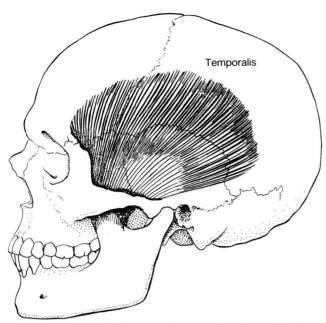

Figure 13–23. Temporalis muscle of mastication.

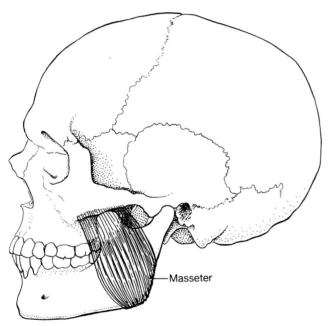

Figure 13–24. Masseter muscle of mastication.

Clinical Application

In no instance does the TMJ operate independently of the muscles that surrounded it. It is the action of these muscles of mastication that in turn function in groups for elevation, protrusion, and lateral motion.

The *temporalis* muscle fibers originate from the floor of the temporal fossa and temporal fascia and insert on the anterior border of the coronoid process and anterior border of the ramus of the mandible (Fig. 13–23). The blood supply is from the superficial temporal and maxillary arteries, and the nerve supply is from the deep temporal branches of the mandibular nerve. Functions of the temporalis muscle are elevation of the jaw, retraction of the mandible, and clenching of the teeth.

The *masseter* muscle has a deep part and superficial part. The superficial fibers originate from the anterior two thirds of the lower border of the zygomatic arch, and the deep fibers from the medial surface of the same arch. The superficial fibers are at right angles to the occlusal plane of the posterior teeth, and the deep fibers are directed down and slightly anteriorly. This muscle inserts into the lateral surface of the coronoid process of the mandible, the upper half of the ramus, and the angle of the mandible. Blood supply is from the superficial temporal and maxillary arteries, and the nerve supply comes from the mandibular division of the trigeminal nerve. The masseter muscle functions to elevate the jaw and clench the teeth (Fig. 13–24).

Functional and Clinical Considerations

The sensations of pain and pressure are important symptoms in temporomandibular disorders. The nature of the transmission of these sensations from this joint is still not fully understood. In view of the previously described innervation of the joint, pain and pressure may be explained by the following malfunctions: (1) changes in occlusion, from various causes, may produce a displacement of the condyle–disc to disc–fossa relation and irritate the peripheral disc areas and associated nerve receptors; (2) inflammation and associated increases in synovial fluid would produce pressure effects and irritation of the specialized nerve endings in the synovial folds; and (3) muscle tensions may act on the nerves not only in muscle per se but also on the endings in the periosteal connective tissue.

Disturbances to the TMJ are, in part, no different from those in other joints. There are dissimilarities in the disorders of the TMJ, however, as a result of its specific anatomic and functional features. The TMJs are bilaterally coupled as a single unit by the mandible, which prevents unilateral motion. Its articular surfaces are covered by articular fibrous tissue rather than hyaline cartilage, and are found in other joints. There is a functional relation with the dentition, the periodontal tissues, muscles of mastication, and the joint. Pathology in one component may affect another, which thereby complicates diagnosis of a disease; thus, the TMJ is exposed to functional changes seen in the oral cavity.

Developmental Disturbances

Although uncommon, developmental disturbances do appear. Condylar aplasia may occur either unilaterally or bilaterally. Usually, it is associated with other anatomically related defects, such as a defective or absent external ear. The intimate relation in the development of the external ear, mandible, and TMJ may clarify why they are related. Underdevelopment or defective formation of the mandibular condyle may be congenital or may be acquired as a result of toxic agents interfering with normal prenatal and postnatal development of the condyle. These defects may result from infections, dietary insufficiencies, hormonal dysfunction, or trauma.

Dislocation

Dislocation, or luxation and subluxation of the TMJ, occurs when the head of the condyle is displaced anteriorly over the articular eminence and cannot be returned voluntarily to its normal position. It may occur after a condylar fracture or, more frequently, in overstretching, usually at the attachment point of the lateral pterygoid into the capsule. It is commonly characterized by sudden locking and immobilization of the jaws when the mouth is open, and it is accompanied by prolonged spasmodic contraction of the temporal, medial pterygoid, and masseter muscles with protrusion of the jaw. The normal positioned relation of the muscles of mastication are shown in Figures 13–21 through 13–24.

Ankylosis

Ankylosis of the TMJ is a debilitating condition involving immobility of the jaw. Causes of ankylosis usually are traumatic injuries or infection in and about the joint. The ankylosis may be of two types: intra-articular and extra-articular. In intra-articular ankylosis, there is progressive destruction of the meniscus, flattening of the fossa, thickening of the condyle, and shrinkage of the capsule with partial or even complete abolition of the joint. Usually, the ankylosis is fibrous, although the fibrous type may ossify. After infection, extra-articular ankylosis leads to "splinting" of the joint by a fibrous or a bony mass external to the joint proper.

Injury to the Articular Disc

Inflammation and, more commonly, malocclusion may result in articular disc injury. The latter usually results from abnormal patterns of mandibular excursion carried out during mastication. During these excessive movements, the capsule is overstretched, which prevents too great an anterior condylar movement. The adaptation of the disc to the condyle is lost, and disc degeneration occurs.

After an acute traumatic injury to the jaw, a *condylar fracture* accompanied by pain, swelling, and limitation of motion over the involved area is not unusual. The condylar fragments usually are displaced anteriorly and medially into the infratemporal fossa because of the pull of the lateral pterygoid muscle.

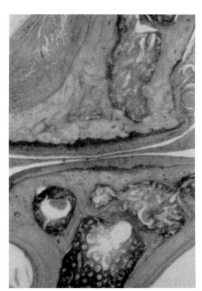

Figure 13–25. Flattened condyle in old age.

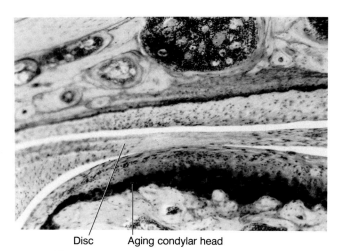

Disc   Aging condylar head

Figure 13–26. Aging condylar head.

Arthritis

Inflammation of the joints, or arthritis, also involves the TMJ. Three types of arthritis occur in the TMJ, the most common of which usually is caused by direct extension of infection into the joint. Such an extension may result from dental infection, infection of the parotid gland, or an ear infection. Rheumatoid arthritis in the TMJ is not common; more common is osteoarthritis. The changes in the articular cartilage consist of a loss of elasticity and surface erosion, with vertical cracks that may extend into the subchrondal bone. There is complete destruction of the chondrocytes. The disc may exhibit cracks and fissures and may be hyalinized or even mineralized. Sometimes, necrosis or destruction of the disc may occur.

Age Changes in Temporomandibular Joint

The TMJ undergoes age changes similar to those that occur in other masticatory structures. The condyle appears flattened in outline (Fig. 13–25), and it is not unusual to find a remnant of condylar cartilage in aged joints. The fibrous covering of the condyle, which consists of dense collagen fiber bundles, is thicker in older specimens than in younger ones. In addition, it is not surprising to see chondroid changes. Osteoporosis of the underlying bone of the condyle is a common feature of the aging TMJ complex. The loss of bone has been reported to be more marked in women than in men over 60 years of age. The osteoporosis may become so advanced that the ramus and condyle of the mandible appear to be a thin shell of cortical bone.

The articular disc becomes thinner and exhibits hyalinization and chondroid changes similar to what has been described for the connective tissue layer of the condyle (Fig. 13–26). In addition, there are small acellular areas where tears appear. Similar alterations are found in the connective tissue capsule.

The synovial folds appear fibrotic, and a thick basement membrane develops that separates the synovial lining cells from the underlying stroma. The walls of blood vessels are thickened. Nerves appear decreased in number in the capsule and peripheral portion of the disc.

These age changes in the various components of the joint could lead to its dysfunction in older individuals. The changes in the connective tissue elements in the capsule and disc could lead to a decrease in the extensibility of the disc and capsule and result in an impairment of motion. The chondroid changes to the collagenous elements of the articular tubercle, articular disc, and condyle may affect the degree of resiliency during masticatory function. The alterations found in the synovial folds may lead to a decrease in the formation of synovial fluid and a loss of lubrication of the two compartments.

Summary

In the adult TMJ, the condyle consists of a fibrous articulating surface, a thin cartilaginous zone overlying the bone of the condyle. The articular disc is characterized by colllagen fibers with a few fibroblasts. The central portion of the disc is very thin. The articulating surface of the glenoid fossa also is fibrous in nature. Synovial membranes and villi are found lining the capsule.

The TMJ is well vascularized. A rich vascular plexus appears from the superficial temporal, anterior tympanic, and ascending pharyngeal arteries to terminate in the articular capsule. These arteries form a "crown" circumferentially around the central region of the disc. There are no blood vessels in this thin portion of the disc. Capillary networks are found in the capsular synovia and villi. The capillaries are adjacent to the synovial membrane, and their positions are important for the production of synovial fluid.

Nerves originating from the auriculotemporal, masseteric, and deep temporal areas can be traced into the capsule, disc, and synovial villi. Nerve fibers end in the capsule as free nerve endings and encapsulated endings. Only free nerve endings are observed in the peripheral portion of the disc. There are no nerves in the thin central portion of the disc. Specialized end-bulbs of varying types are found in the synovial villi. These specialized end-organs may be proprioceptive in function.

Aging changes to the TMJ include chondroid changes to the articular surfaces of the glenoid fossa and condyle as well as to that of the disc. In addition, there is thinning or absence of the cartilaginous zone of the condyle. Finally, there are varying degrees of osteoporosis of the bony portion of the condyle, ramus of the mandible, and temporal bone.

Self-Evaluation Review

1. Describe the function of the superior and inferior TMJ compartments.
2. Compare the actions of the two heads of the lateral pterygoid muscle.
3. Describe the blood supply to the TMJ.
4. How do the heads of the condyles modify from a young adult to an aging person?
5. Define the function of the TMJ capsule and its supporting ligaments.
6, What is meant by the sling muscles? Are these separate muscles able to work in synchrony?
7. In what direction do the TMJ fossa and condyles grow during childhood?
8. Describe the nerve supply to the joint. Where do nerve endings terminate in the joint?
9. How does connective tissue of the perichondrium provide a role in vascularity of the cartilage for the TMJ?
10. Describe the development of new cartilage, its maturation, and its replacement by bone.

Acknowledgments

Dr. Donald Wright contributed Figure 13–5A and B, Dr. C. C. Boyer contributed Figure 13–15, and the now deceased Dr. S. Bernick contributed Figures 13–6 and 13–13, 13–14, 13–17, 13–18, and 13–19.

Suggested Readings

DuBrul EL. The cramiomandibular articulation. In: *Sicher's Oral Anatomy.* 7th ed. St. Louis, Mosby Co.; 1980: chaps4, 16.

Dixon AD. Structure and functional significance of the intra-articular disc of the temporomandibular joint. *Oral Surg.* 1962;15:48.

Griffin CJ, Hawthorne R, Harris R. Anatomy and histology of the human temporomandibular joint. *Monog Oral Sci.* 1975;4:1.

Karakasis D, Tsaknakis A. Aging changes in the articular disk of the temporomandibular joint in the guinea pig. *I Dent Res.* 1976;55:262.

Meikie MC. The role of the condyle in the postnatal growth of the mandible. *Am J Ortho.* 1973;64:50.

Sarnat BG, Laskin DM. *Temporomandibular joint: Biological Basis for Clinical Practice.* Springfield, Ill: Charles C Thomas; 1979.

Thilander B. Innervation of the temporomandibular disc in man. *Acta Odont Scand.* 1964;22:151.

14

Histology of Enamel

James W. Simmelink

Introduction

Enamel is the hard mineralized tissue covering of the tooth crown, is the primary site of attack of dental caries, and is, therefore, of special interest in dentistry. Enamel is unique because it is a mineralized *epithelial* tissue whereas bone, dentin, and cementum are mineralized *connective* tissues. Mature human enamel is the only tissue that is totally acellular. During the development of enamel, its histology is influenced by cells (ameloblasts) that form the enamel tissue as a mineralized secretory product. The products formed by each ameloblast are termed enamel rods or enamel prisms (Fig. 14–1A). The secretory ends (Tomes' processes) of the ameloblasts and the enamel rods that these cells have produced are shown in Figure 14–1B.

As enamel matures, it loses both organic material and water, which results in a product that is primarily composed of inorganic crystals (96% by weight), with only a small amount of water (3%) and organic matrix (less than 1%). Mature enamel is therefore extremely hard and brittle. There is so little organic substance that it can be only partially preserved, even in a carefully prepared, demineralized histological section. The results are seen as organic lamellae projecting into the enamel, as in Figure 14–2, a light micrograph of the cuspal area of a developing, unerupted tooth. The enamel appears as an unstained "enamel space."

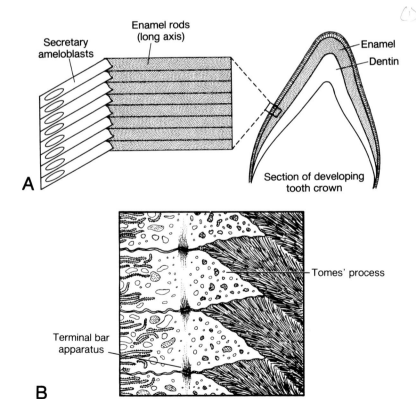

Figure 14–1. (A). Enamel rods, products of ameloblasts. (B). Secretory front of ameloblasts.

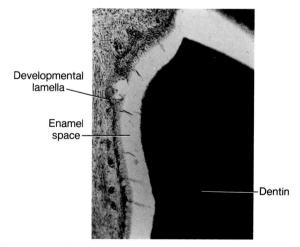

Figure 14–2. Lamellae or organic tracts in enamel.

Objectives

After reading this chapter you should be able to describe the enamel rod configuration and its relation to other rods, be able to discuss its inorganic and organic components and its structural variations, be aware of the changes in enamel in an acidic environment and the effects of fluoride on enamel surface, and be able to describe the coverings (both natural cuticles and plastic sealants) and how they relate to this environment.

Enamel Rods

The mineralized state should be examined for the best understanding of the histology of enamel. Ground sections of teeth that are sufficiently thin for use with light microscopy can be prepared. Sections can be made either sagittally, along the long axis of the tooth, or coronally, through the crown of the tooth (Fig. 14–3). Better resolution of the enamel rods is obtained by using a scanning electron microscope to look at enamel surfaces. Rod morphology is enhanced by a brief acid etching of the enamel. Figure 14–4 is a scanning electron micrograph that shows about 50 enamel rods in their longitudinal axes. The orientation of the rods would appear similar in both of the diagrammed sections in Figure 14–3.

The enamel rod is a long, thin structure extending from the dentinoenamel junction (DEJ) to the surface of the enamel (Fig. 14–4). The length of a rod may be greater than the enamel thickness if it follows an undulating course to the surface. The rods are correspondingly shorter in areas where the enamel is thin, namely the cervical and fissural areas of the crown. The average length of a rod in the mid-crown region is about 2 mm (2000 μm), and its diameter is only about 5 μm. The diameter of a rod primarily corresponds to the diameter of the columnar ameloblast that formed it, but is increased slightly as the rod radiates away from the dentinoenamel junction toward the enamel surface and enlarges its surface area.

In longitudinal section, the parallel rods are unremarkable in outline. When the rods are examined in cross section at higher magnification, however, a keyhole shape can be clearly observed (Fig. 14–5). Rods are seen in cross section at the enamel surface and in facets ground parallel to the enamel surface (Fig. 14–6). Enamel rods have a specific orientation: the top or "head" of the keyhole-shaped rods is oriented toward the cuspal or incisal direction, and the "tail" of the rods is oriented toward the cervix of the tooth.

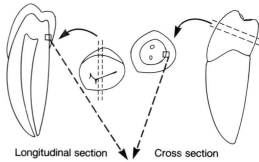

Figure 14–3. Sections of enamel. Arrows point to the location of the section seen in Figure 14–4.

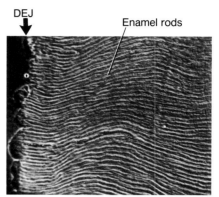

Figure 14–4. Scanning electron micrograph of enamel rods seen after acid etch.

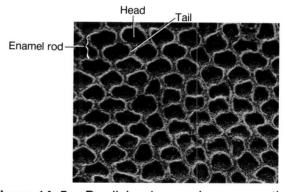

Figure 14–5. Parallel rods seen in cross section.

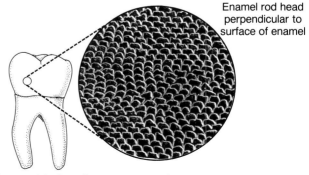

Figure 14–6. Appearance of rods at enamel surface.

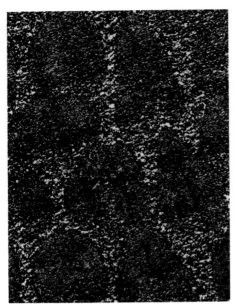

Figure 14–13. Electron micrograph of crystal orientation in cross section of enamel rod. Compare this crystal orientation with that in Figure 14–12B.

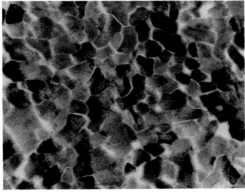

Figure 14–14. Transmission electron micrograph of enamel crystals seen as irregular hexagons in cross section (× 150,000).

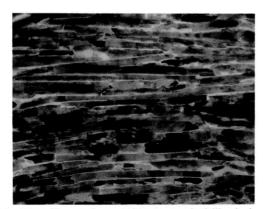

Figure 14–15. Enamel crystals appear lathlike in longitudinal section on transmission electron micrograph.

Enamel Crystals

Inorganic hydroxyapatite crystals, which make up 96% of mature human enamel, are only clearly resolved in the transmission electron microscope. The crystals are about 30 nm thick by 65 nm wide in cross section, and are several micrometers in length. Although they are small in terms of microscopic resolution, they are about 10 times larger than the crystals of mineralized connective tissue. In the enamel, the crystals are primarily oriented with their long dimension paralleling that of the enamel rod (Fig. 14–12B). In the tail portion, however, there is a subtle shift in crystal orientation. In a cross section of enamel rods, the majority of crystals in the rod head area are cut in cross section whereas those in the rod tail area are cut obliquely. In the cutting of thin sections for transmission electron microscopy, the obliquely cut crystals in the rod tail area are usually slightly displaced. The appearance of more white space in the tail area is thus a sectioning artifact (Fig. 14–13). In mature enamel, the space between the crystals is severely limited (less than 2 nm). In cross section, the pattern of hydroxyapatite crystals that normally form as elongated hexagons is necessarily altered, with the crystals taking on an irregular hexagonal shape that occupies nearly all the available space. The transmission electron micrograph shows the crystals in cross section at ×150,000 (Fig. 14–14). In longitudinal section, the crystals have a slatlike appearance with little space between them (Fig. 14–15).

The basic crystallographic formula for the unit cell of hydroxyapatite is $Ca_{10}(PO_4)_6(OH)_2$; crystals in enamel, however, differ from the ideal formula. First, there are vacancies in the crystal lattice, which result in the enamel apatite being slightly deficient in calcium. Second, there are minor ion substitutions in the crystal lattice (e.g., strontium, carbonate, magnesium, lead, and fluoride). Most of the ion substitutions result in a small increase in the solubility of the crystal at an acidic pH. The fluoride ion substitution for the hydroxyl ion is an exception in that it causes a decrease in enamel crystal solubility in acid. This effect is considered to be a major reason for reduction of tooth decay due to fluoridation.

Histology of Dentin

Nicholas P. Piesco

Introduction

Dentin is primarily formed from secretory products of the odontoblasts and their processes. It is the hard tissue that constitutes the body of each tooth serving as both a protective covering for the pulp and as support for the overlying enamel (Fig. 15–1). Unlike enamel, dentin is a vital tissue containing the cell processes of odontoblasts and neurons. The odontoblasts perform a structural role in the formation of the dentin matrix and neurons convey sensory information. The primary component of the dentin matrix, the collagen, imparts the resiliency necessary for the crown (enamel as well as dentin) to withstand the forces of mastication. The color of the crown of the tooth is partially due to the color of the underlying dentin as well as to the thinness and translucency of enamel.

Although dentin resembles bone in composition, it differs from bone in that true dentin contains no trapped cells or blood vessels, and also, unlike bone dentin, is not continuously remodeled. However, dentin does have a limited capacity for repair. New physiological or reparative dentin can only be added on its inner aspect, with the result that as the tooth ages the bulk of dentin increases because the pulp chamber decreases in volume. Unlike bone, coronal dentin is covered with enamel and radicular dentin is covered with cementum.

Objectives

After reading this chapter you should be able to recognize and classify the various types of dentin; discuss the developmental origin of the various types of dentin; list the organic and mineral components of the dentin matrix, and understand the roles of the primary organic components of the dentinal matrix such as structural elements, mineralization activators or inhibitors, and growth factors. Furthermore, you should be able to describe the effects of natural (environmental, physiological, or pathologic) and clinician-induced (iatrogenic) factors that alter dentin composition and permeability.

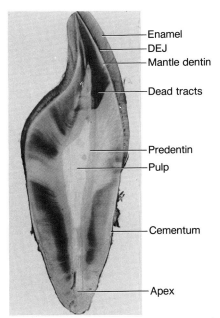

Figure 15–1. Relation between dentin, enamel, and the pulp. DEJ, dentin-enamel junction.

Enamel
DEJ
Mantle dentin
Dead tracts
Predentin
Pulp
Cementum
Apex

Dentin Structure and Classification

Orthodentin, true dentin, is a calcified tissue that lacks cells, contains tubules and is organized by odontoblasts (Fig. 15–2, 15–3). The most prominent feature of dentin is the dentinal tubules. In the crown, the direction of the dentinal tubules extends in an S-shaped curve from the dentin-enamel junction to the mineralization front. The two bends making up the S-shape are called the *primary curvatures*. The first curve bends toward the occlusal or incisal surface of the tooth

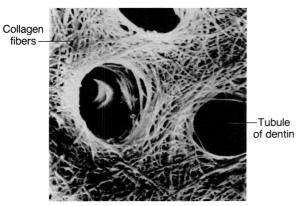

Figure 15–2. Scanning electron micrograph of decalcified dentin showing collagen fibers and dentinal tubules.

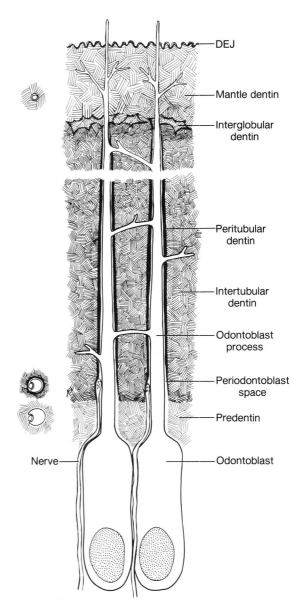

Figure 15–3. Relation between the odontoblastic process and the dentinal tubule.

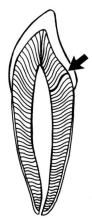

Figure 15–4. "S" curvature of the dentinal tubules.

and the second, toward the apex of the root (Figs. 15–1 and 15–4). These curves become less pronounced in the cervical region and the tubules are rather straight in the root (Fig. 15–4). Smaller *secondary curvatures* are visible microscopically. The primary curvatures represent the path taken during the inward migration of the odontoblasts. The secondary curvatures may be the result of small spiraling undulations of the odontoblast process during matrix formation and mineralization. The tubules, like the odontoblast processes, are tapered and branched. The narrowest part and the most pronounced branching occurs near the dentin-enamel junction. As the odontoblasts produce more dentin matrix, they migrate centrally and become more crowded. Therefore, dentinal tubules are more numerous and closer together nearer the pulp ($40,000/mm^2$) than in the mantle dentin ($20,000/mm^2$).

The orthodentin, or true dentin, matrix can be classified into distinct types of dentin based on location, matrix composition, structure, and developmental pattern (Table 15–1). The nomenclature is not necessarily exclusive and in most instances is self-descriptive.

Table 15–1.
Classification of Dentin by Location, Patterns of Mineralization, and Development

Location	Pattern of Mineralization	Developmental Pattern
Intertubular dentin: found around and between dentinal tubules	*Globular dentin*: formed from calcospherites	*Primary dentin*: formed before and during active eruption
Intratubular dentin: found and formed within dentinal tubules; also called peritubular dentin	*Intraglobular dentin*: hypomineralized dentin between mantle and circumpulpal dentin; normally only found in coronal dentin	*Secondary dentin*: formed when the tooth first comes into occlusion
Mantle dentin: in the crown formed initially; outer coronal dentin	*Tomes granular layer*: hypomineralized zone in root dentin; similar to intraglobular dentin in the crown.	*Tertiary dentin*: formed as a result of a pathologic response
Circumpulpal dentin: nearest to the pulp; formed in crown after mantle dentin has been deposited.	*Sclerotic dentin*: hypermineralized, occluding intratubular dentin	

The first-formed dentin, nearest the dentin-enamel junction (DEJ) of the crown, is called *mantle dentin* (Fig. 15–5). At the DEJ, mantle dentin and enamel interdigitate, giving the DEJ a scalloped appearance. Mantle dentin consists of relatively large collagen fibers that run roughly perpendicular to the DEJ. The highly ordered structure of mantle dentin makes it positively birefringent in polarized light. In the root, unlike the crown, the collagen fibers in the first-formed dentin lie parallel or oblique to the DEJ. Therefore, no true mantle layer exists in root dentin. The bulk of the dentin underlying the mantle dentin is called *circumpulpal dentin* (Fig. 15–5 and 15–6). Collagen fibers throughout this dentin are smaller in diameter and more randomly oriented than in mantle dentin. The region separating these two layers has a characteristically high amount of *interglobular dentin* (Fig. 15–5). Interglobular dentin is formed as the result of the initial rapid mineralization of dentin. Initially, dentin is mineralized by the fusion of numerous *calcospherites*. Calcospherites represent spherical foci of hydroxyapatite formed from calcium phosphate nucleating sites. This mineralization pattern is often referred to as *globular mineralization*. These spherical foci of mineralizing dentin are also termed *globular dentin*. These regions eventually fuse to form a *mineralization front*. Matrix between the fusing calcospherites is often *hypomineralized* (undermineralized). As a result, areas of hypomineralized dentin, called interglobular dentin, persist in the areas between fusing calcospherites. Increased amounts of interglobular dentin can be formed as a result of fluorosis and vitamin D deficiency. The neonatal line is an accentuated line in dentin and enamel (Fig. 15–6).

Dentin surrounding and nearest to each tubule in the circumpulpal dentin is *hypermineralized*, and lacks collagen as an organic component of its matrix. Historically, this dentin has been termed *peritubular dentin* because it seems to surround the tubule. Developmentally speaking, this dentin is really formed within the existing tubule and the term *intratubular dentin* is anatomically more accurate (Figs. 15–7,

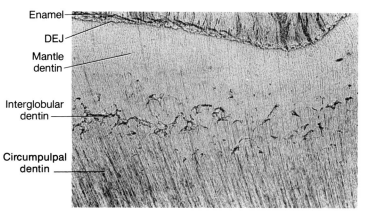

Figure 15–5. Interglobular spaces lie between the mantle dentin (above) and circumpulpal dentin (below) in the crown.

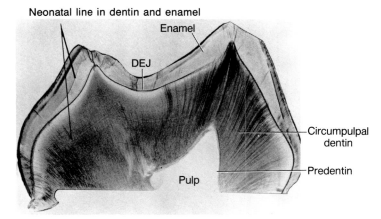

Figure 15–6. Circumpulpal dentin comprises most of the dentin of the tooth.

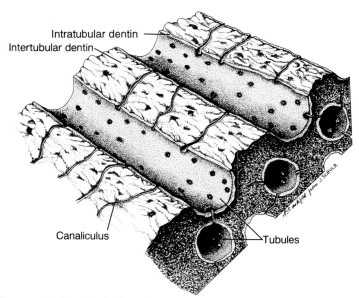

Figure 15–7. Relation of intertubular and intratubular dentin and canaliculi between tubules.

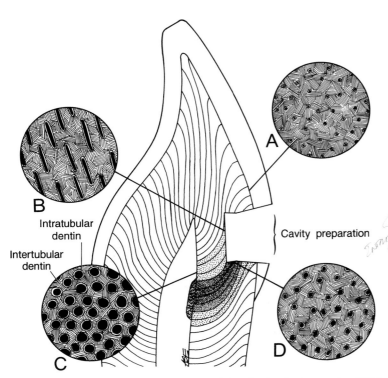

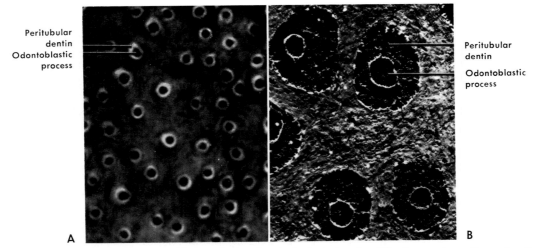

Figure 15–8. Location and size of dentinal tubules at the DEJ (A) and the pulp (C). Relation between tubules in the cavity floor (B and D) and pathway of caries through dentin.

15–8, and 15–9A. The deposition of this form of dentin begins shortly after the formation of the mantle dentin is complete. Organic matrix is deeply basophilic, metachromatic with toluidine and methylene blue (pH 2.6 and 3.6), and stains deeply with alcian blue (pH 2.6), indicating a high content of acidic glycosaminoglycans. The matrix products are synthesized in the cell body of the odontoblast, and transported via the cytoskeletal network through the odontoblast process, and are liberated laterally into the dentinal tubule. Note the difference in the size of the tubule in Fig. 15–8A,B,C. The tubule size increases as it approaches the pulp at the expense of the intertubular matrix. Intratubular dentin is found throughout the dentin matrix except in areas of interglobular dentin and in about the first 100 μm of mineralized dentin (mantle dentin). In both of these areas, the tubule lacks this hypermineralized layer. Upon demineralization, intratubular dentin mostly disappears, leaving only traces of organic material (Fig. 15–9B). The remainder of the dentin matrix, that lies between the tubules, is described as *intertubular dentin.* The zone between the intertubular dentin and intratubular dentin is hypomineralized and has been referred to as the sheath of Neuman (Fig. 15–9B). Although no true sheath seems to exist, the boundary between these two distinct matrices is distinct (differing in mineral and collagen content). The boundary may mark the previous outer extent of the dentinal tubule. Historically, the *sheath of Neuman* referred to the space between the odontoblast process and the wall of the dentinal tubule by demineralization. Therefore, it was formerly equated with the intratubular dentin space. However, with

Figure 15–9. Microscopic appearance of intratubular (peritubular) dentin. (A). Ground section of soft Roentgen-ray analysis showing increased mineral density in the intratubular zone. (B). Electron micrograph of a demineralized section showing both the loss of mineral and low organic content of intratubular dentin.

increased formation and mineralization of intratubular dentin, the tubule may eventually become occluded. The resulting dentin is the termed *sclerotic, transparent,* or *translucent dentin* (Figs. 15–10 and 15–11). When immersed in water, the high mineral content of sclerotic dentin gives it a transparent or glassy appearance (Fig. 15–11).

Dentin deposition begins with the formation of the pulp chamber and continues as long as the pulp remains vital. Dentin can be classified as *developmental* when it is formed during development as a result of embryonic interactions, or *physiological* when it is formed as the result of responses to the environment. *Primary dentin* is developmental dentin and is formed before and during eruption. *Secondary* and *tertiary* dentin may be thought of as physiological dentin. They are formed as the result of normal physiological and pathologic stimuli, respectively. *Secondary dentin* normally begins to be formed when root development is completed and during and after the teeth come into occlusion. However, in impacted (unerupted) third molars secondary dentin deposition has been observed. The rate of secondary dentin deposition is generally slower than primary dentin deposition, and depends on diet and occlusal forces to which the crown is subjected. Abrasive foods and greater chewing forces provide a stronger stimulus for dentin deposition. There is an abrupt change in the course of the dentinal tubules in the shift from primary to secondary dentin deposition, the

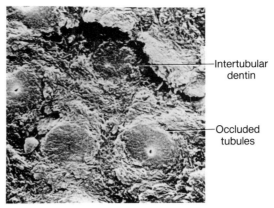

Figure 15–10. Scanning electron micrograph showing the closed ends of sclerosed or occluded dentinal tubules.

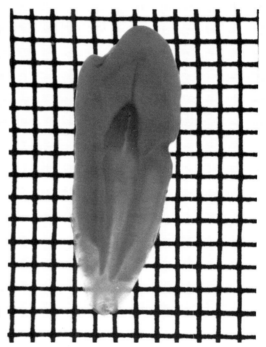

Figure 15–11. Sclerotic dentin in the apical area of root dentin in a hemisectioned tooth. Note the translucency of the sclerotic dentin, which is caused by the filling of dentinal tubules with sclerotic dentin.

tubules being more irregular in secondary dentin (Fig. 15–12). It should be obvious that secondary deposition does not occur uniformly in all areas of the crown. The areas subjected to the most stimulus have higher rates of dentin deposition. The pulp chamber, which roughly outlines the shape of the crown during development and the formation of primary dentin, assumes a different shape because of the asymmetrical deposition of secondary dentin. The junction between primary and secondary dentin can be distinguished by a slight change in the direction of the dentinal tubules (Fig. 15–12). With increased deposition, the pulp chamber becomes reduced in size and there is crowding of odontoblasts. Some odontoblasts may disappear and their tubules may become occluded (sclerotic). As mentioned previously, tubules are believed to become sclerotic by the progressive deposition of intratubular dentin. Electron micrographs have revealed mineralization occurring within the odontoblast process during the formation of sclerotic dentin. This is not a normal process and is most likely a result from cell injury or death. Calcium that enters the damage process and precipitates because of the presence of phosphates (such as ATP and ADP) in the cytoplasm.

Unlike secondary dentin, which is formed as a result of normal physiological stimuli, *tertiary* or *reparative dentin* is formed as a result of a pathological process, caries. Deep caries stimulate odontoblasts to form dentin at a rapid rate (see Fig. 15–15). Operative procedures, which are needed to restore decayed tooth surfaces, can also provide a stimulus or damage to the underlying odontoblasts. When the odontoblast layer has been destroyed, cells in the underlying pulp migrate to this site and differentiate and rapidly deposit an

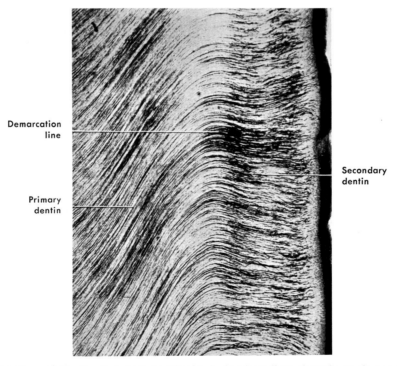

Demarcation line

Primary dentin

Secondary dentin

Figure 15–12. Ground section of dentin showing dentinal tubules bending sharply as they pass into secondary dentin. The dentinal tubules are somewhat irregular in secondary dentin, which is closer to the pulp.

which is about 20 to 25 nm wide. This space is comparable to a synaptic cleft in thickness as found elsewhere in the body. However, other features of a synapse (specializations of the pre- and postsynaptic membrane and the presence of synaptic vesicles) are either lacking or are poorly developed. It is not known whether this cellular relation functions as a rudimentary synapse. Some nerve endings in the dentinal tubules have singular enlargements whereas others have alternating dilations and constrictions with the odontoblast processes. Both types exhibit a similar vesiculated appearance and contain a few mitochondria, and both have a characteristic cleft surrounding them (Figs. 15–21 and 15–22).

Another feature of the dentinal tubule is the presence of an organic coating or inner lining consisting mostly of glycosaminoglycans. The coating has the appearance of a membrane, in decalcified stained sections and by light microscopy, and can easily be confused with the outer cell membrane of the odontoblastic process. This layer represents hypomineralized intratubular dentin, and has been termed the *internal hypomineralized layer*. More recently the term *limiting membrane* or *lamina limitans* has been applied to this layer.

Incremental Nature of Dentin Deposition

The daily deposition of dentin can be measured through the use of labeling agents. A labeling agent is a substance that is visibly incorporated into the dentin matrix. This agent is given initially, and after a period of time (a week to 10 days), the process is repeated. The tooth is removed some days later, sectioned, and microscopically examined. The distance between the two labeled bands divided by the time represents the amount of matrix formed per unit time, usually days. Labels that are commonly used to bind to hydroxyapatite are fluorescent markers such as tetracyclines, or calcium stains such as procion and alizarin red. Radioactive precursors that are incorporated into the dentin matrix have also been given to measure matrix synthesis. Microradiographs, through their demonstration of alternating densities in the mineralization pattern of dentin, also indicate the incremental nature of dentin deposition (Fig. 15–23). Based on these measurements, dentin is believed to be deposited at a rate of about 4 to 8 μm per day. Dentinogenesis is thought to occur in a rhythmic manner, possibly due to the circadian rhythmic activity of neurons that control the flow of nutrients

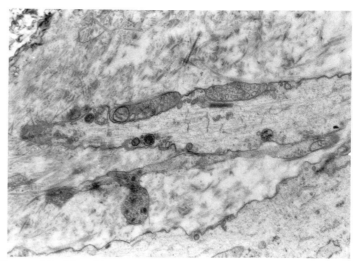

Figure 15–22. Nerve endings in the dentinal tubule parallel the odontoblast process. Below is a nerve ending extending lateral to the tubule in a canaliculus at right angles.

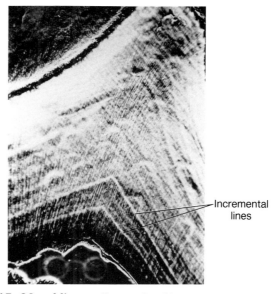

Incremental lines

Figure 15–23. Microradiograph of incremental lines in dentin that depict the rhythmic recurrent deposition of mineral.

Clinical Application

Enclosure of the dental pulp in a mineralized space means that during acute inflammation there is an increse in pulpal pressure. This can cause compression of nerves as well as venules. The resulting pressure and ischemia is painful and can be damaging to the pulp.

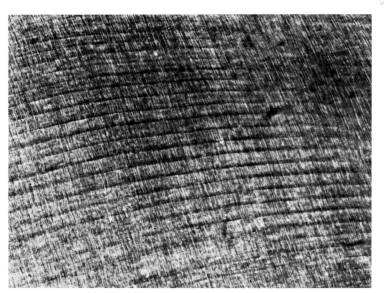

Figure 15–24. Ground section showing the daily incremental deposition of dentin (imbrication lines of von Ebner).

to odontoblasts. The *imbrication lines of von Ebner* represent daily changes in odontoblast activity (Fig. 15–24). More pronounced incremental lines, *contour lines of Owen*, represent normal physiological alterations in the pattern of mineralization that occur at less frequent intervals (Fig. 15–25). Exaggerated contour lines may be the result of a sudden change or pathologic process. The *neonatal line* represents an exaggerated contour line of Owen and is representative of the changes in physiology (nutritional, hormonal, etc.) that occur at birth. These neonatal lines are seen in the primary teeth and the first permanent molars. The dentin distal (nearer the DEJ) to this line was formed before birth, and that proximal (nearer the pulp) was formed after birth.

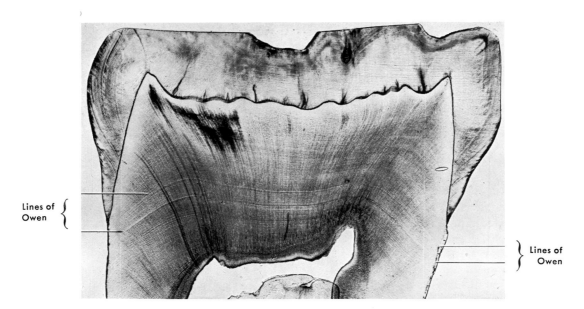

Lines of Owen

Lines of Owen

Figure 15–25. Ground section showing accentuated incremental lines, contour lines of Owen.

There are no reversal lines because dentin does not remodel in the same manner as bone. For odontoclastic activity to occur, the odontoblast layer would have to be disrupted. Bone resorption is mediated by osteoblasts. Factors that cause bone resorption, such as parathyroid hormone and interleukin-1β, do so indirectly by binding to receptors on osteoblasts, causing them to retract from bone surfaces. Because odontoblasts have branched processes that extend great distances into the dentin and are tightly joined to each other by terminal bars and other junctions, no easy way exists for them to separate from the predentin surface to allow for odontoclasia. Furthermore, these cells may be incapable of responding to these hormones because of a lack of receptors. However, there is evidence of minimal remodeling by odontoblasts. Endocytic activity has been demonstrated along the odontoblast process in dentinal tubules as well as at the mineralization front. Ultrastructural evidence of intracellular collagen degradation also suggests that odontoblasts may participate in predentin matrix turnover to a minimal degree.

Dentin Matrix Composition: Inorganic and Organic Constituents

Mature dentin is about 70% mineral, 20% organic matrix, and 10% water on a weight basis, and about 50% mineral, 30%, and 20% organic on a volume basis. Dentin does not have a uniform composition throughout the tooth. It can vary in hardness and mineral content in different areas of the tooth as a result of sclerosis. The relatively high organic content in comparison with enamel enables dentin, unlike enamel, to deform slightly under compression. Another factor contributing to the resiliency of the dentin may be the fluid within the dentinal tubules (vide infra). The fluid-filled dentinal tubules may function as "hydraulic shock absorbers" dissipating the forces of mastication. Dentin, therefore provides a "cushion" for the overlying brittle enamel.

Inorganic Matrix

Although trace amounts of calcium carbonate, fluoride, magnesium, zinc, and other minerals (e.g., metal phosphates and sulfates) are found in dentin, *hydroxyapatite*, $CA_{10}(PO_4)_6(OH)_2$, is the principal inorganic component of the dentin matrix. Hydroxyapatite crystals are in the form of flattened plates having the dimensions of approximately 60–70 nm in length, 20–30 nm in width, and 3–4 nm in thickness. The calcium:phosphate ratio (by weight) varies in peritubular (1:2.14) and intertubular (1:2.10) dentin, but overall averages 1:2.13. Extensive sclerosis or deposition of intratubular dentin (sclerosis) may occur with aging, making the dentin brittle and less resilient.

Table 15-2.
Comparison of Hardness of Enamel and Types of Dentin

Matrix	Knoop Hardness Number
Enamel	343
Orthodentin	68
Sclerotic dentin	80
Carious dentin	25

The high mineral content of dentin makes it harder than cementum or bone, although softer than enamel. In the laboratory, hardness can be measured by Knoop hardness test (KHN), in which a small diamond point is dropped from a known distance onto a polished dentin surface. These indentation tests have shown that the average KHN (Knoop hardness number) is approximately 68 for dentin and approximately 343 for enamel, making enamel five times harder than dentin (Table 15–2). Basically, there is little or no difference in the range of KHN between teeth of different types or between root and coronal dentin of the same tooth. Variations may occur, however, under the various environmental influences discussed previously. Sclerotic dentin is harder, having a KHN of approximately 80. Carious dentin or dead tracts are partially demineralized and have a reduced KHN of approximately 25.

Organic Matrix

The bulk of the organic matrix of dentin, about 91 to 92%, consists of *collagen* (Fig. 15–2). Most of the collagen is type I with minor amounts of type V. Although type III collagen may be found in the pulp and in the predentin matrix of developing teeth, its presence in mature dentin has not been demonstrated.

The noncollagenous macromolecules of dentin can be classified into seven broad categories (Table 15–3): *phosphoproteins, proteoglycans, γ-carboxyglutamate-containing (Gla) proteins, miscellaneous acidic glycoproteins, growth-related factors, lipids, and serum-derived proteins.*

Table 15-3.
Organic Components in Dentin and Their Possible Functions

Component	Comments	Function
Collagen	Major organic component (91–92%). Type I predominates with minor amounts of type V; type III is found in the pulp and during early dentin matrix formation.	May play a role in initiating mineralization. Provides the structural framework for dentin, giving it strength and resilience.
Phosphoproteins	Major noncollagenous protein; deposited at the mineralization front; not found in predentin.	May play an important role in mineralization.
Proteoglycans	Dermatin, chondroitin and keratin sulfates; decorin and biglycan are present.	Some inhibit mineralization and others bind calcium nonspecifically. Thus, their presence may control the mineralization process. Those that associate with collagen may control fibrilogenesis.
γ-Carboxyglutamate-containing proteins, matrix Gla, and bone Gla (osteocalcin) proteins	Carboxylation reaction is vitamin K-dependent.	Role in mineralized tissues is uncertain, but they can bind calcium, suggesting that they may initiate or control the mineralization process in some way by regulating local calcium levels.
Acidic glycoproteins	Osteopontin, 65 and 90 kDa glycoproteins.	Osteopontin may be associated with the odontoblast process, serving as a link between matrix and cell membrane. Roles of other proteins are unknown.
Growth factors	Transforming growth factor-β, cartilage inducing factors, insulinlike growth factors and platelet-derived growth factors.	May control the proliferation and differentiation of new odontoblasts following injury or a pathologic process. Stimulate repair.
Lipids	No unique lipids are found in dentin.	Phospholipids may be involved in the initiation of mineralization.

Pulpal Architecture

The dental pulp can be divided into several compartments based on its location within the pulp chambers. The average volume of the dental pulp is 0.02 cc, with the molar pulps having four times the volume of incisor pulps (Fig. 16–2). The coronal pulp extends occlusally into the pulp horns of each crown. Apically, the coronal pulp extends into the radicular or root pulp. The floor of the coronal pulp in multirooted teeth is the furcation zone. Accessory canals, formed by a defective root sheath, penetrate the apical root dentin and cementum in permanent teeth and the furcation zone in primary teeth. Fibroblasts, blood vessels, and nerves can usually be found within the accessory canals. At the apical foramen, the pulpal tissue becomes continuous with the tissue of the periodontal ligament. As the erupting tooth enters functional occlusion, the cell-free and cell-rich zones become defined (Fig. 16–3). The cell-rich zone may be absent in older teeth. The cell-free zone separates the cell-rich and odontoblastic layers. The cell-rich zone is thought to contain progenitor odontoblasts that can be induced to differentiate into mature odontoblasts in response to wounding. The most peripheral aspect of the coronal pulp is lined by the columnar-shaped odontoblasts whereas the odontoblasts in

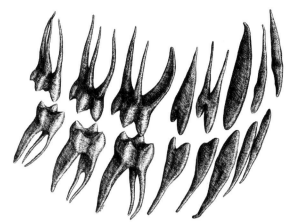

Figure 16–2. Pulp organs of permanent human teeth. Upper row, maxillary arch; left central incisor through third molar. Lower row, mandibular arch; left central incisor through third molar.

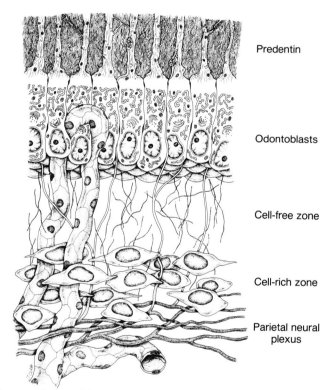

Predentin

Odontoblasts

Cell-free zone

Cell-rich zone

Parietal neural plexus

Figure 16–3. Diagram of odontogenic zone with odontoblasts, cell-free and cell-rich zones, and parietal layer of nerves.

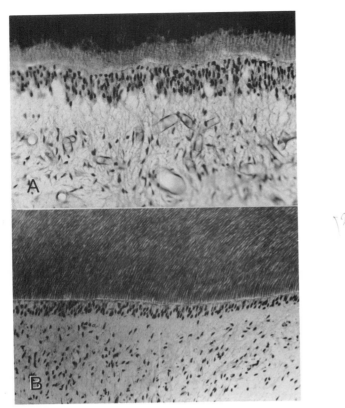

Figure 16–4. (A). Columnar odontoblasts in coronal area. (B). Cuboidal odontoblasts in radicular pulp.

the radicular pulp and furcation zones are cuboidal, or exhibit a flattened morphology (16–4). The pulp proper, or central pulp, contains the large blood vessels of the pulp and nerve trunks. The veins in the pulp range from 100 to 150 μm in diameter and arterioles, 50 to 150 μm in diameter. Myelinated and nonmyelinated nerves are normally found in close association with the blood vessels (Fig. 16–5).

Cells of the Pulp

The most predominant cell type in the dental pulp is the fibroblast, but the pulp also contains odontoblasts, blood cells, Schwann cells, endothelial cells, and undifferentiated mesenchymal cells. Cells involved in the immune response, such as macrophages, mast cells, antigen processing cells (dendritic cells), and plasma cells can also be found in the pulp during periods of inflammation.

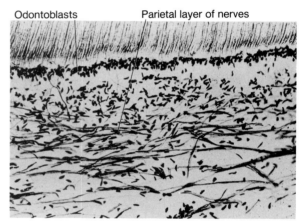

Odontoblasts   Parietal layer of nerves

Figure 16–5. Photomicrograph of a sliver-stained section of a human tooth demonstrating the odontogenic zone including the parietal plexus of nerves.

Odontoblasts

Odontoblasts are terminally differentiated, polarized pulpal cells derived from the cranial neural crest, which are found in a peripheral layer closely associated with the predentin (Fig. 16–6). The major function of odontoblasts is the synthesis and secretion of the fibers and extracellular matrix (ECM) of the predentin and biomineralization of the dentin (Fig. 16–7). The cell body of the odontoblast contains all of the organelles that are paramount to the cells role in protein synthesis (Fig. 16–8). The nucleus of the odontoblast is basally located, with the RER and Golgi apparatus located supranuclear. Numerous mitochondria and lysosomes are found throughout the cytoplasm. The major protein produced by the odontoblast is type I collagen and is secreted into the extracellular space at the predentin interface. Type I trimer and type V collagens have also been reported to be a minor component of the extracellular matrix. Noncollagenous components of the extracellular matrix of predentin and dentin, including proteoglycans, glycosaminoglycans, phosphoproteins, and γ-carboxyglutamate-containing proteins, are also synthesized and secreted by odontoblasts.

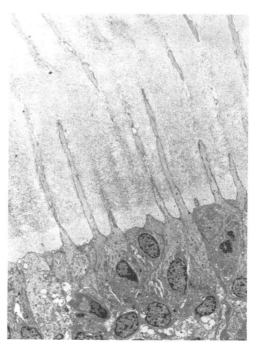

Figure 16–7. This low-magnification transmission electron micrograph shows the odontoblastic layer. The majority of the odontoblasts demonstrate a normal distribution of organelles and processes extending into the predentin and dentin. Tight-junctional complexes can be seen at the neck of the odontoblast at the level of the cell and the predentin matrix.

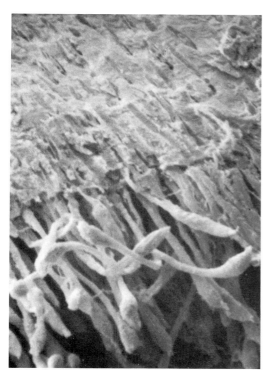

Figure 16–6. This high-magnification scanning electron micrograph demonstrates intact human odontoblasts and odontoblastic processes attached to the fractured surface of the predentin and dentin. Cut odontoblastic tubules containing odontoblast processes can be seen above the cells.

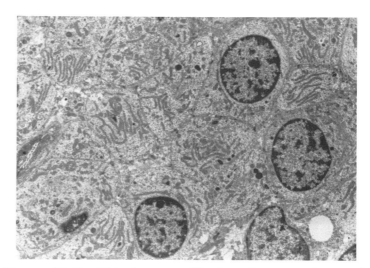

Figure 16–8. This low-magnification electron micrograph demonstrates a cross-sectional view of the odontoblastic layer. The odontoblasts contain organelles typical of protein synthetic activity, including abundant rough endoplasmic reticulum, ribosomes, and mitochondria.

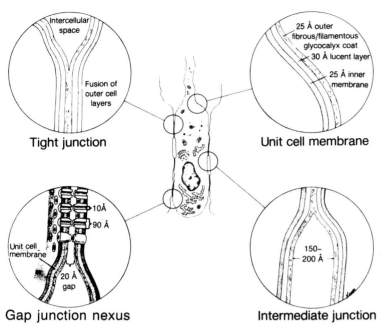

Figure 16–9. Diagram of odontoblasts, cell membranes, and types of junctional complexes.

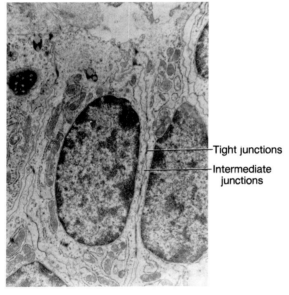

Figure 16–10. Ultrastructure of junctional complexes of odontoblasts in region of nuclei.

The odontoblast also has a process extending from the cell body to the DEJ contained within a dentinal tubule. The odontoblast exhibits multiple processes at the time of terminal differentiation. By the time mantle dentin layer has been completed, the cells normally exhibit only one main process. There are multiple lateral odontoblast processes contained within the dentin that are maintained through the life of the odontoblast. The odontoblast process may also contain mitochondria, secretory granules, microtubules, and intermediate filaments.

Odontoblasts are intimately associated with adjacent odontoblasts through a series of junctional complexes including desmosomes, and tight, intermediate, and gap junctions (Fig. 16–9). The tight and intermediate junctional complexes are important for maintaining the integrity of the odontoblast layer and preventing the ingress of foreign material—that is, toxins and bacterial products, from the oral cavity (Fig. 16–10). The tight junction provides mechanical attachment between adjacent odontoblasts. Intermediate junctions have been shown to extend around the perimeter of the odontoblasts as narrow bands. The gap junctions are areas of reduced electrical resistance that also allow selective exchange of substances between odontoblasts. Gap junctions are characterized as circumscribed structures with 2-nm tubular channels surrounded by rings of proteins of adjacent plasma membranes that traverse the gap between cells and link the interior of adjacent odontoblasts. Each half of the gap junctional complex consists of a symmetrically equivalent hexamer of approximately 27-kD, and is termed a connexin. Various mechanisms have been proposed to explain how gap junctions are regulated, including changes in pH, calcium concentrations, and voltage changes. Opening of the gap junction allows small molecules and ions, such as c-AMP and Ca^{2+}, to diffuse between the cells and initiate a cascade of events leading to an increase or decrease in cell activity. Gap junctions between odontoblasts have been demonstrated ultrastructurally by using special staining techniques and immunohistochemistry, and by freeze fracture. It has been suggested that gap junctions play an important role in the regulation of cell growth and differentiation as well as coordinating cellular activity between odontoblasts—for example, dentinogenesis.

As the tooth ages, the odontoblasts change shape from cuboidal to ovoid and become quiescent. Some odontoblasts are lost and not replaced. The functioning odontoblasts continue to produce predentin throughout the life of the tooth, although at a much reduced rate. Odontoblasts retain the ability to upregulate protein synthetic activity in response to trauma after aging; however, the response is initiated slower. The odontoblast cell layer becomes discontinuous, and the cells vary in the amount of ECM being produced and subsequently mineralized in the older tooth.

Fibroblasts and Undifferentiated Mesenchymal Cells

Fibroblasts are the most numerrous cells found in the dental pulp. They are stellate-shaped cells with long cytoplasmic extensions that contact adjacent fibroblasts or odontoblasts through gap-junctional processes. Fibroblasts synthesize and secrete type III collagen and other ECM components of the pulp, including proteoglycans and glycosaminoglycans. The fibroblast is also responsible for degrading the ECM, and can simultaneously synthesize and degrade the pulpal ECM. Collagen is the most abundant connective tissue protein and occurs in several specific isotopes, types I through XII. Each is recognized as a specific genetic product differing in amino acid and palpated composition. In the pulp, type III is the most abundant with other types, such as IV and V, as minor constituents. As the dental pulp ages, there is a reduction in the numbers of fibroblasts and a concomitant increase in the number and size of the collagen fibrils, fibers, and bundles.

Fibroblasts or undifferentiated mesenchymal cells also have an important role in wound healing mechanisms in the pulp. The fibroblasts of the cell-rich zone are thought to differentiate into odontoblasts after the right stimulus—for example, growth factor, a bone morphogenic protein, cytokine, or inflammatory mediator, released during wounding from the exposed predentin or dentin, or inflammatory cells that have migrated to the wound site.

There are many other cells found in a vital dental pulp, and some are associated with a diseased pulp.

Perivascular cells are found in the dental pulp closely associated with the vasculature. These cells have been reported to be important in wound-healing mechanisms associated with pulpal repair mechanisms. Perivascular cells have also been shown to proliferate in response to an iatrogenic exposure of the dental pulp, and are thought to possibly provide replacement cells for the odontoblast layer in wounds where the cell-rich layer has been destroyed.

Endothelial cells line the lumen of the pulpal blood vessels and contribute to the basal lamina by producing type IV collagen, an afibrillar collagen. They have been shown to proliferate after a pulp exposure in an attempt to neovascularize the wounded area during the process of wound healing.

Class II antigen processing cells have been demonstrated by immunohistochemical methods in both the normal and inflamed pulp (Fig. 16–11). These cells are commonly called dendritic cells because of multiple, long cytoplasmic processes that bind antigens and process them for presentation to macrophages and lymphocytes. Dendritic cells have been found within the walls of periapical granulomas after pulpal necrosis.

Clinical Application

Pulp stones are a normal resident of the mature dental pulp. In most cases pulp stones are asymptomatic unless they impinge on the pulpal blood supply or neurovascular bundle. However, if a patient presents with clinical symptoms that require endodontic therapy, a pulp stone that obstructs the root canals could potentially interfere with treatment.

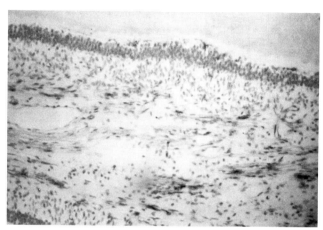

Figure 16–11. Immunohistochemical localization of dendritic cells in the deep pulp under a pulp exposure and at the odontoblast–dentin interface where a series of dendritic cells were also localized.

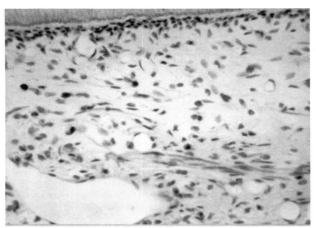

Figure 16–12. Immunohistochemically-stained T-lymphocyte in an inflamed dental pulp.

Other vascular-derived cells found in the pulp during an inflammatory condition include mast cells, B- and T-lymphocytes, polymorphonuclear neutrophils, and macrophages (Figs. 16–12 and 16–13). These blood cells are of paramount importance in fighting infection in the pulp because of the substances they contain: histamine, serotonin, cytokines, growth factors, and other cellular mediators.

Schwann cells envelope nerve processes with a myelin sheath. The myelin is a lipid-rich substance produced by the Schwann cell and contained within the cytoplasm. It requires many Schwann cells to cover an individual axon, and therefore only a small portion of each axon is covered by one Schwann cell. The joint where two axons meet is called a node of Ranvier. Myelinated nerves contain many wrappings of myelin whereas unmyelinated nerves are covered by a single wrapping of the Schwann cell's cytoplasm.

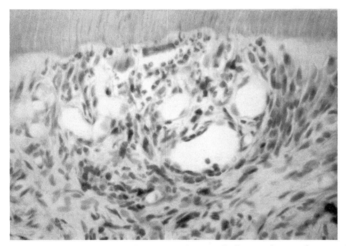

Figure 16–13. B-lymphocytes in an inflamed monkey pulp underlying a cavity preparation.

Pulp stones (denticles) can be found in the dental pulp as a normal consequence of aging (Fig. 16–14). True pulp stones contain dentinal tubules within a mineralized matrix and are surrounded by odontoblastlike cells. False pulp stones are composed of a mineralized matrix arranged in a series of concentric lamellae (Fig. 16–15). Flattened or spindle-shaped cells are occasionally seen on the surface of the tissue. Pulp stones can be found embedded within the dentinal matrix, attached to the predentin and dentin, or lying free within the stroma of the pulp proper. Pulp stones are usually asymptomatic unless they impinge upon a nerve or blood vessel. Pulp stones can cause problems during endodontic procedures when they lie over or within the radicular pulp. Occasionally, diffuse calcifications can be found in the coronal or radicular portion of the dental pulp, and are usually associated with the vasculature in a linear arrangement. These dystrophic calcifications are thought to be initiated by microtrauma to pulp in the areas where they are found.

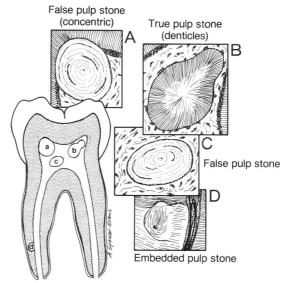

Figure 16–14. Diagram of pulp stones (denticles). (A). False attached denticle. (B). True denticle with tubules. (C). False, free denticle. (D). Embedded denticle.

Clinical Application

The placement of a hard-set, calcium hydroxide–containing material over deep cavity preparations or after a pulp exposure is standard clinical dental practice. How the hard-set, calcium hydroxide–containing materials function to aid pulpal healing is not known. Recent work suggests that pulp-capping materials that combine growth factors with an inert carrier can be equally, if not more, efficacious in promoting pulpal healing.

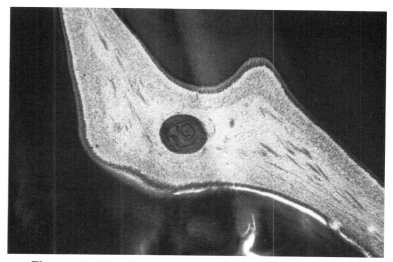

Figure 16–15. Photomicrograph of a false, free pulp stone in coronal pulp.

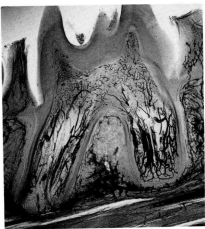

Figure 16–16. The vascular organization in the pulp (India-ink injection of vessels).

Vasculature of Pulp

Blood vessels enter the pulp through the apical foramen in a connective tissue compartment known as the central core (Fig. 16–16). The venules are between 100 to 150 μm and the arterioles are approximately 50 to 150 μm in diameter. Branches of smaller vessels are given off as the blood vessels proceed toward the coronal pulp and pulp horns (Fig. 16–17). The terminal capillaries and venules anastomose in deep to the odontoblast layer, where they provide nutrients and oxygen needed for cellular metabolism (Fig. 16–18). The capillary loops are dense in the coronal and pulp horn aspect of the pulp and less dense in the radicular pulp. Continuous and fenestrated capillaries are present in the odontoblastic layer. The fenestrated capillaries have small pores that contain only a thin membrane covering composed of endothelial cell cytoplasm and a basement membrane (Fig. 16–19). These pores allow for a rapid outward transport

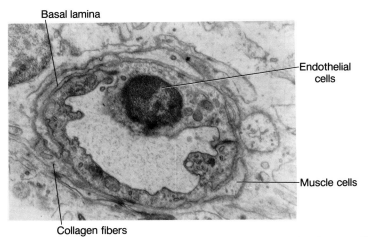

Figure 16–17. Transmission electron micrograph of a small arteriole in pulp, with endothelial cells and a cytoplasmic extension of a smooth muscle cell.

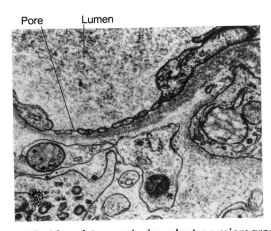

Figure 16–19. A transmission electron micrograph of a fenestrated capillary in the odontogenic zone.

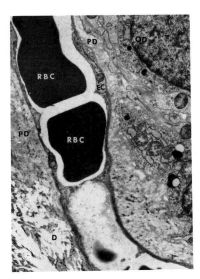

Figure 16–18. Transmission electron micrograph of capillary coursing among odontoblasts. D, dentin; EC, endothelial cell; OD, odontoblast, PD, predentin; RBC, red blood cell.

of substances and cells into the extracellular space, as well as removal of metabolic waste during times of pulpal insult. Arteriovenous and venous–venous shunts are also present in the pulp for rapid transfer of blood (Fig. 16–20). Both the arteriovenous shunt and the fenestrated capillaries have been suggested to function in reducing interstitial pressure in the pulp during inflammation. After dental operative procedures the capillaries underlying a cavity preparation will become leaky, allowing plasma and vascular cells into the extracellular spaces. Lymphatic vessels have also been reported to be located in the dental pulp. The lymphatic vessels are thin-walled tubular structures that usually do not contain cellular elements.

During the aging process, the blood vessels of the pulp exhibit changes similar to those seen in the rest of the body. Accumulations of cholesterol can be seen in the walls of the vessels. These cholesterol deposits can cause a localized inflammatory response, which in turn causes the intimal surface of the pulpal vessel to become adherent, allowing erythrocytes to adhere to the walls of the vessels. The reduced diameter of the vessels decreases the blood flow to those areas of the pulp, resulting in hypoxia. Eventually, the thrombus formed by the accumulation of erythrocytes can dislodge and cause an embolus, which will cause a localized pulp necrosis when it occludes a terminal capillary within the odontoblast region or pulp proper.

Nerves in the Pulp

The sensory and postganglionic sympathetic nerves that innervate the dental pulp (Fig. 16–21) originate in the trigeminal and superior cervical ganglia and enter the teeth

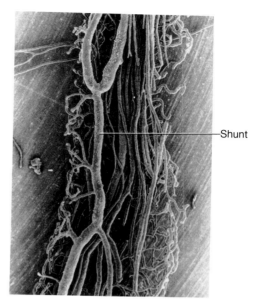

Figure 16–20. A scanning electron micrograph of a vein-to-vein shunt in the coronal pulp.

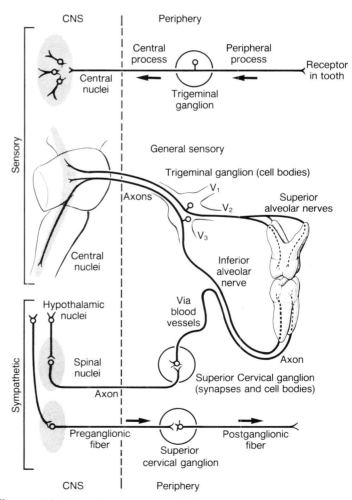

Figure 16–21. A summary of the sensory and autonomic nerve supply to the dental pulp.

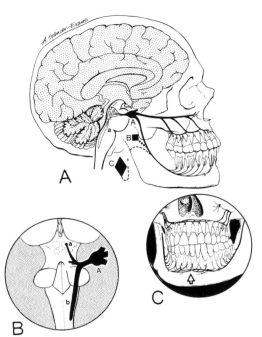

Figure 16–22. Peripheral and central innervation to teeth. (A). Pathways of the trigeminal nerve. A, trigeminal ganglion; B, otic ganglion; C, superior cervical sympathetic ganglion; a, brainstem trigeminal nuclear complex. (B). Trigeminal ganglion (A), with mesencephalic nucleus (a) and brainstem trigeminal nuclear complex (b). (C). Transmedian collateral innervation.

through the apical foramen. From the neural receptor in the pulp, the central process of a trigeminal sensory neuron traverses the trigeminal ganglion located in the floor of the middle cranial fossa (Fig. 16–22). The central process then synapses on a second-order neuron located in the subnucleus caudalis of the brainstem trigeminal complex. The majority of second-order neurons then decussate and ascend to synapse on neuronal cell bodies located in the ventroposterio-medial nucleus of the thalamus. The third-order neurons ascend to the area of the postcentral gyrus concerned with the orofacial region. The majority of sensory stimuli to the teeth are perceived by the patient as pain, although recent reports suggest that other sensory modalities may also be discerned, such as pressure and temperature. The mandibular teeth are innervated by the inferior alveolar nerve originating from the third division of the trigeminal ganglion. The maxillary teeth are innervated by the anterior, middle, and posterior superior alveolar nerves. The postganglionic sympathetic nerves form a plexus on the external carotid arteries and subsequently follow the terminal branches of this artery into the pulps of the mandibular and maxillary teeth.

Clinical Application

The dental pulp has an inherent capacity to respond to environmental or iatorogenic trauma resulting from bacterial insult or operative procedures. Some of the mechanisms the pulp has available to meet these challenges include various antigen-processing cells such as macrophages and class II dendricytes, fenestrated capillaries, arteriovenous and venous–venous shunts, a lymphatic circulation, and an effective vascular supply.

Branches of the inferior and superior alveolar nerves and sympathetic nerves enter the apices of the teeth as myelinated A-β and A-δ fibers or unmyelinated c-fibers. The myelinated fibers are associated with nociception and the unmyelinated c-fibers, with postganglionic sympathetic nerves. Two or three branches enter the premolars and molars, and single trunks usually enter the incisors and canines. Some terminal branches from the nerve trunks are given off within the radicular pulp, but most of the branches terminate in the coronal pulp, in the pulp horns, and within the dentinal tubules. As the nerve trunks reach the subodontoblastic region they form a plexus in the coronal pulp. The myelinated nerves then lose the myelin sheath and, together with the sympathetic nerves, enter the cell-rich layer, traverse the cell-free and odontoblast layers, and enter the predentin. Nerve terminals are found in all parts of the dental pulp, but the densest area of innervation is in the pulp horns (Fig. 16–23). The pulp horns are the most clinically susceptible areas for environmental trauma, which may explain the density of innervation. Approximately every 10th dentinal tubule contains a nerve terminal in the pulp horn region of the coronal pulp (Fig. 16–24). The nerves extend nearly 200 μm into the dentinal tubules through the predentin and dentin (Fig. 16–25).

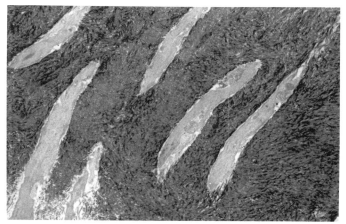

Figure 16–24. A transmission electron micrograph demonstrating a series of dentinal tubules in a pulp horn containing nerves and odontoblastic processes.

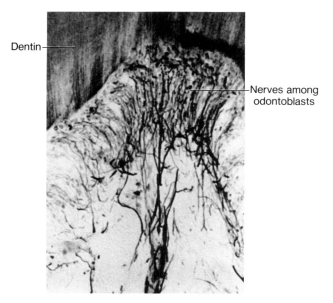

Dentin

Nerves among odontoblasts

Figure 16–23. Nerves in the odontogenic zone of the pulp.

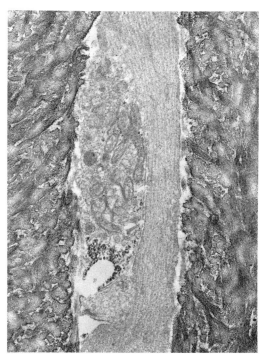

Figure 16–25. High-magnification transmission electron micrograph showing a nerve terminal and odontoblast process in a dentinal tubule.

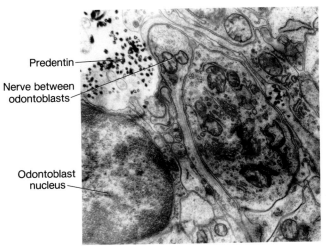

Figure 16-26. Ultrastructure of unmyelinated nerve extending between odontoblasts into predentin.

The majority of the nerves located within the odontogenic zone of the mature dental pulp are unmyelinated A-δ or c-fibers and are thought to be nociceptive fibers or post-ganglionic sympathetic fibers. These fibers are located below and between the odontoblasts and are also located in the dentinal tubules of predentin juxtaposed to the odontoblast process. Most of the terminals associated with the odontoblast and the odontoblast process contain a variety of electron-dense and/or electron-lucent vesicles (Fig. 16-26). The majority of nerve terminals located in the coronal or root pulp are associated with the vasculature and contain dense core vesicles that stain positively for catecholamines. These nerve terminals are thought to be postganglionic sympathetic terminals for the regulation of pulpal blood flow (Fig. 16-27). There are terminals located in the odontogenic zone that contain a homogeneous population of dense core vesicles and are associated with capillaries (Fig. 16-28A and B).

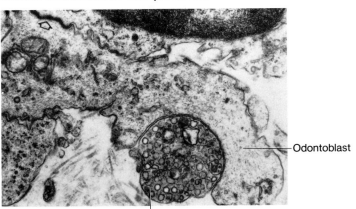

Figure 16-27. Ultrastructure of nerve ending indenting an odontoblastic process. Arrow, Gap junction between adjacent odontoblasts.

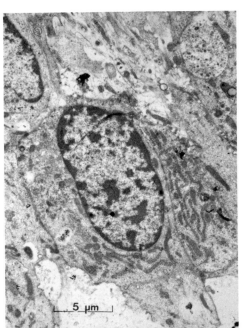

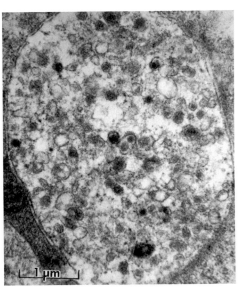

Figure 16-28. Ultrastructural transmission electron micrograph of odontoblasts (A) with a large nerve terminal (B) containing various sizes and types of membrane bounded vesicles.

However, their vascular stimulation function is unclear because capillary diameter is regulated by local humoral factors such as bradykinin and prostaglandins elaborated by cells involved in the inflammatory response. Several authors have reported that these dense core–containing terminals located in the odontoblastic region have a role in modulating the response of the sensory nociceptors by regulating the vascular supply to these terminals. Other investigators suggest that these nerve terminals have a role in modifying the response of the odontoblast to insult, in recruitment of progenitor cells after pulp exposure or deep cavity preparation, or in the regulation of odontoblast metabolism (Fig. 16–29).

Many anatomic variations of nerves and nerve terminals have been reported to exist in the dental pulp as described morphologically, neurohistochemically, and immunohistochemically. These variations have raised questions as to the functional significance of these findings. Neurotransmitters such as calcitonin gene-related peptide (CGRP), enkephalin, neuropeptide Y, vasoactive intestinal peptide (VIP), substance P, somatostatin, serotonin, acetylcholine, and norepinepherine have been reported to be associated with nerves innervating the dental pulp. Presumably, these putative neurotransmitters are contained in the vesicles of the nerve terminals adjacent to the odontoblasts. However, there are no ultrastructural studies characterizing the contents of the vesicles within nerve terminals juxtaposed to the odontoblasts of the dental pulp or in the dentinal tubules located within the predentin or dentin. Do these different conformations of nerve terminals and different neurotransmitters function only during the transmission or modulation of nociceptive mechanoreception, or do they have other roles, such as modifying the responsiveness of the odontoblasts to iatrogenic or environmental insult? The answer to these questions are unknown at present, but recent evidence suggests that CGRP-containing nerves in the periosteum and marrow of bones can increase osteoblastic activity. CGRP-containing nerves have also been found in the dental pulp in close proximity to odontoblasts, which were in the process of forming reparative dentin.

Reports of adrenergic sympathetic nerves located in the dental pulp of various species of animals suggest that the sympathetic nerve supply to the dental pulp has multiple functions. One function that is well established is the response of the vasculature of the dental pulp to sympathetic stimulation. Many investigators have shown that the adrenergic sympathetic nerves function to control intravascular and interstitial pressures within the pulpal tissues. Electrical stimulation of the superior sympathetic trunk and/or ganglion results in a decrease in pulpal blood flow, but does not result in a change in diameter of the blood vessels located in the dental pulp. The use of sympathomimetics decreases the flow rate. Several investigators have reported changes in the pulpal blood flow rate after injection of specific cholinergic agonists, suggesting that there is a population of autonomic nerves in the dental pulp that use acetylcholine as the postganglionic neurotransmitter. These studies corroborate light-microscopic studies in which acetylcholine esterase has been localized

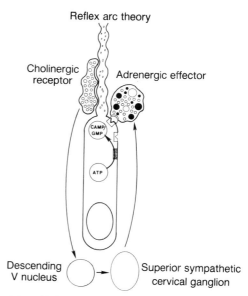

Figure 16–29. Schematic of reflex arc theory. Cell movement or deformation of the nerve terminal may stimulate the sensory terminal (cholinergic) to conduct an impulse to the main sensory nucleus in the central nervous system. A descending pathway may stimulate sympathetic stimuli to the effectory (adrenergic) on or near the odontoblast, which effects response of dentinogenesis and reparative dentin formation.

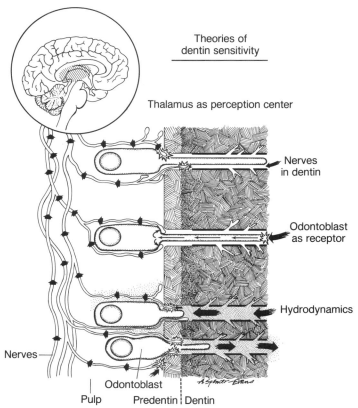

Figure 16–30. Summary of information on function according to three theories of dentinal innervation.

in the odontogenic zone and adjacent subodontoblastic plexus where the nerve supply is most dense. These results present a perplexing problem that needs to be further elucidated, considering there are very few morphological reports in the literature of a parasympathetic nerve supply to the dental pulp.

Theories of Pain Transmission through Dentin

At present there are three major theories that have been suggested to explain how pain is transmitted through the dentin (Fig. 16–30). Confusion arises as a result of several factors, including the lack of synaptic specializations between nerves and odontoblasts, the multiplicity of neurotransmitters found in the dental pulp, and the technical difficulties in recording electrophysiologically from an intact pulp. Currently, the hydrodynamic theory predominates, although each theory has positive and negative points.

Hydrodynamic Theory

The movement of the fluid contained in the dentinal tubules, in response to iatrogenic or environmental trauma, is the basis of the hydrodynamic theory. When the fluid in the dentinal tubules, a derivative of the blood plasma, is perturbed, the nerve terminals within the dentinal tubules and the odontoblast layer are deformed and initiate an action potential. Numerous studies have demonstrated that rapid movement of the dentinal fluid will cause pain whether the stimulus is osmotic, chemical, temperature-related, or mechanical.

Transduction Theory

The transduction theory is based on several experimental criteria that suggest that the odontoblast can transduce a mechanical stimulus and transfer that signal to a closely opposed nerve terminal. Support for this theory is from reports showing odontoblasts to be derived from neural crest cells, to be closely associated with nerve terminals, and to contain gap junctions that electronically couple adjacent odontoblasts. Arguments against the odontoblast transduction theory are that there have been no reports of synaptic specializations between odontoblasts and nerve terminals, and therefore no means of chemical transmission, and that odontoblasts are not excitable cells, and therefore are unable to produce an electrical response.

Direct Innervation Theory

The direct innervation hypothesis is the oldest theory of dentinal innervation and is based on the belief that dentinal nerve terminals extend to the dentino-enamel junction. When the dentin is penetrated the nerve terminal is deformed directly by mechanical perturbation and initiates an action potential. Presently, the evidence suggests that nerve terminals extend between 200 and 300 μm into the predentin–dentin, which is too close to the pulp to support this theory.

Pulp Response to Environmental and Iatrogenic Trauma

Caries

Dentin affected by a carious insult will initiate an inflammatory response from the dental pulp as a result of invasion of the pulpal tissue by bacterial toxins (Fig. 16–31). Initial disruption of the odontoblasts due to edema breaks down the junctional complexes between odontoblasts and allows access of the pulpal tissue by the bacteria (Fig. 16–32). The capillaries begin to leak plasma, and vascular cells will become extravasated (Fig. 16–33). The acute inflammatory cells release various chemotaxic factors, cytokines, and growth factors. The inflammatory response consists of a rapid accumulation of neutrophils, histiocytes, and monocytes. Prolonged inflammation results in a chronic inflammatory response that includes B- and T-lymphocytes and plasma cells. With the presence of chronic inflammation, focal necrotic lesions develop that may lead to total pulpal necrosis possibly due to anaerobic bacterial invasion and the subsequent release of degradative enzymes by these virulent bacteria.

Healing after Cavity Preparation

Experimental evidence suggests that wound healing in the rat dental pulp begins after mechanical or thermal trauma caused by the cavity preparation injures the odontoblast, opens the dentinal tubules, and displaces the nerves and nerve terminals that are adjacent to the odontoblasts and odontoblast processes within the dentinal tubules. The distortion of the nerve terminals causes them rapidly to release neuropeptides that are contained within their vesicles, such as substance P and VIP. Disruption of the odontoblastic layer and injury to the cells as a result of the cavity preparation initiate chemotactic signals recruiting inflammatory cells to the area. The inflammatory cells respond by releasing various cellular mediators—histamine, serotonin, and prostaglandins—into the surrounding tissue, thus potentiating the

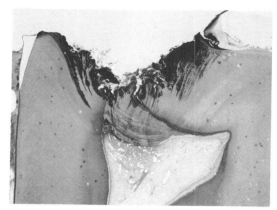

Figure 16–32. Histology of caries in dentin with underlying reparative dentin and inflammatory pulp response.

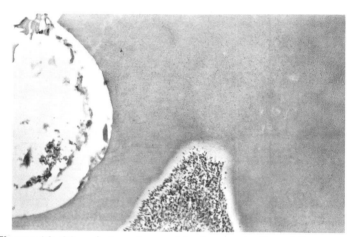

Figure 16–33. Autoradiographic demonstration of the pattern of labeling of I^{125}-fibrinogen 10 min after a class V cavity preparation was completed.

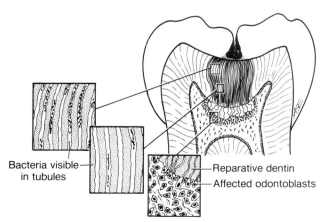

Bacteria visible in tubules

Reparative dentin
Affected odontoblasts

Figure 16–31. Diagram of dental caries in tubules and inflammatory pulp exposure.

Clinical Application

The high density of nerves in the dental pulp has been reported to function in the transmission of nociceptive stimuli (pain) and in regulating the response of the odontoblast and pulp to trauma. Various investigators have shown that mitotic activity and reparative dentinogenesis can be altered when the sensory or postganglionic sympathetic nerves are resected. The nervous system has also been reported to modulate immunologic responses in various tissues. The regulation of vascular tone by the postganglionic sympathetic nerves is also important in maintaining interstitial fluid pressure in the pulp as well as in modulating the response of the nociceptive nerve terminals within the dental pulp.

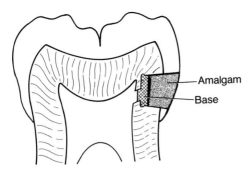

Figure 16–34. Diagram of cavity preparation and exposure of pulp.

Amalgam
Base

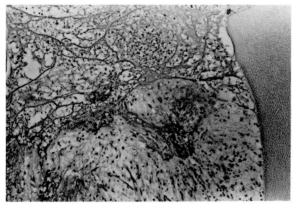

Figure 16–35. Pulp exposure with blood clot after 2 days.

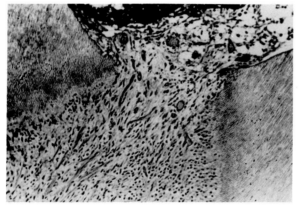

Figure 16–36. Pulp exposure in rhesus monkey after 4 days. Observe granulation tissue near exposure site.

Clinical Application

Today, individuals retain their teeth for long periods of time. Periodontal disease is currently prevalent. The gingiva and epithelial attachment migrate down the root surface of the teeth, exposing the cementum and root dentin, resulting in an increased of root caries. Root odontoblasts have recently been reported to respond to root caries in the aging pulp in a manner similar to coronal odontoblasts, except that it takes longer to initiate reparative dentinogenesis and to complete the reparative process.

inflammatory response. The junctional complexes between adjacent odontoblasts are disrupted, allowing an influx of ionic calcium from the extracellular dentinal fluid into the injured odontoblast, and possibly from intracellular sequestration because of injury, causing disruption of gap-junctional complexes. The intercellular spaces become filled with fluid and proteins derived from the plasma leaking from the permeable capillaries, effectively preventing intercellular communication. Concomitantly, the clotting cascade is initiated, decreasing the permeability of the dentin and preventing further ingress of irritants into the dental pulp. Within 1 day, in shallow cavity preparations, the odontoblasts reorganize and re-establish their plasma membranes that were damaged during the operative procedure. These odontoblasts begin to secrete collagen and other extracellular matrix components in an attempt to repair the damage effectively. However, at 3 days, their metabolic functions are not synchronous because the tight- and gap-junctional complexes have not been re-established between adjacent cells. At 5 days after the initial trauma, the gap junctions and tight-junctional complexes re-establish, and reparative dentinogenesis has reached the point where the amount of extracellular matrix produced by the odontoblasts begins to decrease. By 14 days, the inflammatory response is resolved, the odontoblast cell layer is re-established, and reparative dentinogenesis and new collagen formation are diminished to the level of the controls.

Immediate Pulp Exposure and Direct Pulp Capping

Numerous studies have demonstrated that the dental pulp has an inherent capacity to respond to wounding in the absence of other inflammatory insults (Fig. 16–34). Experimental evidence has shown that using clinically acceptable criteria, an uninflamed and exposed dental pulp will form a dentin bridge by 2 weeks in a human and by 9 days in the monkey.

When an experimental pulp exposure is completed in a previously healthy tooth, portions of the odontoblast layer and underlying cell-free and cell-rich layers and pulp proper are destroyed. Nerves and blood vessels are cut and extravasation of erythrocytes and plasma causes tissue edema and increased interstitial pressure in the surrounding pulp tissue. At 2 days after pulp capping with a calcium hydroxide containing medicament and restoration to the surface, the exposure site contains a clot composed of fibrin, platelets, and red blood cells (Fig. 16–35). Some polymorphonuclear leukocytes migrate from the blood vessels into the reorganizing pulp proper surrounding the exposure site. Fibroblasts begin to migrate into the periphery of the subjacent injured pulp (Fig. 16–36). The clot begins to reorganize. The previously terminally injured odontoblasts have completely degenerated whereas the adjacent uninjured pulp appears normal.

By 5 days after pulp exposure, the clot has been phagocytosed and stellate-shaped fibroblasts can be seen migrating into the injured area along the axial walls of the cut dentin and in the area below the exposure site (Fig. 16–37). Neoangiogenesis and a predominance of fibroblasts describe the granulation tissue occupying the wound site. Pulp tissue can be seen adjacent to the overlying medicament. Late in this stage of pulpal healing, the fibroblasts become oriented parallel to the medicament interface.

At 7 to 9 days, the fibroblasts begin to enlarge and polarize with their nucleus oriented basally (Fig. 16–38). These odontoblastlike cells then reorganize perpendicular to the pulp-capping material. By 12 days, the cells have deposited and mineralized the secreted extracellular matrix, reparative dentin (Fig. 16–39). As reparative dentin formation continues the tissue begins to resemble normal circumpulpal dentin and contains odontoblast processes. Ths process continues until healing has been completed.

The clinical success of direct pulp capping depends on several factors including prevention of bacteria and bacterial products from entering the pulp during the operative procedures. Successful treatment includes the formation of a permanent dentinal bridge by replacement odontoblasts that act, along with the restorative material, to prevent leakage of oral contaminants from affecting the pulp. The formation of a dentinal bridge is similar to reparative dentin formation under a cavity preparation or in the pulp horns resulting from occlusal attrition or trauma.

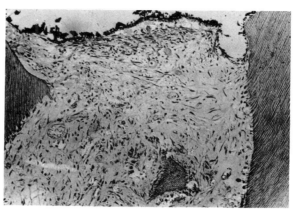

Figure 16–37. Pulp exposure, granulation tissue, and pulp growth into exposure site in rhesus monkey after 5 days.

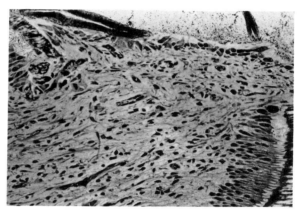

Figure 16–38. Pulp exposure after 9 days. Note organization of cells along the exposure site.

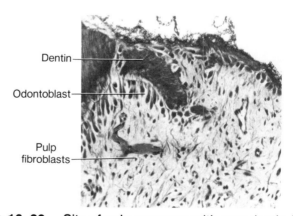

Figure 16–39. Site of pulp exposure with new dentin formation after 12 days.

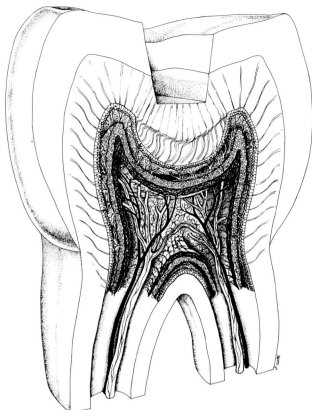

Figure 16–40. Summary of diagram of cavity preparation with underlying reparative dentin. Pulp organization with odontoblasts, cell-free and cell-rich zones, and parietal layer of nerves. Large myelinated nerve trunks appear in the central pulp and nonmyelinated nerves appear on vessel walls.

Summary

The dental pulp consists of a loose connective tissue enclosed by rigid predentin and dentin lining the coronal and radicular pulp. The most peripheral aspect of the dental pulp contains four layers of cells including the odontoblast layer, the cell-free zone, the cell-rich zone, and the parietal plexus of nerves. Deep within these four layers is the pulp proper, composed of fibroblasts and an extracellular matrix. The pulp is densely innervated with sensory and postganglionic sympathetic nerves. Some nerves are associated with maintenance of vascular tone whereas other nerves are associated with the conduction of nociceptive stimuli. The most dense innervation is in the pulp horns. Of the three theories of dentinal sensitivity, the hydrodynamic theory is the most viable. Arterioles, venules, and lymphatics vessels are also present. The pulp has an inherent capacity to respond to environmental as well as iatrogenic trauma resulting from restorative procedures by the upregulation of odontoblastic activity and the production, secretion, and subsequent mineralization of reparative dentin (Fig. 16–40).

Self-Evaluation Review

1. What embryonic cell layer gives rise to odontoblasts?
2. Describe and discuss the junctional complexes between odontoblasts.
3. Discuss the pulpal fibroblast and how it functions during maintenance and repair of the dental pulp.
4. What vascular structures are important in reducing interstitial pressure during pulpal injury?
5. Which pulpal nerves function in maintenance of vascular tone? How are pulpal capillaries controlled?
6. Which theory of pain transmission through dentin is the most popular? Give reasons to support your answer.
7. Discuss inflammation in the dental pulp, including the types of cells and sequence of events leading to pulpal healing.
8. Describe the aging process in the dental pulp.
9. Name three neurotransmitters found in the dental pulp and give their functions.
10. Compare and contrast the extracellular matrix of predentin and dentin.

Suggested Readings

Avery JK, Chiego DJ Jr. Cholinergic system and the dental pulp. In: Inoki R, Kudo T, Olgart LM, eds. Dynamic Aspects of the Dental Pulp—Molecular Biology, Pharmacology and Pathophysiology New York: Chapman Hall; 1990:297–332.

Avery JK, Cox CF, Chiego DJ Jr. The ultrastructure and physiology of dentin. In: Linde A, ed. *Dentin and Dentinogenesis.* Cleveland, Ohio:CRC Press; 1984:19–46.

Avery JK, Cox CF, Chiego DJ Jr. Presence and location of adrenergic nerve endings in the dental pulps of mice. *Anat Rec.* 1980; 198:59–71.

Byers MR, Neuhaus SJ, Gehrig JD. Dental sensory receptor structure in human teeth. *Pain.* 1982;13:221–235.

Chiego DJ Jr. An ultrastructural and autoradiographic analysis of primary and replacement odontoblasts following cavity preparation and wound healing in the rat molar. *Proc. Finn. Dent. Soc.* 1993;88:243.

Chiego DJ Jr, Fisher MA, Klein RM, Avery JK. Effects of denervation on 3H-fucose incorporation by odontoblasts in the mouse incisor. *Cell Tiss. Res.* 1983;230:197–203.

Chiego DJ Jr, Klein RM, Avery JK, Gruhl IM. Denervation induced changes in cell proliferation in the rat molar after wounding. *Anat Rec.* 1986;214:348–352.

Chiego DJ Jr, Klein RM, Avery JK. Neuroregulation of protein synthesis in odontoblasts of the first molar of the rat after wounding. *Cell Tiss. Res.* 1987;248:119–123.

Chiego DJ Jr. Cox CF, Avery JK. H3-HRP analysis of the nerve supply to primate teeth. *J Dent Res.* 1980;59:736–744.

Chiego DJ Jr, Klein RM, Avery JK. Tritiated thymidine autoradiographic study of the effects of inferior alveolar nerve resection on the proliferative compartments of the mouse incisors formative tissues. *Arch Oral Biol.* 1981;26:83–89.

Contos JG, Corcoran JF, LaTurno SA, Chiego DJ Jr, Regezi JA. Langerhans cells in apical periodontal cysts. *J Endodont.* 1987;13:52–55.

Fitzgerald M, Chiego DJ Jr, Heys DR. Autoradiographic analysis of odontoblast replacement following pulp exposure in primate teeth. *Arch Oral Biol.* 1990;35:707–715.

Heys DR, Fitzgerald M, Heys RJ, Chiego DJ Jr. Healing of primate dental pulps capped with Teflon. *Oral Surg Oral Med Oral Pathol.* 1990;69:227–237.

Holland GR. Lanthanum hydroxide labeling of gap junctions in the odontoblast layer. *Anat Rec.* 1976;186:211–216.

Inoki R, Kudo T, Olgart LM, eds. *Dynamic Aspects of Dental Pulp: Molecular Biology, Pharmacology and Pathophysiology.* New York, NY: Chapman Hall; 1990.

Linde A, ed. *Dentin and Dentinogenesis.* Vol. I and II. Boca Raton, Fla: CRC Press; 1984.

Kim S. Regulation of pulpal blood flow. *J Dent Res.* 1985;65:602–606.

Klein RM, Chiego, DJ Jr, and Avery JK. Effects of chemical sympathectomy on cell proliferation in the progenitive comparment of the neonatal mouse incisor.. *Arch Oral Biol.* 1981;26:319–325.

Pashley DH. Dentin-predentin complex and its permeability: physiological overview. *J Dent Res.* 1985;64:613–620.

Rutherford RB, Wahle J, Tucker M, Rueger D, Charette M. Induction of reparative dentine formation in monkeys by recombinant human osteogenic protein-1. *Arch Oral Biol.* 1993;38:571–576.

Turner DF, Marfurt CF, Sattelberg C. Demonstration of physiological barrier between pulpal odontoblasts and its perturbation following routine restorative procedures: a horseradish peroxidase tracking study in the rat. *J Dent Res.* 1989;68:1262–1268.

Ushiyama J. Gap junctions between odontoblasts revealed by transjunctional flux of fluorescent tracers. *Cell Tissue Res.* 1989; 258:611–616.

Comparison of Primary and Permanent Teeth

David C. Johnsen

Introduction

A comparison of the morphology and histology of primary and permanent teeth is important, as they differ in a number of ways. Clinical problems in the developing jaw of the growing child, as compared with the jaw in the adult, are related to characteristics of developing primary and permanent teeth and their supporting structures. As described in Chapter 7, there are differences in the number of teeth; there are 20 in the primary dentition and 32 in the permanent dentition. As also discussed previously, the anterior 20 permanent teeth replace the primary dentition and are thus defined as successional. These teeth are closely related in the timing of their exfoliation and in the development of the successional dentition. The remaining 12 permanent teeth develop posterior to the 20 primary teeth as the jaws continue to grow in length (Fig. 17-1). Both primary and permanent teeth proceed through the same stages of development. This chapter describes differences in tooth size, shape of crowns, roots, and pulp chambers, the microscopic structure of enamel and dentin, as well as interdental spacing, tooth inclination, and arch shape.

Objectives

After reading this chapter you should be able to discuss the similarities and differences between primary and permanent teeth and to describe how these characteristics relate to clinical treatment.

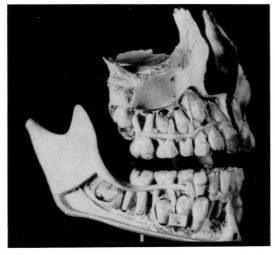

Figure 17-1. Mixed dentition period as seen in the cadaver specimen of a child about 9 years of age.

Root Resorption and Pulp Degeneration

Another major difference between primary and permanent teeth is that the roots of primary teeth normally resorb (fig. 17–24). The process occurs simultaneously with the eruption of the permanent teeth. In the absence of a permanent tooth, primary tooth resorption still occurs, but it occurs much more slowly. The primary tooth roots have a higher susceptibility to resorption than do permanent teeth. The primary tooth roots have pressure from the permanent tooth exerted on their roots, but this is not the total cause of this susceptibility to resorption. As stated previously, even when a permanent tooth is missing, the primary tooth roots will gradually resorb. The process of resorption is accompanied by gradual changes in the pulp. Figures 17–25 and 17–26 show the pulp during root resorption. The first sign is reduction in the number of cells in the pulp; nerve trunks degenerate into patches of myelin, and some fibrosis occurs. Blood vessels remain until the tooth is exfoliated.

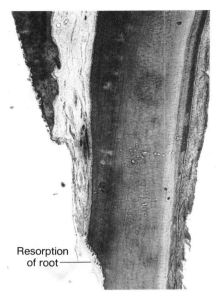

Figure 17–25. Pulp changes during primary tooth root resorption. There is a reduction in cells, nerves, blood vessels, and various intercellular components.

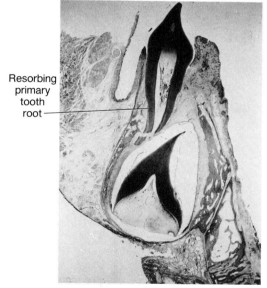

Figure 17–24. Relation between exfoliating primary tooth and erupting permanent crown.

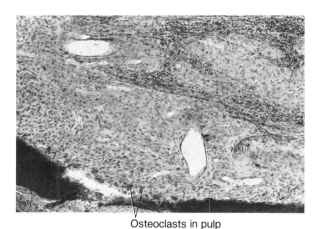

Figure 17–26. Histological appearance of root resorption by osteoclasts.

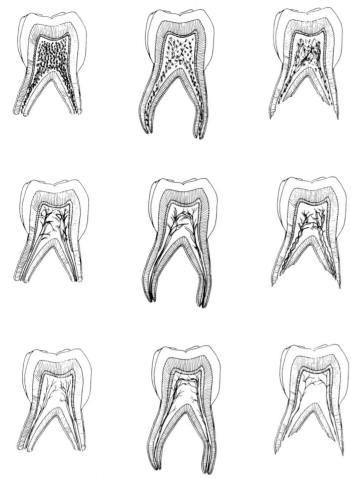

Figure 17–27. Pulp changes in life cycle of primary tooth. (A). Decrease in number of cells. (B). Development of vascular, and (C), development of and loss of nerves. At left is the root formation stage, center, root completion stage, and at right, root resorption stage.

Clinical Application

Primary and permanent teeth differ in their response to trauma. Although both have similar kinds of outcomes when a blow is struck, such as causing tooth fracture, the permanent tooth has an additional sequela. When the primary tooth is dislodged, the permanent tooth may be damaged sufficiently to cause enamel hypoplasia or white spots.

Cellular and fibrillar changes occur during the three phases in the root life of primary teeth: formation, completion, and resorption. During root formation, the young primary tooth pulp is highly cellular. As the roots are completed, fewer cells and more fibers are evident. The proliferation of fibers continues during the root resorption phase, and fiber bundles may be seen (Fig. 17–27).

The blood vessels that enter the pulp chamber through the forming roots are initially associated with the odontoblastic layer. They will later form a subodontoblastic network. As the roots are resorbed, these blood vessels exhibit some degenerative changes, although most are maintained until the tooth is lost.

Nerve fibers gradually organize in the pulp chamber of the primary tooth. As the tooth reaches occlusion, the nerve fibers form a plexus underlying the odontoblastic layer; this plexus is termed the *parietal layer of nerve fibers*. These nerve fibers are lost during resorption of the primary tooth roots, which makes teeth insensitive to pulpal pain at the time of exfoliation.

The periodontal support of primary and permanent teeth is similar in basic architecture. Healthy gingiva of permanent teeth has been observed to be redder than the gingiva around primary teeth.

Sequela to Injuries

The differences between permanent and primary teeth extend to the area of dental trauma. Primary and permanent teeth differ in their response to trauma in one clinically significant aspect. Although both primary and permanent teeth can have similar kinds of outcomes when struck (fracture of the tooth, fracture of the crown, dislodgement of the tooth, etc.), the permanent tooth has the additional sequelae of the indirect effect of a blow to the primary tooth. Early in enamel formation, there can be interruption of the enamel formation in the form of a mark on the tooth at the point where the root tip of the primary tooth strikes the facial surface of the developing permanent tooth crown. The clinical appearance can be a "white spot" or a frank enamel hypoplasia. Intrusion of the primary tooth can also displace the developing crown of the permanent tooth before root formation. The reason for the relative ease of displacement of the crown before root formation is that there is no ligament to stabilize the position of the permanent tooth crown. Once root formation begins, the periodontal ligament has a stabilizing effect on the orientation of the tooth. Once the permanent tooth crown is rotated in its sac, the permanent tooth root continues to develop in its original orientation. The result is a disfigured angulation (or dilaceration) between the crown and root of the permanent tooth. Recognition of such disfigurements resulting from trauma can lead to clearer planning for treatment for the affected tooth.

Susceptibility to Enamel Defects

Enamel of primary and permanent teeth differ in their susceptibility to tooth defects. The greater susceptibility of the enamel from permanent teeth to hypomineralization is associated with the different environment for the tooth after birth. Permanent teeth are more susceptible to hypomineralization or "white spot" defects. Although the teeth are not at increased risk for dental caries or abrasion, there can be aesthetic concers. Inference has been made to the apparent incresed prevalence of white-spot lesions of incisors to the increased use of fluorides from multiple sources. It is interesting that the defects for the permanent teeth are located in the outer portions of the tooth enamel. Removal of the outer portion of enamel, either mechanically or with inorganic acid, can result in removal of the "white-spot" lesion. The technique has been described as microabrasion. Primary teeth, on the other hand, form for the most part before birth and in relative isolation from the mother. Primary teeth are therefore less likely to have defects unless there is a significant systemic insult affecting the unborn child.

Clinical Application

Enamels of primary and permanent teeth differ in their susceptibility to tooth defects. The permanent teeth are more susceptible to hypomineralization or "white spots" than are primary teeth. Because these defects are in the outer enamel they can be removed by mechanically or by inorganic acid. This is known as microabrasion.

Summary

For the practitioner, primary and permanent teeth have several significant gross differences. Primary teeth are fewer and smaller in all dimensions that are their successors, with one exception. Primary molars have a greater mesiodistal dimension than do succeeding premolars. Primary tooth crowns have a short and thick-set apperance and exhibit contour, especially near the cervical region. Primary molars form line contacts, whereas permanent molars form point contacts. Although primary and permanent teeth have similar processes of tissue formation, primary teeth take less time to form than do permanent teeth. Enamel and dentin are thinner in primary teeth than in permanent teeth. Primary tooth enamel is more opaque than permanent tooth enamel and has a neonatal line. Surface enamel is more likely to be prismless in primary than permanent teeth; however, much variability occurs in primary teeth, from tooth to tooth and for different sites on the same tooth. Tooth pulps of primary molars are relatively large in the coronal portion and become ribbonlike to accommodate to the flat roots (Fig. 17–28).

Primary and permanent dentitions have several differences that influence tooth alignment in the arch. Interdental spacing is greater in the primary than the permanent dentition. Primary anterior teeth are more upright than the more labially inclined permanent anterior teeth. Arch shape in primary and permanent teeth is similar in the anterior portion, but the permanent dentition extends further posteriorly.

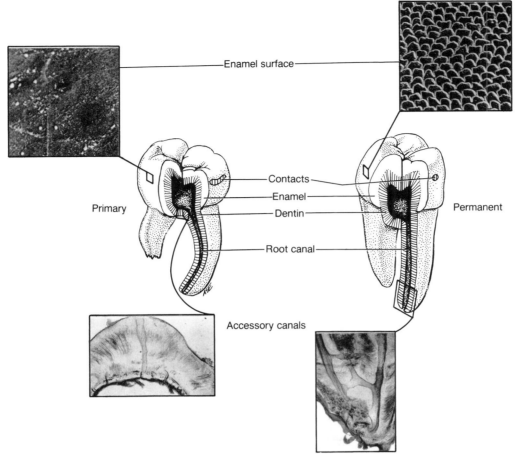

Figure 17-28. Summary comparison of primary and permanent teeth. Enamel thickness, enamel surface characteristics, contact points, dentin hardness, pulp size, root canal and root curvature, and location of accessory canals.

Self-Evaluation Review

1. State differences in shape between the root canals of primary and permanent molars and the potential clinical significance.
2. Describe the difference in duration of tooth tissue formation between the primary and permanent dentitions.
3. State the differences in the enamel and dentin thicknesses of primary and permanent teeth.
4. Discuss the differences between the enamel surfaces of the primary and permanent teeth, and the potential clinical significance of these differences.
5. Explain the potential effect on the permanent tooth as a result of trauma to the primary tooth.
6. State differences and similarities of dentin hardness at various depths for primary and permanent teeth.
7. State differences in the sites of accessory canals in primary and permanent molars.

8. Discuss the clinical significance of crown contour, pulp size, and shape in the preparation of an interproximal cavity in a primary and permanent first molar.
9. State four principal factors that influence tooth alignment in the arches of primary and permanent dentitions.
10. Define "incisor liability" and "leeway space." State the clinical significance of each.

Acknowledgments

Figure 17–6 is provided courtesy of Joe Camp, DDS. Figures 17–7 and 17–21 are provided courtesy of David Scott, DDS, and Figue 17–11 is provided courtesy of Rod Owen, DDS.

Suggested Readings

Avery JK. A possible mechanism of pain conduction in teeth. *Ann Histochem.* 1963:59–64.

Croll TP. Enamel microabrasion for removal of superficial dysmineralization and decalcification defects. *J Am Dent Assoc.* 1990;120:411–415.

Enlow DH. *Handbook of Facial Growth.* Philadelphia, Pa: WB Saunders, 1975.

Gutmann Jr. Prevalence, location and patency of accessory canals in the furcation region of permanent molars. *J. Periodontics,* 1978:21–26.

Johnsen DC, Johns S. Quantitation of nerve fibers in the primary and permanent canine and incisor teeth in man. *Arch Oral Biol.* 1978;23:825.

Karus BS, Jordan RE. *The Human Dentition Before Birth.* Philadelphia, Pa: Lea & Febinger; 1965.

Pinkham JR. *Pediatric Dentistry.* Philadelphia, Pa: WB Saunders; 1994.

Rapp R, Avery JK, Strachan DS. The distribution of nerves in human primary teeth. *Anat Rec.* 1967;159:89–103.

Wheeler RC. *A Textbook of Dental Anatomy and Physiology.* 4th ed. Philadelphia, Pa: WB Saunders; 1965.

Yoshida H, Yakushijim, Sugihara A, Tanaka K, Taguchi M, Machida Y. Accessory canals at floor of the pulp chamber of primary molars. *J Tokyo Dent Coll Soc.* 1975;580–585.

SECTION V

Structure of the Soft Tissues

CHAPTERS 18–23

18

Histology of the Oral Mucosa and Tonsils

Donald S. Strachan

Introduction

The oral mucosa consists of two layers: an epithelium (stratified squamous epithelium) and an underlying layer of connective tissue, which is the lamina propria. Mucosa forms the lining of the oral cavity and shows regional modifications corresponding to functional needs. The palate and gingiva function in mastication and are kertinized. The dorsal (superior) surface of the tongue relative to its taste and masticatory functions is specialized. Epithelium of the tongue is also keratinized, and there are numerous taste buds located in this epithelium. The remainder of the oral mucosa functions as a lining. The epithelium of the oral cavity is continually being replaced by basal cells that divide, migrate to the surface, and eventually are worn off during normal function of speech and mastication. Beneath select areas of the oral mucosa is a loose connective tissue, the submucosa.

The tonsils are found posterior to the oral and nasal cavities and form a ring of tonsillar tissue in this area. There are three tonsils: palatine, pharyngeal, and lingual. All contain lymphatic tissue and function in the production of lymphocytes, which are important in processing antigens for the production of immunocompetent T-cell and B-cell lymphocytes for the immune system.

Objectives

After reading this chapter you should be able to discuss the following material by: (1) describing the structure and function of the various types of oral mucosa with a detailed description of the keratinocytes and the nonkeratinocytes; (2) explain how epithelial cells can be replaced (turnover) and understand the basic process of keratinization; (3) identify and describe the various papillae of the tongue; and describe the morphology of the three types of tonsils and discuss the functions of the tonsils.

Development and Structure of Oral Epithelium

The epithelium of the oral cavity is derived from the embryonic ectoderm and is stratified squamous throughout. As is true of stratified squamous epithelium elsewhere, the cells vary from cuboidal or low columnar at the connective tissue interface to flat squamous cells at the surface. Most of the mucosal surfaces of the oral cavity is lined by a nonkeratinized stratified squamous epithelium, except for the gingiva, hard palate, and dorsal surface of the tongue, where the epithelium is keratinized. From the underlying connective tissue of the lamina propria to the surface, the four layers in the nonkeratinized epithelium are: stratum basale (basal layer), stratum spinosum, stratum intermedium (intermediate layer), and stratum superficiale (superficial layer). In keratinized epithelium there are also four layers (strata). The first two layers are the same as nonkeratinized epithelium (stratum basale and stratum spinosum), and the next two layers are stratum granulosum (granular layer) and stratum corneum (keratinized layer) (Fig. 18–1). Four layers of the epithelium can be clearly seen at the ultrastructural level in Figure 18–2.

Stratum Basale

The cells of the stratum basale are cuboidal or low columnar and form a single layer of cells resting on the basal lamina at the interface of the epithelium and lamina propria (Figs. 18–2 and 18–3). The epithelia of the oral mucosa are in a contant state of renewal, and the basal cells show the most mitotic activity.

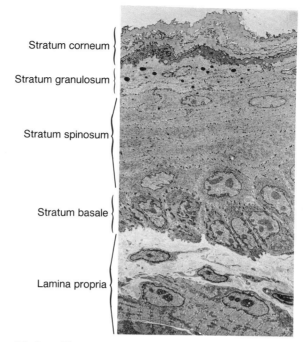

Figure 18–2. Electron micrograph of keratinized oral mucosa.

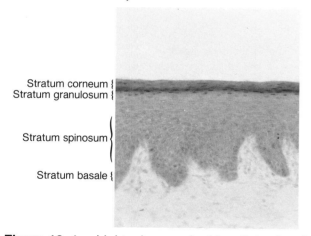

Figure 18–1. Light micrograph of keratinized oral mucosa. The lamina propria is below the stratum basale.

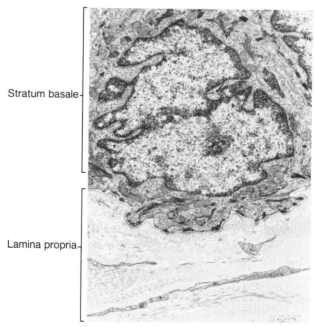

Figure 18–3. Stratum basale cell. Note the interface with connective tissue of the lamina propria.

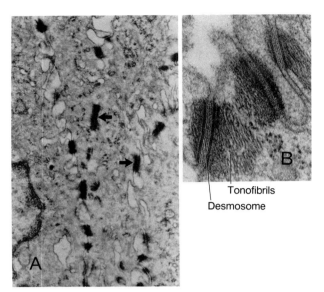

Figure 18-4. (A). Cell-to-cell junctions between epithelial cells. These are termed desmosomes (arrows). (B). Desmosomes under high magnification. These are adhesion discs between plasma membranes. Desmosomes are anchored by tonofilaments located in the cell.

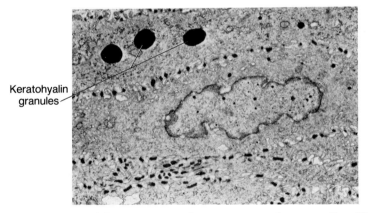

Figure 18-5. Ultrastructure of stratum granulosum cells with keratohyalin granules.

Clinical Application

For the clinician, astute observation and interpretation of the status of the oral mucosa and the tongue have long been known to give a sensitive diagnosis of systemic disease and nutritional deficiencies. The oral mucosa can change in relation to smoking, age, disease, and various other factors.

Stratum Spinosum

The stratum spinosum usually is several cells thick and mitotic figures can occasionally be seen in the layer adjacent to the basal cell layer. The stratum basale and the first layer(s) of the stratum spinosum are sometimes referred to as the *stratum germinativum*. This zone gives rise to new epithelial cells. The cells of the stratum spinosum are shaped like a polyhedron, with short cytoplasmic processes. At the point where the processes of neighboring cells meet, mechanical adhesions (desmosomes) coupling the cells together can be seen (Fig. 18-4). Under the light microscope, the normal appearance of these stratum spinosum cells usually is accentuated by shrinkage artifacts produced during routine fixation, staining, and mounting. This has caused some observers to refer to this layer as the prickle-cell layer (Fig. 18-2). These cells have an abundance of intracytoplasmic fibrils (tonofibrils) that project toward and attach to the desmosomes (Fig. 18-4). In the upper layers of the stratum spinosum, the cells contain a unique cytoplasmic inclusion in the form of dense spherical granules (Fig. 18-5). Because of the intimate association of these granules with the cell membrane, they are often referred to as membrane-coating granules. These granules fuse with the cytoplasmic membrane of the cell and exteriorize their contents into the intercellular spaces. Morphological differences have been shown between the membrane-coating granules in keratinized and in nonkeratinized epithelium. The precise nature and function of these granules is not yet known.

Stratum Granulosum

The cells of the stratum granulosum layer are flat and stacked in a layer three to five cells thick. This layer is prominent in keratinized epithelium but deficient or nonexistent in nonkeratinized epithelium. The cells of this layer have many dense, relatively large (0.5 to 1 μm) keratohyaline granules in their cytoplasm. Many microfilaments are in close association with these granules (Fig. 18-5). Viewed under the light micrscope the granules are basophilic (blue with a hematoxylin stain), and viewed under the electron microscope they are dense (appearing black). They are closely associated with ribosomes. There are many microfilaments throughout the cells of this layer. The keratohyaline granules help to form the matrix for the numerous keratin fibers found in the superficial layers. Recently, many studies have shown great heterogenity in the types of cytokeratins synthesized in the oral epithelium of various locations. Variations in the cytokeratin patterns have been shown in pathologically changed oral mucosa. Some 27 cytokeratins have been identified.

Stratum Corneum

The junction between the nucleated cells in the stratum granulosum and the superficial layer of keratinized cells (stratum corneum) is abrupt, as can be seen in Figure 18–6. The cells of the stratum corneum are very flat, devoid of nuclei, and full of keratin filaments surrounded by a matrix. Figure 18–7 shows the abrupt change between the stratum corneum (above, only four cell layers thick in this figure) and a stratum granulosum cell (below). Note the interdigitation between cells in this electron micrograph. Greater magnification of two adjacent cells in the stratum corneum (Fig. 18–8) shows the abundance of keratin fibers throughout these cells.

The cells of the stratum corneum are squamous (flat), and superficially have various shapes. These surface cells are continually being sloughed and are replaced by the continual migration of cells from the underlying layers. Figure 18–9 shows the surface of the stratified squamous epithelium of the hard palate; the boundaries between cells are prominent and the surface of the cells appears pitted.

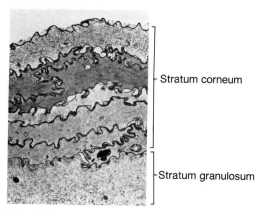

Figure 18–7. Ultrastructure of stratum corneum with interdigitation between cells.

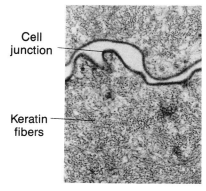

Figure 18–8. Ultrastructure of stratum corneum. Note the cell junctions and keratin fibers.

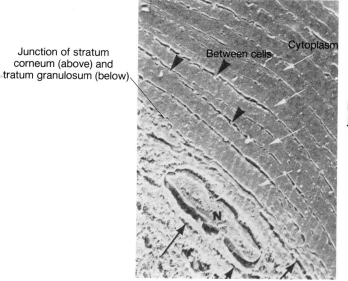

Figure 18–6. Ultrastructure of cells of stratum corneum (black arrows). Spaces between cells (black arrowheads) and cell cytoplasm (white arrows) in cells of stratum corneum. N, nucleus.

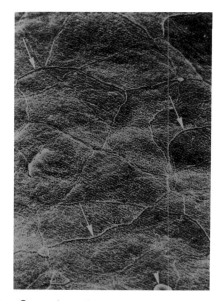

Figure 18–9. Scanning electron micrograph of surface view of epithelial cells. Note the cell junctions (arrows).

Turnover of Oral Epithelium

Consistent with the day-to-day function of the oral epithelium and the histological description presented previously, there is a high turnover rate of the cells of the oral epithelium. The concept of cells undergoing mitosis in the basal cell layer and eventually migrating to the free surface is sometimes difficult to appreciate on a static diagram or histological slide. The dynamic nature of this epithelium is best appreciated when the cells are labeled experimentally with radioactive thymidine, which "tags" DNA at synthesis. With sampling of tissue at various times, the labeling substance appears first in the basal cell layer and later in the stratum corneum (Fig. 18–10). The technique used to view the labeled DNA is termed radioautography. Different areas of the oral epithelium change at varying rates. Sulcular epithelium takes 10 days to renew, whereas the general oral mucosa takes approximately 12–13 days. The basal cells move away from the basal layer perpendicularly and toward the surface of the epithelium.

Functional Characteristics

The surface of stratified squamous epithelium, depending on the location and functional requirements of the oral mucosa, has various characteristics. As the cells migrate from the basal cell layer to the surface layer, differentiation produces a surface layer that is either keratinized, parakeratinized, or nonkeratinized.

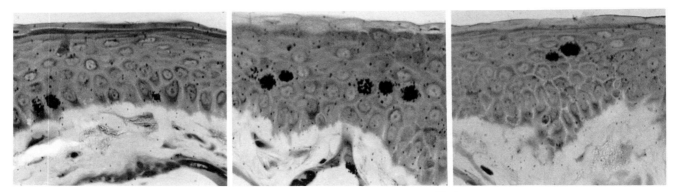

Figure 18–10. Turnover of epithelial cells revealed by |³H|thymidine labeling.

Keratinized

As described previously, the keratinized surface results when the cells have lost their nuclei and the cytoplasm has been displaced by large numbers of the keratin filaments. This surface can only be present where there is a well-defined *stratum granulosum*. The surface of the gingiva and palate is usually of the keratinized type, as it is associated with "masticatory function" (Fig. 18–11).

Parakeratinized

In perakeratinized epithelium, the surface cells have dark-staining pyknotic nuclei and the cytoplasm contains little if any keratin filaments. The stratum corneum and stratum granulosum are not found in parakeratinized epithelium. Like nonkeratinized epithelium, the keratinized epithelium is composed of four layers. Usually, this epithelium is associated with the gingiva (Fig. 18–11).

Nonkeratinized

In nonkeratinized epithelium, the surface cells retain their nuclei and the cytoplasm does not contain keratin filaments. The stratum corneum and granulosum is absent; this epithelium is composed of four layers (stratum basale, stratum spinosum, stratum intermedium, and stratum superficiale). This type of epithelium is associated with the "lining mucosa" in the oral cavity (Fig. 18–11).

Junction of Epithelium and Connective Tissue

The interface between the lamina propria and the epithelium is an interesting area (Fig. 18–12). Connective tissue, with its inductive properties, exerts control over the overlying epithelium. When viewed by light microscopy, the interface tissue termed the *basement membrane* can be observed. Electron microscopic magnification reveals the basement membrane to be composed of three parts: (1) the lamina lucida, which is less dense and is toward the epithelial side; (2) the lamina densa (basal lamina), the middle of the three parts; and (3) the lamina reticularis, which is less dense than the lamina densa and is located next to the lamina

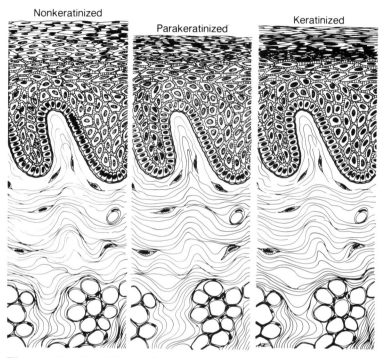

Figure 18–11. Illustration of three functional types of oral epithelium.

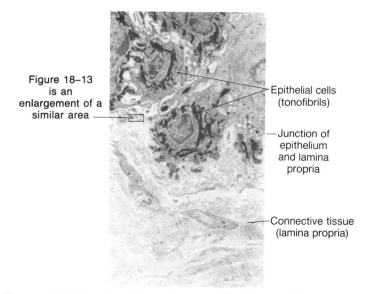

Figure 18–12. Junction of oral epithelium and connective tissue.

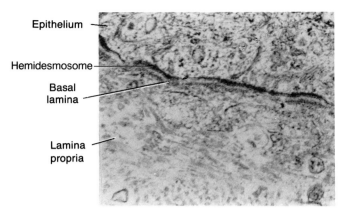

Figure 18–13. Junction of oral epithelium (above) and connective tissue (below) separated by basal lamina and hemidesmosomes.

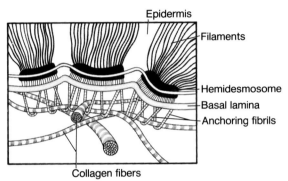

Figure 18–14. Diagram of hemidesmosome.

propria. Type IV collagen and laminin, a glycoprotein, are major components of the lamina densa. The lamina reticularis contains fine reticular fibers. Basal cells of the epithelium are not attached to the connective tissue proper, but rather, form mechanical adhesions with the basal lamina. These attachments are *hemidesmosomes* (Fig. 18–13). Hemidesmosomes are composed of an attachment plaque that possesses intracellular modifications of tonofilaments that penetrate the plasma membrane of the cell, which terminate in the basal lamina (Fig. 18–13 and 18–14). Fine collagen fibers attach to this lamina on the connective tissue side (Fig. 18–14). These fibers are anchoring fibers, composed of type VII collagen. This complex of fibers is found at intervals along the basal cell plasma membrane of the epithelial–connective tissue interface.

Lamina Propria

The lamina propria is the connective tissue layer immediately below the epithelium (Fig. 18–13), which can be divided into the papillary layer and reticular layer. In the papillary layer, fingerlike projections of connective tissue extend into the deep surface of the epithelium (Fig. 18–15). The length of the papillae varies with location and functional requirements. An increase in the number and length of the papillae is seen in areas where mechanical adhesion between the epithelium and lamina propria is required (masticatory mucosa). In areas of lining mucosa, the reticular or subpapillary layer predominates (Fig. 18–15). The blood supply

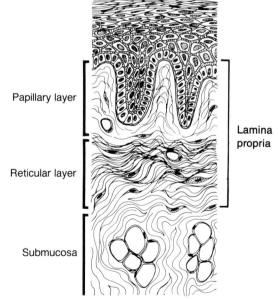

Figure 18–15. The lamina propria consists of the papillary layer and reticular layer, below which is the submucosa.

The blood supply consists of a deep plexus of large vessels in the submucosa, which gives rise to a secondary plexus in the papillary layer of the lamina propria. Capillary loops extend into the connective tissue papillae. The epithelium is avascular; therefore, its metabolic needs must come via the vessels of the lamina propria. The amino acids, peptides, carbohydrates, lipids, inorganic compounds, and salts required for the nutrition of the epithelium diffuse from the capillary beds through the connective tissue and basement membrane to enter the epithelium. In addition to the fibroblasts, cells of blood vessels and lymphatics (endothelial, pericytes, and smooth muscle cells), and nerves (Schwann cells), many other cells are found in the lamina propria. Some of these cells are normal residents and others are present because of inflammation or trauma. Mast cells, macrophages, fat cells, plasma cells, eosinophils, undifferentiated cells, and other cells can be found in this tissue. Lymphocytes are a common cell found in the lamina propria of the gingiva. Lymphocytes are also found many times in the epithelium itself, presumedly in transit to the surface.

Submucosa

In most areas of the mouth the submucosa is absent or limited and serves primarily as an attachment for the lamina propria to the underlying bone or skeletal muscle. Like the lamina propria, the submucosa is a connective tissue compartment composed of cells and intercellular elements. The submucosa is found in the cheeks, lips, and parts of the palate, and is a less dense component than the lamina propria. It functions in nutrition and defense, containing numerous large blood vessels, nerves, and lymphatics. The submucosa is also the site containing adipose tissue and minor salivary glands in the oral cavity (Fig. 18–16 and 18–17). In the bony areas with no submucosa, fibers of the lamina propria attach tightly to bone. The mucosa and lamina propria in these areas is generally referred to as a mucoperiosteum.

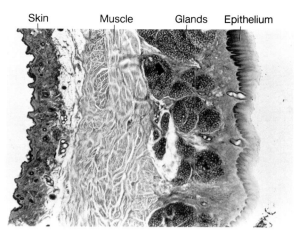

Figure 18–16. Full thickness of cheek. Skin is on the left; oral mucosa is on the right.

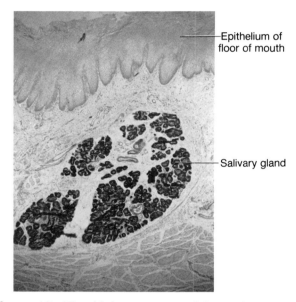

Figure 18–17. Lining mucosa of floor of mouth.

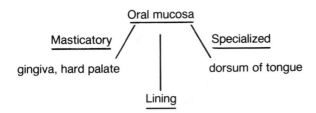

Figure 18–18. Classification of oral mucosa.

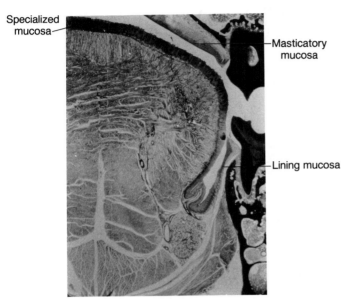

Figure 18–19. Cross section of tongue. Note the lining mucosa below and beside the tongue, the specialized mucosa over it, and the masticatory mucosa in the palate.

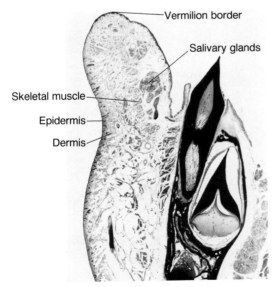

Figure 18–20. Lip with skin on outer surface and lining mucosa on inner surface.

Functional Types of Oral Mucosa

The three functional types of oral mucosa are the *lining* mucosa, *masticatory* mucosa, and *specialized* mucosa. These terms provide functional descriptions of the oral mucosa in specific locations (Fig. 18–18). Each type of oral mucosa can be recognized on visual inspection of the oral cavity. In Figure 18–19, a cross section through the molar area of the oral cavity, each of the three types of oral mucosa can be observed.

Lining Mucosa

The lining mucosa covers all soft tissues of the oral cavity except the gingiva, hard palate, and dorsal surface of the tongue. The epithelium is nonkeratinized stratified squamous epithelium, and the lamina propria contains the typical collagen, elastic, and reticular fibers found in other supporting connective tissues. These collagenous fibers are not as thick and tightly organized as the ones found in other types of oral mucosa. Lining mucosa is smooth and shiny. Oral epithelium is less pigmented than the epithelium of the skin and varies in color from light pink to darker pink or red. The hues are influenced by the underlying capillary network in relation to the free surface and by the amount of melanin pigment in the epithelial cells. The submucosa associated with most of the lining mucosa is loosely organized and allows for free mobility of the mucosa in relation to the underlying tissue.

Lip. Figure 18–20 is a microscopic section of the lip in which the following structures can be identified: skin with hair follicles, sweat glands, mucous membrane, skeletal muscle, salivary glands, submucosa, and lamina propria. Near the inner surface of the lips and cheeks are many small salivary glands. Their ducts may be seen clinically by everting the lip and drying the surface. Small droplets of saliva will eventually be visible.

Vermilion Border. The junction between the skin and mucous membrane is known as the vermilion border, which is apparent where the epithelium changes from the keratinized stratified squamous epithelium of the skin to the moist stratified squamous epithelium of the oral cavity. The epithelium is thin, especially where the connective tissue papillae are close to the surface (Fig. 18–21). The red blood cells in the capillaries show through the thin epithelium, contributing to the vermilion color. Note the ink-injected specimen (Fig. 18–22). The thin epithelium in this region contains a protein, *eleidin*, which is more transparent than the protein *keratin*. The appearance of the vermilion border is therefore due to several factors: (1) vascularized connective tissue papillae situated close to the surface; (2) the thin epithelium; and (3) the transparent nature of eleidin in the epithelium, revealing the vermilion color of the red blood cells.

Frequently, ectopic (out of place) sebaceious glands are seen in the vermilion border at the corners of the mouth or, more laterally, in the cheeks opposite the molar teeth. These are termed *Fordyce's spots*. The presence of sebaceous glands at these sites is considered normal and should not be construed as a pathologic entity (Fig. 18–23).

Soft Palate. The oral surface of the soft palate is covered by lining mucosa, which is more pink than the hard palate. This results from the highly vascularized lamina propria. A layer of elastic fibers separates the lamina propria from the underlining submucosa, the latter which contains both muscles and mucous glands. Above the muscles are mixed glands that underlie the respiratory epithelium of the nasal cavity (Fig. 18–24).

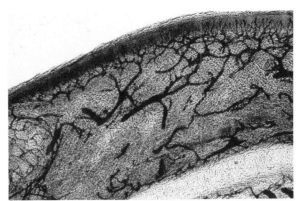

Figure 18–22. Blood vessels (injected) in connective tissue papillae of vermilion border of lip. This illustrates the close relation of the vasculature to the surface of the vermilion border.

Clinical Application

Infections are few after oral surgical procedures; scarring is almost absent; and the healing capacity of the oral mucosa is greater when compared with skin. Orthognathic surgery to move segments of the mandible and maxilla can be done from an intraoral approach to take advantage of these characteristics.

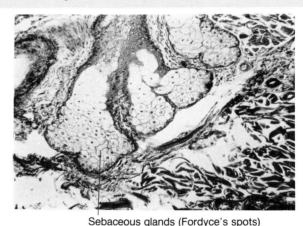

Sebaceous glands (Fordyce's spots)

Figure 18–23. Fordyce's spot (sebaceous gland) found at borders of mouth.

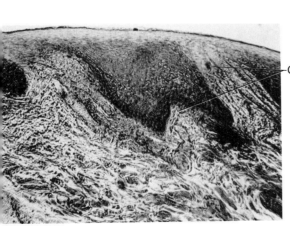

Connective tissue papillae

Figure 18–21. Vermilion border with its covering of clear eleidin.

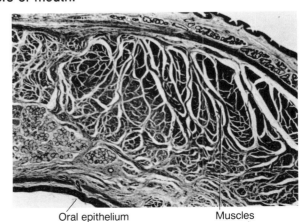

Oral epithelium   Muscles

Figure 18–24. Sagittal section of soft palate (anterior on the left). Note the muscle and glands in the submucosa. The respiratory epithelium of the nasal cavity is above.

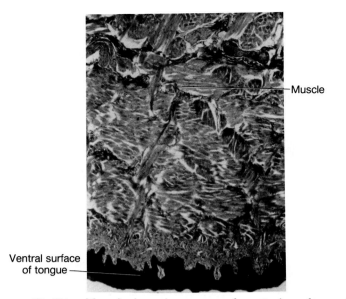

Figure 18–25. Muscle in submucosa of ventral surface of tongue.

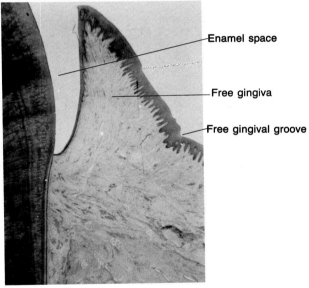

Figure 18–26. Boundary of gingiva. The enamel was lost during the decalcification process resulting in the enamel space.

Ventral Surface of the Tongue. This lining mucosa contains both a lamina propria and submucosa. The mucous membrane is smooth and thin with short but numerous connective tissue papillae. The submucosa is not clearly distinguishable, as it merges with the connective tissue that lies between the muscle bundles of the ventral tongue (Fig. 18–25).

Cheek. The lining mucosa of the cheek is stratified squamous and nonkeratinized epithelium. The underlying submucosa contains fat cells and small, mixed salivary glands intermingled with connective tissue fibers that bind the mucous membrane to the underlying musculature. The presence of these mixed glands lodged between the muscle bundles in the submucosa is a characteristic of the cheek (Fig. 18–16).

Floor of the Mouth. The mucous membrane of the floor of the mouth is thin and loosely attached to the underlying structures. The connective tissue papillae are short, and there is adipose tissue in the underlying submucosa as well as the sublingual mucous glands (Fig. 18–17).

Masticatory Mucosa

Masticatory mucosa covers the gingiva and hard palate. In an edentulous mouth, masticatory mucosa covers the chewing surfaces of the dental arches. The epithelium is keratinized or parakeratinized. The connective tissue of the lamina propria contains collagenous fibers that bind the epithelium tightly to the underlying bone and are thicker and more organized than those fibers in the lining mucosa.

Gingiva. The gingiva is more often parakeratinized than keratinized and has no submucosal layer. The attached gingiva is normally stippled. Keratinized epithelium of the gingiva is represented by a thin, dark-stained border that changes at the junction with the nonkeratinized surface of the alveolar mucosa (Fig. 18–26). This continues as the lining of the vestibule. The enamel was lost because of decalcification. The gingiva is discussed in more detail in Chapter 19.

Hard Palate. The oral surface of the hard palate is covered with masticatory mucosa. The epithelium is bound to the underlying bone in anterior regions of the palate by connective tissue. In the anterior lateral regions of the hard palate the submucosa contains fatty tissue. The lateral regions of the posterior parts contain the palatine glands, which extend posteriorly into the soft palate (Fig. 18–27). These glands are pure mucous glands containing only mucous acini. The glands associated with the lingual tonsil are the only other pure mucous glands associated with the oral cavity and the oropharynx. Although the surface of this mucosa appears to be uniform, it may be subdivided into several zones according to the nature of its submucosa. The midline of the hard palate is termed the *median raphe*. No submucosa is found in this area, and there is only dense fibrous attachment to the underlying bone (Fig. 18–28). This combination of epithelium and lamina propria is given the name *mucoperiosteum*. In the lateral regions of the palatal mucosa, both fatty and glandular tissue make up the submucosa.

Rugae appear in the anterior region of the hard palate, anterior to the *fatty* zones on either side of the midline. Rugae appear as a series of ridges running across the anterior palate (Fig. 18–27). They do not cross the midline but are easily seen and palpated, and can be felt with the tongue. In the midline, the papillae located about 1 cm posterior to the anterior incisors are the incisive papillae.

Three prominent palatal rugae appear in this sagittal section in Figure 18–29. Histologically, the palatal rugae are folds of epithelium that contain a dense connective tissue lamina propria. The connective tissue fibers pass directly from the papillary layer of the lamina propria into the underlying bone. These are termed *traction bands* which make the rugae immovable structures.

Figure 18–29 is a histological cross-section of the palate at low magnification. Note that in the *median raphe* bone underlies the mucosa, so that no submucosa is found. Thus,

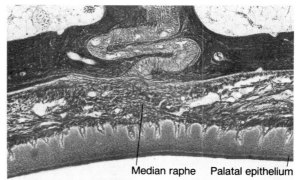

Figure 18–28. Median raphe. There is no submucosa along the median raphe.

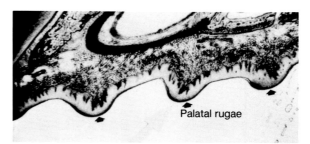

Figure 18–29. Rugae (arrows) of anterior palate, which are supported by connective tissue fibers.

Clinical Application

The integrity of the interface between the oral epithelium and the post that extends from osseointegrated implants will determine the longevity of the implant. Much of the science and therapy of periodontics is focused on the integrity of the interface between the gingiva and the tooth.

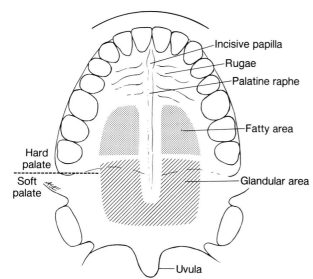

Figure 18–27. Diagram of regions of palate. Observe the location of the glandular and fatty zones.

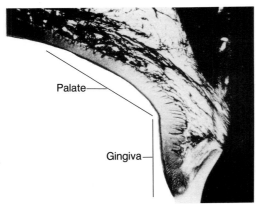

Figure 18–30. Lateral hard palate. There is no submucosa adjacent to the teeth.

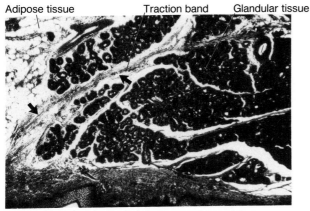

Figure 18–31. Hard palate, with junction of fatty zone on left and glandular zones on right. Arrows, traction band.

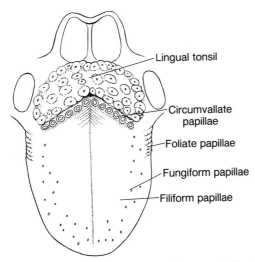

Figure 18–32. Diagram of tongue, with specialized mucosa shown on dorsum of tongue.

the dense lamina propria is directly attached to the underlying bone. This combination of epithelium and lamina propria is given the name *mucoperiosteum*. In the lateral regions of the palatal mucosa, both fatty and glandular tissue make up the submucosa.

Figure 18–30 is a view of the lateral region of the palate near the maxillary molar tooth. There is no submucosal layer adjacent to the teeth overlying the alveolar bone, and the fibers of the lamina propria of the palate and gingiva are continuous. Observe the keratinized epithelium of the palate continuous with the gingiva.

Figure 18–31 is a histologic section in the sagittal plane of the junction of the anterior fatty and posterior glandular zones of the hard palate. The anterior adipose tissue is on the left. Observe the lobules of dark-stained mucous cells on the right. Note the collagen bundles extending through the submucos to the periosteum above; these are termed *traction bands*. They firmly attach the oral mucosa to the underlying bone. The arrows point to a traction band. The adipose tissue and glands are within the submucosa; the dark staining lamina propria and epithelium are seen at the bottom of the picture.

Specialized Mucosa of Tongue

Specialized mucosa covers the dorsum (superior surface) of the body or papillary portion of the tongue (Fig. 18–32). Epithelium on the anterior portion of the tongue is modified keratinized stratified epithelium covered with papillae. The great majority of papillae are the pointed *filiform papillae*, keratinized extensions of the epithelial cells. Among the numerous filiform papillae are seen occasional fungiform papillae covered normally with a nonkeratinized epithelium. The connective tissue under the epithelium binds this mucosa to the underlying skeletal muscle of the tongue. At the posterior limit of the body of the tongue is a row of rounded papillae, the circumvallate papillae, and along the sides of the tongue are rows of foliate papillae (Fig. 18–32). Beneath the specialized epithelial layer of the tongue body is a layer of connective tissue, the lamina propria. Connective tissue fibers of the lamina propria extend from the mucosa to deep within and between the muscle bundles of the tongue.

Filiform Papillae. Filiform papillae, the most numerous papillae of the tongue, are pointed keratinized projections formed by overlapping sheets of the surface epithelial cells. Figure 18–33 is a light transmission micrograph, and Figure 18–34 is a scanning electron micrograph of these papillae. The papillae project toward the oropharynx. They are not associated with taste buds, are easily seen without magnification, and contribute to the rough surface of the tongue.

Fungiform Papillae. Fungiform papillae can also be seen with the naked eye. There are fewer fungiform papillae than filiform papillae, and the fungiform papillae are scattered over the surface of the tongue. They are about 2 mm in diameter, have a smooth surface, and are rounded elevations above the surface of the tongue. They contain taste buds on their superior surfaces. Their surface is not keratinized. Figure 18–35 shows a light micrograph, and Figure 18–36 is a scanning electron micrograph of a fungiform papilla situated on the surface of the tongue.

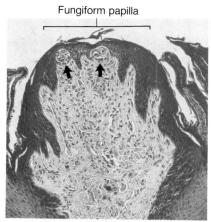

Figure 18–35. Light transmission micrograph of fungiform papilla. Two taste buds are located in the oral surface of this papilla (arrows).

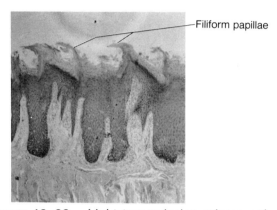

Figure 18–33. Light transmission micrograph of filiform papillae which are pointed keratinized projections on surface of tongue.

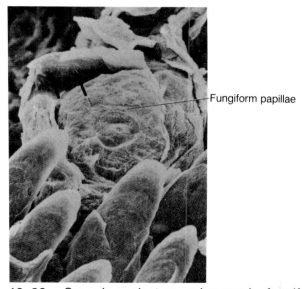

Figure 18–36. Scanning electron micrograph fungiform papilla surrounded by filiform papillae. The arrows point to exfoliating epithelial cells.

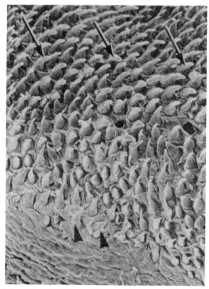

Figure 18–34. Scanning electron micrograph of filiform papillae (arrows and arrowheads).

18: Histology of the Oral Mucosa and Tonsils   **311**

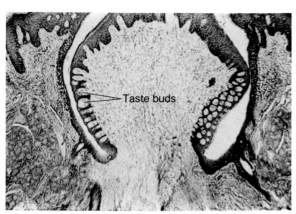

Figure 18–37. Circumvallate papillae with numerous taste buds in trench on wall of papilla.

Circumvallate Papillae. The circumvallate papillae are located at the junction of the anterior two thirds and the posterior one third, of the tongue. They can be located by observing Figure 18–32. There are eight to 12 in number, and they are located at the junction of the base and body of the tongue. These are larger than the fungiform papillae and do not project above the surface of the tongue (Fig. 18–37). Taste buds line the lateral walls of the papillae. Ducts of the underlying serous glands open into the trenches surrounding the papillae, and they function to flush out these areas to allow renewal of taste.

Foliate Papillae. The foliate papillae are located in furrows along the posterior sides of the tongue, (Fig. 18–32). Although they are not as prominent in the human tongue as in lower animals, the four to 11 vertical furrows containing the foliate papillae may be lined with taste buds.

Clinical Application

One method of drug delivery is through the oral mucosa and into the underlying vascular system. Nitroglycerine tablets for relief of angina pectoris, placed under the tongue, are quickly absorbed through the thin nonkeratinized epithelium and into the large veins of the ventral surface of the tongue.

Intraepithelial Nonkeratinocytes

The epithelium of the oral mucosa contains several types of nonkeratinocytes. In contrast to the keratinocytes, when viewed in the light microscope, nonkeratinocytes have a clear halo around their nuclei and have thus been termed clear cells. These cells are comprised of four different types: Langerhans cells, Merkel cells, melanocytes (pigment-producing cells) and lymphocytes (Figs. 18–38 to 18–41). These cells possess none of the characteristic features of epithelial cells except for the Merkel cells, which are joined to neighboring keratinocytes by desmosomes.

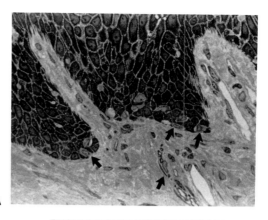

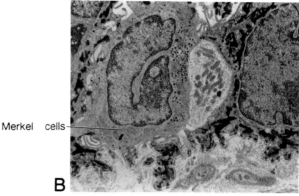

Figure 18–39. (A). Merkel cells located in region of stratum basale. They are lighter staining than are epithelial cells (upper arrows). The axon is noted by the lower arrow. (B). Ultrastructure of Merkel cell reveals dense vesicles in the cytoplasm of the cell adjacent to a nonmyelinated nerve terminal.

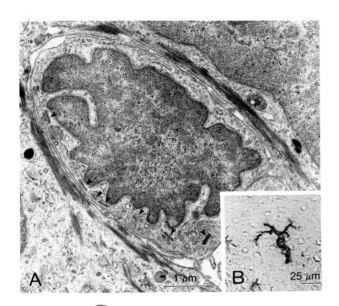

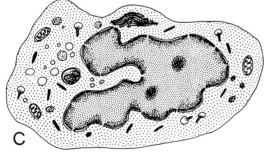

Figure 18–38. (A). Ultrastructure of Langerhans cell. Note the convoluted nucleus and lack of desmosomes. (B). Light micrograph of Langerhans cell. Observe the dendritic nature of the cell. (C). Diagram of Langerhans cell. Note the rodlike Langerhans granules.

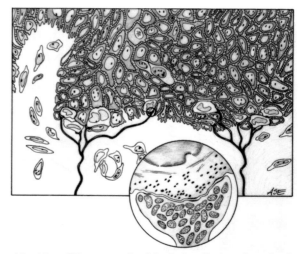

Figure 18–40. Diagram of a Merkel cell showing the location and appearance of these cells in the oral epithelium. Note their relation to the nerves. The inset shows nerve terminal with vesicles in Merkel cell adjacent to nerve.

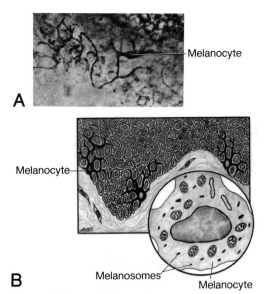

Melanocyte

Melanocyte

Melanosomes

Melanocyte

Figure 18–41. (A). Dendritic melanocyte located in stratum basale. The cell stains positive to dopa oxidase. (B). Diagram of several melanocytes in basal region of oral epithelium. Inset reveals the melanosome granules observed in this cell.

Langerhans Cells

Langerhans cells were first described over a century ago. They are related to similar cells found in the spleen, lymph nodes, and thymus, and also to the cells of the epidermis. These cells have long, thin extensions of the cytoplasmic membrane, called dendrites. Langerhans cells are found in the stratum spinosum and, occasionally, in the stratum basale (Fig. 18–38). They can be distinguished from keratinocytes by the absence of desmosomes and tonofilaments, and from melanocytes by the absence of premelanosomes (Fig. 18–38A to C). The cells contain a unique organelle, the rod- or racquet-shaped Birbeck granule, which allows for positive identification at the ultrastructural level (Fig. 18–38A). Langerhans cells are antigen-presenting cells. They engulf antigens from the external environment, and the intracellular lysosomes split the antigens into peptide components. These fragments are then transferred to T-lymphocytes, which are important cells in the immune system.

Merkel Cells

Merkel cells are situated in the basal layer of the gingival epithelium (Fig. 18–39), and possess occasional desmosomes and tonofilaments, which suggests that they may be of epithelial origin. They are usually associated with an axon terminal, and contain round, electron-dense granules polarized in the cytoplasm between the nucleus and associated axon (Fig. 18–40). The Merkel cell and associated axon terminal form a complex that serves as a *touch receptor*. Merkel cells are usually found in groups or clusters.

Melanocytes

Melanocytes are melanin-producing cells located in the basal layer of the gingival epithelium. These cells arise from the neural crest, and unlike their neighboring keratinocytes, lack tonofibrils, desmosomes, and hemidesmosomes (Fig. 18–41). Although these cells are highly dendritic in nature, this feature is rarely apparent in thin histological sections. The most characteristic feature of the melanocyte is the melanosome granule found within the cytoplasm (Fig. 18–41). Melanosomes are also found in the cytoplasm of keratinocytes. It is thought that the melanocytes inject melanosomes into keratinocytes. A more heavily pigmented gingiva is due to the production of melanin and its subsequent uptake by the epithelial cells. There is great variability in the location and distribution of melanin in the oral cavity.

Lymphocytes

Lymphocytes are found in all epithelia associated with the oral cavity, nasal cavity, and digestive tract. They are more numerous in gingival epithelium, and are described in Chapter 19.

Tonsils

Posteriorly the nasal cavity joins with the pharynx as the nasopharynx, and the oral cavity joins the pharynx as the oropharynx. At these junctions, tonsilar tissue is found as a wide circular band (Waldeyer's ring). The pharyngeal tonsil is in the superior aspects of the nasopharynx. In the oropharynx, the palatine tonsils are located laterally, and completing the ring inferiorly is the lingual tonsil (Fig. 18–42). The tonsils are part of the lymphatic system, which includes the lymph nodes, thymus, spleen, and diffuse lymphatic tissue. Tonsils, having a free surface covered by epithelium, are continuous with clefts or grooves. The tonsils contain many lymphocytes (which appear generally in nodules), some plasma cells, macrophages, and reticular cells. Lymphatic nodules with germinal centers are common both to the lingual and palatine tonsils. Tonsils and lymph nodes have efferent lymphatic vessels draining them. The tonsils do not have afferent lymphatic vessels whereas lymph nodes do. Tonsils have a connective tissue capsule of variable density and have associated glands underlying them. Figure 18–43 shows a clinical view of the palatine tonsils.

Development

The tonsilar ring corresponds to the anterior limit of the embryonic foregut; hence, the epithelium that gives rise to tonsils of endodermal in origin. Tonsils develop by diffuse proliferation of the basal cells of the endodermal epithelium, with simultaneous subepithelial condensation of mesenchyme (Fig. 18–44A). The epithelial areas later evolve into nodular projections that extend into both the lamina propria and the oral cavity. These nodules become the foci of lymphocytic infiltration (Fig. 18–44B). The nodules grow into lymphoid tissue by mitotic division of existing lymphocytes accompanied by differentiation of mesenchymal cells. Additional lymphoid tissue aggregates around the crypt, completing the formation of the nodules (Fig. 18–44C). Connective tissue forms a capsule along the base of the glands and sends supporting projections into the folds of lymphatic tissue.

Growth of the tonsils is very rapid from birth to 3 years and then again from 7 to 12 years. Thereafter, the tonsils atrophy. The pharyngeal tonsils can occupy up to one half the available space of the nasopharynx during childhood growth.

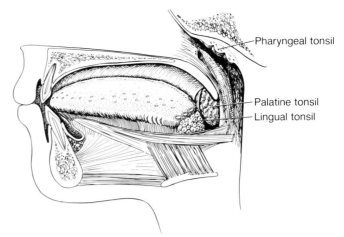

Figure 18–42. Diagram of location of three tonsillar groups: pharyngeal, palatine, and lingual.

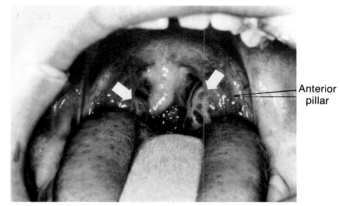

Figure 18–43. Clinical view of palatine tonsils (arrows). These tonsils are infected and appear swollen.

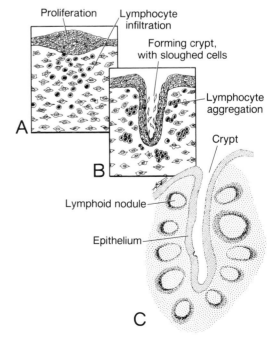

Figure 18–44. Diagram of development of tonsils. (A). Proliferation of epithelium. (B). Development of crypts. (C). Organization of lymphoid nodules.

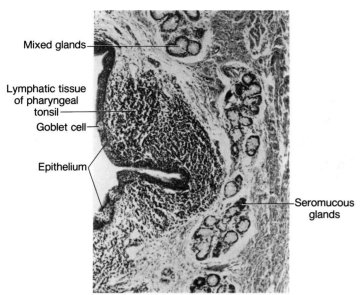

Mixed glands

Lymphatic tissue
of pharyngeal
tonsil

Goblet cell

Epithelium

Seromucous
glands

Figure 18–45. Histological appearance of pharyngeal tonsils with folds in epithelium and with adjacent diffuse lymphatic tissue and seromucous glands underlying them.

Types

Pharyngeal Tonsil. The pharyngeal tonsil is located in the midline, in the posterior wall of the superior portion of the nasopharynx (Fig. 18–42). It may extend laterally around the opening of the auditory tube in the region of the torus tubarius (a raised projection above and to the sides of that opening). Tonsilar tissue in that location is referred to as the tubal tonsil. The pharyngeal tonsil when enlarged is referred to as the adenoids. This tonsil is covered by pseudostratified columnar epithelium (respiratory epithelium) with occasional patches of stratified squamous epithelium. The epithelial cells lining this surface are ciliated and contain numerous goblet cells (Fig. 18–45). There are no crypts associated with this tonsil; there are, however, folds in the mucosa. The pharyngeal tonsils are not highly characterized by lymphoid nodules and germinal centers, but occasionally these structures do occur. In general, the lymphoid tissue is diffusely arranged, as seen in Figure 18–46. In the lamina propria underlying the tonsil are mixed glands that drain on the surface of the respiratory epithelium (Fig. 18–45). Deep to the lamina propria, the periosteum is attached to the sphenoid bone adjacent to the sinuses.

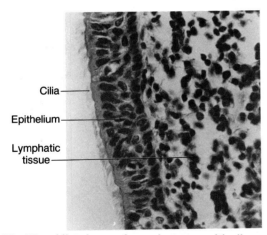

Cilia

Epithelium

Lymphatic
tissue

Figure 18–46. Histology of respiratory epithelium overlying pharyngeal tonsils. At times, this epithelium may appear to be squamous.

Palatine Tonsils. The palatine tonsils are largest in children, protruding into the oropharynx as large masses between the palatoglossus muscle (anterior pillar) and the palatopharygeus muscle (posterior pillar) (Fig. 18–43). Most people refer to the palatine tonsils as "the tonsils." When patients have their "tonsils out," these are the tonsils that are excised. Another name for the palatine tonsil is the faucial tonsil. The stratified squamous epithelium overlying these tonsils is similar to that of the adjacent oropharynx and the oral cavity. The area immediately beneath the epithelium contains numerous lymphatic nodules with germinal centers (Fig. 18–47). Septae of connective tissue support the masses of lymphatic tissue. Numerous branching crypts are present in the tonsilar tissue, and seromucous glands are found in the adjacent lamina propria. These crypts may contain plugs of dead lymphocytes and desquamated epithelium. The seromucous gland ducts do not open into the crypts; however; they open onto the surface of the epithelium. The lack of flushing action in the crypts may account for an accumulation of foreign debris, causing inflammation of the tissues.

The epithelium in many areas of the crypts is discontinuous, and between the epithelial cells are cords and networks of lymphocytes and other nonepithelial cells. This type of epithelium is referred to as *reticulated epithelium*. There are intraepithelial passages from the lumen to the follicular tissue in the lamina propria. Not only are there disruptions in the surface epithelium, there are discontinuites in the basement membrane. The cells close to the surface of the epithelium are M-cells (membrane cells) that initiate the action of processing antigens that come from the outside environment by way of the oral and nasal cavities. Dentritic cells similar to Langerhans cells and other macrophages are present. Antigens are phagocytized by the cells, and the lysosomes of the cells break down the antigens into smaller peptides. These smaller fragments are then transferred to T-cells to start the complex coding of antibodies for the immune system of the body. The cells that process the antigens are called *antigen presentor cells*. These cells in the tonsils are part of a large family of antigen presentor cells found throughout the body.

Lingual Tonsils. The lingual tonsil is located on the posterior third of the tongue, extending from the circumvallate papillae posteriorly to the base of the epiglottis (Fig. 18–42). The surface epithelium of this tonsil is nonkeratinized stratified squamous epithelium similar to oral epithelium elsewhere. There are several dozen or more nonbranching crypts associated with this tonsil (Fig. 18–48). A connective tissue capsule, some adipose tissue, and mucous glands are found under this tonsil. Most of their ducts enter the crypts and aid in the removal of trapped foreign material. Accumulation of debris or infection is rare in these tonsils because they are washed by saliva as well as the mucous secretion that empties into the crypts. Underlying these mucous glands are the skeletal muscles of the tongue.

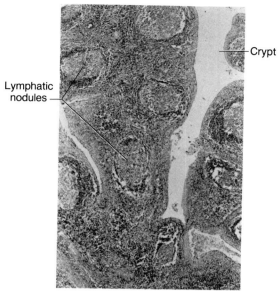

Figure 18–47. Histology of palatine tonsil tissue. Observe the overlying squamous epithelium, deep branching crypts, and organized lymphoid nodules.

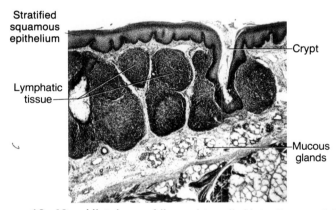

Figure 18–48. Histology of lingual tonsil. Note the overlying stratified squamous epithelium, short crypts, and lymphoid nodules. Mucous glands open into the crypts.

In Figure 18–48, which shows a section of lingual tonsil, the opening and base of a crypt lined by nonkeratinized stratified squamous epithelium can be seen. Note the pure mucous acini of the glands and the well-organized lymphatic nodules. The apical cytoplasm is clear because the mucous is removed during tissue preparation.

Function

One function of tonsils is in the formation of lymphocytes. Because of their location at the entrance of the alimentary and respiratory tracts, they are continuously exposed to a multitude of natural and foreign substances during breathing and eating. The lymphocytes protect the body against invasion of microorganisms. Allergens passing through the epithelium can be sensed by immunogenic cells of the lymphatic tissue, which start the complex process of coding for antibody production.

Table 18–1 provides comparative information regarding morphological features of the three tonsils.

Table 18–1.
Comparison of Tonsils

	Location	Lymphatic Tissue Organization	Epithelial Covering	Crypts or Folds	Capsules and Septa	Associated Glands and Ducts	Lymphatic Drainage
Palatine	Posterior lateral oral cavity between anterior and posterior faucial pillars	Arranged in rows of nodules with germinal centers	Nonkeratinous stratified squamous epithelium	Numerous and deep branching crypts	Fibrous connective tissue capsule under tonsil, thin connective tissue septa between segments	Mixed glands underlie tonsil, ducts open on free surface of epithelium, not in crypts	Drain to deep cervical nodes
Lingual	Dorsum of base of tongue	Row of nodules with terminal centers	Nonkeratinous stratified squamous epithelium	Wide-mouthed deep crypts with few branches	Thin capsule underlying gland, with few trabeculae separating lobules	Mucous glands open in crypts as well as on free surface of epithelium	Drain to deep superior cervical nodes
Pharyngeal	Medial posterior nasopharynx behind ostium of auditory tube	Aggregations of lymphoid tissue, few nodules and, occasionally, germinal center	Pseudostratified ciliated columnar epithelium with patches of stratified squamous epithelium	Folds of epithelium and lymphoid tissue, without crypts	Thin indistinct connective tissue capsule, occasionally with septa	Seromucous glands open on free surface or in folds	Drain to retropharyngeal nodes

Summary

Oral mucosa consists of the epithelium and lamina propria lining all the surfaces of the oral cavity. There is continual turnover of the epithelial cells, with mitotic figures found in the basal layers. Migration of the cells to the surface occurs to replace the surface cells lost in the normal functions of mastication, speech, and swallowing. Both keratinized and nonkeratinized epithelia are found in the oral cavity, and have a basal layer of cells (stratum basalis) next to the lamina propria. These epithelia are characterized by prominent and numerous desmosomes between the cells. In keratinized epithelium, there is a stratum granulosum with prominent spherical keratohyalin granules in these cells. The superficial layer of keratinized epithelium is the stratum corneum. These cells are full of keratin, and the nuclei have disappeared. In nonkeratinized epithelium the stratum granulosum is absent, and in the superficial layers the nuclei are still present and the cells do not have the concentration of keratin found in keratinized epithelium.

The oral mucosa can be divided into three functional types: masticatory mucosa, specialized mucosa, and lining mucosa. The *masticatory mucosa* is a keratinized epithelium found on the gingiva and covering the hard palate. The *specialized mucosa* covers the dorsal surface of the tongue. The *lining mucosa* covers the remainder of the oral cavity and is a nonkeratinized epithelium.

The *lamina propria* varies extensively in the different areas of the mouth and may be tightly bound to underlying bone or freely movable as in the lips, vestibule, and cheeks. The presence of a submucosa varies, being absent in the gingival areas and large areas of the hard palate (anterior and midline).

The tonsils form a ring of lymphatic tissue at the posterior border of the oral and nasal cavities. The pharyngeal tonsil, which is also referred to as the adenoids, is located in the nasopharynx. The epithelium of this tonsil is composed of "respiratory epithelium" because it is ciliated at the luminal ends of the cells. Seromucous glands and diffuse lymphatic tissue are found in the lamina propria. The mucosa is folded, and there are no crypts.

The palatine tonsils are located bilaterally between the anterior and posterior pillars at the posterior border of the oral cavity. These tonsils have deep branching crypts, and the surface epithelium is nonkeratinized stratified squamous epithelium. Many lymphatic nodules are located in this tonsil.

The lingual tonsil is situated on the posterior surface of the tongue in the oropharynx above the epiglottis. Several dozen single (nonbranching) crypts are found in it, and the epithelium is nonkeratinized stratified squamous epithelium. Lymphatic nodules along with many pure mucous glands are found in the lamina propria.

Self-Evaluation Review

1. Describe the process of keratinization.
2. What are the locations of masticatory, lining, and specialized mucosa?
3. Describe the junctions of epithelium and lamina propria as seen in the electron microscope.
4. What is the junction between the free and attached mucosa termed?
5. Name several cells found in the lamina propria.
6. Which of the nonkeratinocytes have dendrites?
7. Give a function for each of the nonkeratinocytes.
8. What is the name of the isolated sebaceous glands in the cheek?
9. In what area of the mucosa are the glands located deep among muscle fibers.
10. What are the three main groups of tonsils? Where are they located?
11. The tonsilar tissue originates from what embryonic tissue?
12. What are the functions of the tonsils?
13. What is the term applied to the tonsilar ring?
14. What tonsilar group has deep crypts?
15. What tonsilar group is referred to as "the tonsils" by nonmedical people?

Acknowledgments

Figures 18–2 through 18–8 are provided courtesy of Dr. D. Mac-Callum, University of Michigan. Figures 18–6, 18–9, 18–34, and 18–36 are provided courtesy of Dr. M. Pirbazari. Figures 18–12, 18–13, and 18–39 are provided courtesy of Dr. D. Turner, University of Michigan. Figure 18–38B is provided courtesy of Dr. Ian MacKenzie, University of Iowa. Figure 18–10 is provided courtesy of Dr. S. S. Han, University of Michigan.

Suggested Readings

Barrett AW, Beynen AD. A histochemical study on the distribution of melanin in human oral epithelium. *Arch Oral Biol.* 1991;36:771–774.

Breustedt A. Age-induced changes in the oral mucosa and their therapeutic consequences. *Int Dent J.* 1983;33:272–280.

Dreizen S. The mouth as an indicator of internal nutritional problems. *Pediatrician.* 1989;16:139–146.

Harris D, Robinson JR. Drug delivery via the mucous membranes of the oral cavity. *J Pharm Sci.* 1992;81:1–10.

Hoefsmit ECM, Arkema JMS, Betjes MGH, et al. Heterogeneity of dendritic cells and nomenclature. In: Kamperdijk EWA, Nieuwenhuis P, Hoefsmit ECM, eds. *Dendritic Cells in Fundamental and Clinical Immunology.* New York, NY: Plenum Press; 1993.

Karchev T. Specialization of tonsils as analyzers of the human immune system. *Acta Otolaryngol (Stockholm).* 1988;Suppl. 454:23–27.

MacKenzie IC, Binnie WH. Recent advances in oral mucosal research. *J Oral Pathol.* 1983;12:389–415.

Perry ME, Jones MM, Mustafa Y. Structure of the crypt epithelium in human palatine tonsils. *Acta Otolaryngol (Stockholm).* 1988; Suppl. 454:53–59.

Regauer S, Seiler GR, Barrandon Y, Easley KW, Compton CC. Epithelial origin of cutaneous anchoring fibrils. *J Cell Biol.* 1990;111:2109–2115.

Riebel J, Sorensen CH. Association between keratin staining patterns and the structural and functional aspects of palatine tonsil epithelium. *APMIS* 1991;99:905–915.

Schroeder HE. *Differentiation of Human Oral Stratified Epithelia.* Basel, Karger, 1981.

Schroeder HE. *Oral Structural Biology.* New York, NY: Thieme; 1991.

Schulz J, Ermich T, Kasper M, Raabe G, Schamann D. Cytokeratin pattern of clinically intact and pathologically changed oral mucosa. *Int J Oral Maxillofac Surg.* 1992;21:35–39.

Slipka J. Palatine tonsils—their evolution and ontogeny. *Acta Otolaryngol (Stockholm).* 1988; Suppl. 454:18–22.

Squire CA. Zinc iodide-osmium staining of membrane-coating granules in keratinized and nonkeratinized mammalian oral epithelium. *Arch Oral Biol.* 1982;27:377–382.

Squier CA. Oral mucosa. In: Ten Cate AR ed. *Oral Histology, Development, Structure and Function.* St Louis, Mo: Mosby; 1989:341–382.

Squier CA. The permeability of oral mucosa. *Crit Rev Oral Biol Med.* 1991;2:13–32.

Yamamoto Y, Okato S, Takahashi H, Takeda K, Magati S. Distribution and morphology of macrophages in palatine tonsils. *Acta Otolaryngol (Stockholm).* 1988; Suppl. 454:83–95.

Histology of Gingiva and Epithelial Attachment

James K. Avery

Introduction

The gingiva is that portion of the oral mucosa located around the necks of teeth, extending apically over the alveolar bone, and ending at the mucogingival junction. Like the palatal mucosa, it is keratinized and functions during mastication. The gingiva traditionally is divided into three zones (Fig. 19–1): (1) the free or marginal zone, which circles the tooth and defines the gingival sulcus as that space between the tooth and the free gingiva; (2) the attached zone, which is joined to the tooth by a unique junctional epithelium and is firmly attached to the underlying alveolar bone; and (3) the interdental zone, which occupies the space between two adjacent teeth apical to the contact area. The free gingiva often is separated from the adjacent attached gingiva by a minute intervening groove, termed the *free gingival groove*, which runs parallel and slightly apical to the free gingival margin (Fig. 19–1).

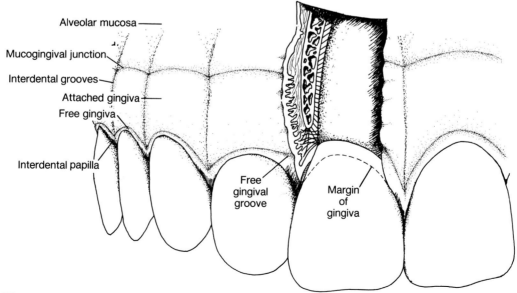

Alveolar mucosa

Mucogingival junction

Interdental grooves

Attached gingiva

Free gingiva

Interdental papilla

Free gingival groove

Margin of gingiva

Figure 19–1. Diagram of the anatomy of the gingiva illustrating the location of the attached and the free gingiva.

Objectives

After reading this chapter you should be able to describe the histological structure of the gingiva in a young adult or in an aging person, discuss cellular turnover in this tissue, and describe the vascular and neural components and the mechanism of attachment of the gingiva to the surface of the tooth.

Development

The gingiva develops as a coalescence of oral and enamel organ epithelia (Fig. 19–2A). As the tooth emerges into the oral cavity, the reduced enamel organ epithelium covering the surface of the tooth fuses with the oral epithelium (Fig. 19–2B). With further tooth eruption, the reduced enamel epithelium separates from the primary cuticle on the surface of the enamel (Fig. 19–2C). The resulting cuff of epithelium and connective tissue surrounding the neck of the tooth becomes the gingiva. The reduced enamel organ epithelium continues its apical separation along the enamel surface until the tooth reaches occlusion. At that point, the gingiva covers only the cervical portion of the crown (Fig. 19–2). Thereafter, the epithelial attachment is limited to a zone at the cementoenamel junction.

Free Gingiva

The *free* or *marginal gingiva* can be clearly defined by four distinct boundaries: (1) *coronally,* by the gingival margin; (2) *apically,* by the free gingival groove (in the absence of this groove, the apical boundary would correspond to a line opposite the bottom of the gingival sulcus, which is usually about 1.0 to 1.5 mm apical to the free gingival margin); (3) along the *inner* margin or tooth surface, by the gingival sulcus; and (4) on its *outer* surface, by the vestibular and oral cavities (Figs. 19–3 and 19–4). The free gingival mucosa is composed of stratified squamous epithelium with a dense

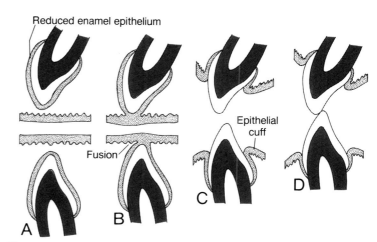

Figure 19–2. Development of gingiva from oral and reduced enamel organ epithelium.

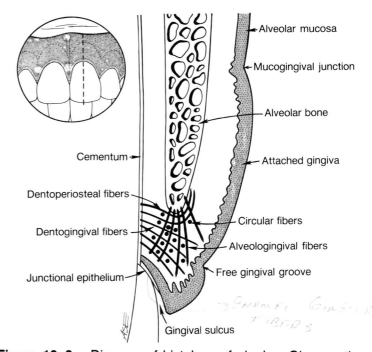

Figure 19–3. Diagram of histology of gingiva. Observe the fiber groups and their origins and insertions.

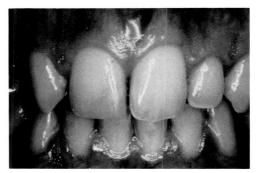

Figure 19–4. Appearance of normal gingiva.

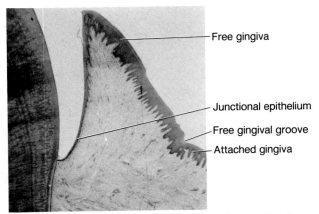

Figure 19–5. Histological components of sulcular, free, and attached gingiva.

OR ORTH KERATINIZED

Table 19–1.
Composition of Surface Epithelium of Free Gingiva Cell

Gingival Epithelium	Percent of Cases	Surface Nucleus Present	Stratum Granulosum
Keratinized	15	No	Present
Nonkeratinized	10	Yes	None
Parakeratinized	75	Partially	None

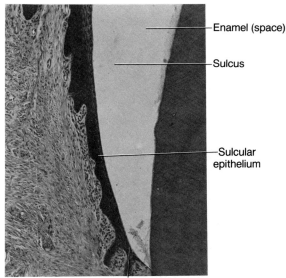

Figure 19–6. Histology of zone of junctional or epithelial attachment.

underlying connective tissue stroma (lamina propria) (Fig. 19–5). The outer surface epithelium interdigitates with the underlying connective tissue, forming long interconnected rete ridges separated by thin connective tissue plates and papillae. This surface epithelium may be composed of keratinized epithelium, parakeratinized epithelium, or nonkeratinized epithelium (Table 19–1). In keratinized epithelium, there is a distinct stratum granulosum layer. In nonkeratinized epithelium, the cells lack the keratohyalin protein. The epithelial lining of the gingival sulcus (sulcular epithelium) differs from that of the surface epithelium in that it is thinner, lacks prominent epithelial rete ridges, and lacks signs of keratinization (Fig. 19–6).

Attached Gingiva

The attached gingival mucosa lies between the free gingival mucosa and the alveolar mucosa. It is separated from the former by the free gingival groove and from the latter by the mucogingival junction (Fig. 19–3). The mucogingival junction is the transition site from the keratinized epithelium of the attached gingiva to the nonkeratinized alveolar mucosa (Fig. 19–1). In a healthy mouth, the attached gingiva shows signs of stippling (orange-peel appearance) which is not found in other areas of the oral mucosa. The absence of stippling, which is brought about by edema of the tissue, can be an initial sign of pathology. A unique feature of the attached gingiva is the junctional epithelial or the epithelial attachment.

Junctional Epithelium

The junctional epithelium forms the floor of the gingival sulcus and exends apically in apposition to the surface of the enamel to form a seal between the epithelium and the tooth (Figs. 19–5 through 19–7). The cells of the junctional epithelium, or the epithelial attachment, have several identifying characteristics that distinguish them from epithelial

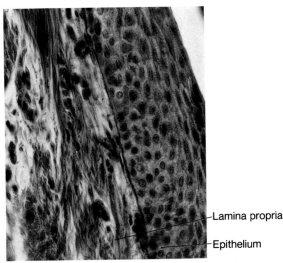

Figure 19–7. Higher magnification of zone of epithelial attachment.

cells in other areas of the gingiva: (1) They have a smaller tonofilament-to-cytoplasmic ratio. (2) The number of mechanical adhesion sites, *desmosomes* between these cells, is approximately four times less in these cells than in other areas of gingival mucosa, which allows molecules of high molecular weight, as well as whole cells, to migrate into the surface of the mucosa. (3) The organelles involved in protein synthesis and glycosylation (i.e., rough endoplasmic reticulum and Golgi apparatus) are more highly developed in these cells. The attachment of the epithelial cells to the tooth surface is an interesting and important feature of these cells. This attachment is structurally similar to the interface between epithelium and connective tissue elsewhere in the body. Epithelial attachment cells probably function much like basal epithelial cells, producing a basal lamina-like secretion or cuticular substance on the surface of the tooth. This structure may be added to by salivary glycoprotein and bacterial deposition. The junctional epithelial cells are attached to the cuticle by cell surface modifications, the hemisdesmosomes (Figs. 19–8 and 19–9). A hemidesmosome consists of an attachment plaque that is approximately 20 nm thick and appears continuous with the inner part of the epithelial cell membrane. Tonofilaments insert into the hemidesmosome plaque. *Lamina lucida* and *lamina densa* regions are also seen. Cellular fibrils penetrate into the subjacent zona lucida and zona densa to facilitate attachment to the surface of the tooth (Fig. 19–9). This attachment is dynamic in that the epithelial cells are continuously being renewed and new desmosomes and hemidesmosomes are being formed.

Junctional Epithelium Turnover

The junctional epithelium has a high rate of cell turnover. In approximately 6 days, cells of the stratum basale migrate to the surface and are sloughed. Cells from other areas of the oral cavity have schedules of maturation that differ in length of time. During outward migration, the cells maintain their attachment to the tooth surface (Fig. 19–10). The responsible mechanism is probably similar to the one involved in wound healing, in which the epithelial cells migrate on the wound surface, forming and maintaining an attachment to the underlying basal lamina. Disturbance of the epithelial attachment will lead to a resulting deepening of the gingival sulcus. This can be due to a number of factors: (1) effects of an inflammatory process on the cells of the epithelial attachment or the adjacent connective tissue; (2) immunologic response to bacterial antigens; and (3) mechanical irritation resulting from instrumentation or from food impaction or plaque and calculus formation.

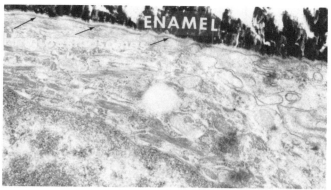

Figure 19–8. Ultrastructure of epithelial attachment with hemidesmosomes (arrows).

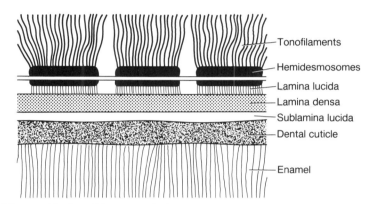

Figure 19–9. Diagram of ultrastructure of attachment of hemidesmosomes to enamel.

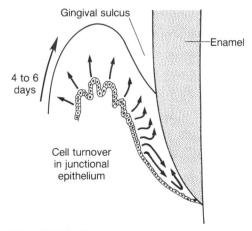

Figure 19–10. Epithelial cell turnover in gingiva. Note the direction of cell migration.

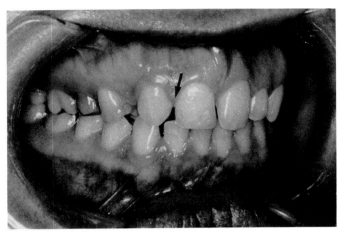

Figure 19–11. Clinical view of interdental papilla (arrow).

Interdental Papilla

Those parts of the gingiva that appear between the teeth as wedge-shaped zones, extending high on the interproximal areas of the crowns on the labial and lingual surfaces, are interdental papillae (Fig. 19–11, arrow). This tissue fills the space created by the constricted cervical regions of adjacent crowns. *Interdental grooves* extend vertically toward the interdental papillae and correspond to the depressions between the roots of adjacent teeth.

Col

Interproximal to the vestibular and oral cavity surfaces of the interdental papilla is a concave area termed the *col* (Fig. 19–12). In the area of the col, the gingival epithelium is thin and nonkeratinized (Fig. 19–13). The morphology of the col differs between the anterior and the posterior teeth. Anteriorly it is shaped like a pyramid, whereas posteriorly it is flattened. In Figure 19–12, the contact point between teeth and the shape of the col in both normal and inflamed gingiva are indicated. When the gingiva is inflamed and hyperemic, the col is exaggerated. The col usually exhibits signs of inflammation (Fig. 19–14), probably because it is difficult to keep the interproximal area clean because plaque and calculus form there. The epithelium of the col often sends numerous extensions into the underlying connective tissue (Fig. 19–14). With age, the vestibular and oral interdental peaks descend and the area of the col flattens.

Clinical Application

The dorsal surface of the tongue is characterized by the presence of many fine papilla, some of which help break up food particles. Some contain organs of taste reception. In general, they help move food around the mouth during mastication.

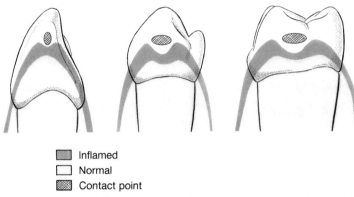

▨ Inflamed
☐ Normal
▧ Contact point

Figure 19–12. Diagram of positional relation of col in health, and disease. Observe that the results of inflammation accentuate the col.

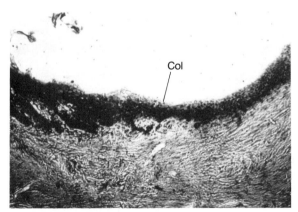

Figure 19–14. Histology of col as thin layer of epithelium, with inflammatory cells and epithelial cell invasion of connective tissue.

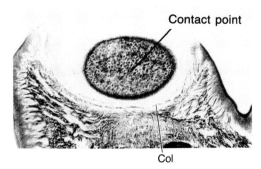

Figure 19–13. Epithelial lining of col. Observe the contact point of the tooth above the col.

Keratinocytes

The keratinocyte is the predominant cell type that forms the epithelium of the gingival mucosa. In keratinized epithelium, these cells are organized into four distinct layers (Fig. 19–15). Just above the lamina propria is the basal cell layer (Fig. 19–15A). These cells are cuboidal or low columnar, and their oval nuclei usually are oriented at right angles to the plane of the epithelium–connective tissue junction. The second layer, or stratum spinosum, is composed of four to five layers of cells (Fig. 19–15B). The lower cells of this layer are shaped like a polyhedron and are separated from one another by large expanses of intercellular fluid. Bridging the intercellular spaces are cytoplasmic extensions joined to each other by desmosomes. The superficial layers of the stratum spinosum contain cells that become flattened and less distinct. The third layer is the stratum granulosum (Fig. 19–15C). The cells of this layer contain irregular keratohyalin granules. These granules are highly characteristic of this level of the surface epithelium, but their exact origin and nature are not fully understood. The fourth and most superficial layer is the stratum corneum (Fig. 19–15D). Keratinized cells represent the final stage of the differentiation process. The multiple layers of these closely bound cells form a functional barrier to the passage of materials.

Intraepithelial Nonkeratinocytes

In addition to the keratinocytes, there are melanocytes, Langerhans cells, Merkel cells, lymphocytes, and leucocytes, in the gingiva. Collectively, these cells constitute only a minor population and are localized in the basal and prickle cell layers. In routine histological sections stained with hematoxylin and eosin, the cytoplasm of these cells appears vacuolated. Therefore, these cells are often referred to as "clear cells." They are mentioned only briefly here, as they are also described in Chapter 18.

Melanocytes

Melanocytes are highly specialized dendritic cells of neural crest origin. The function of these branched cells is to synthesize the pigment melanin, which is packaged in numerous, small, intracytoplasmic structures named melanosomes. The melanosomes are then transferred to the surrounding epithelial cells. The actual number of melanocytes does not seem to vary among individuals, although there are regional differences within the same individual. The variation in color among races is generally attributed to the functional nature of these cells (Fig. 19–16).

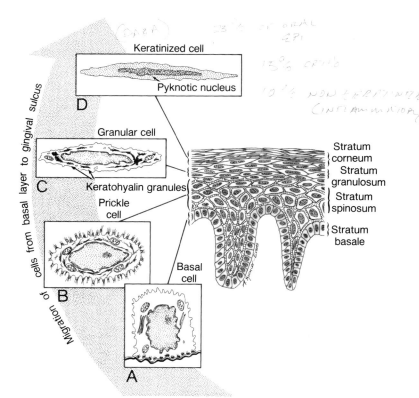

Figure 19–15. Maturation of keratinocytes in oral mucosa. A, basal; B, spinosum; C, granulosum; D, corneum.

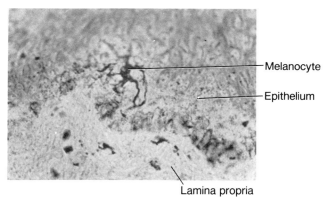

Figure 19–16. Nonkeratinocyte. Note the appearance of dendritic melanocyte in the stratum basale.

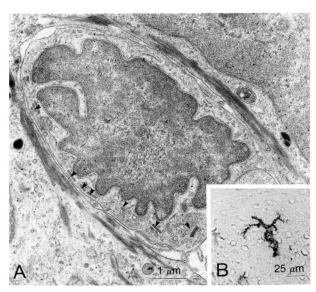

Figure 19–17. Nonkeratinocyte with Langerhans cell. (A). Electron micrograph of rod-shaped inclusions (arrows) in cytoplasm. (B). Light micrograph of dendritic Langerhans cell (stained with ATPase).

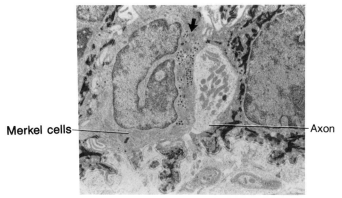

Merkel cells——————⎯⎯⎯⎯⎯⎯⎯⎯——Axon

Figure 19–18. Merkel cell containing dark-staining vesicles in cytoplasm (arrow) adjacent to nerve axon.

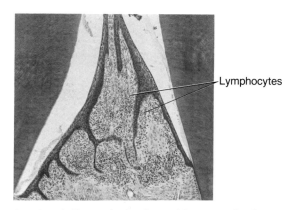

⎯Lymphocytes

Figure 19–19. Inflamed gingiva with many leukocytes and lymphocytes in connective tissue.

Langerhans Cells

Langerhans cells are similar in appearance to the melanocyte. Usually, it lacks melanosomes, having instead a unique rod-shaped membrane-limited inclusion termed the Birbeck granule. Current evidence indicates that these cells may process antigens and act locally as part of the immune system (Fig. 19–17). These cells probably arise from the bone marrow, and they may migrate from the gingiva to regional lymph nodes.

Merkel Cells

Merkel cells are located in the basal cell layer of the gingival epithelium and appear individually or in clusters. These cells appear similar to keratinocytes, possessing tonofilaments and desmosomes. Merkel cells contain dense-cored granules and usually are associated with small, unmyelinated axons. The Merkel cell and its associated axon function as an intraepithelial tactile receptor (Fig. 19–18).

Lymphocytes

Lymphocytes found in gingival epithelium are associated with an inflammatory process. They may be found anywhere in the gingival epithelium but most often are in the area of the junctional epithelium (Fig. 19–19).

Leucocytes

Leucocytes are found in the gingival epithelium, usually in the sulcular and attachment epithelium. These cells move between the epithelial cells and through its surface and become salivary corpuscles. They contribute protein and immunochemical substances to the sulcular fluid.

Epithelium–Lamina Propria Junction

Along the basal surface of the epithelium, the cells of the stratum basale are continuously dividing while maintaining close contact with the underlying connective tissue. Between the connective tissue and the basal cell layer of the epithelium is a basal lamina. Hemidesmosomes of the epithelial cells attach to this lamina (Fig. 19–20). Hemidesmosomes are composed of an attachment plaque that possesses intracellular modifications of tonofilaments that penetrate the plasma membrane of the cell to terminate in the basal lamina (Fig. 19–21). The basal lamina is composed of two layers, a lamina lucida and a lamina densa. Fine collagen fibers attach to the lamina on the connective tissue side. For further details regarding hemidesmosomes, refer to Chapter 18.

As is true throughout the body, connective tissue plays a role in maintaining the epithelium. In addition, the nature of the epithelium is largely dependent on the adjacent, underlying connective tissue. Recombination experiments have shown that epithelium transplanted to a site other than its own will soon take on characteristics of the new site. For example, if gingival epithelium is transplanted to an alveolar mucosa, a loss of keratinization will occur. If the underlying connective tissue is transplanted with the epithelium, however, the original characteristics will be maintained. The interface of the epithelium of the gingiva and lamina propria is characterized by projections of the connective tissue into the overlying epithelium. Characteristics of these projections varies with age (Fig. 19–22). In the young adult aged 20 years, ridges of connective tissue appear (Fig. 19–22A). In the adult about aged 40 years, there are no ridges and individual papillae appear (Fig. 19–22B). In a 60-year-old, the papillae decrease in number and are shorter and broader (Fig. 19–22C). Figure 19–23A through C, illustrates the relation between the lamina propria and the epithelium at 20, 40, and 60 years in the human.

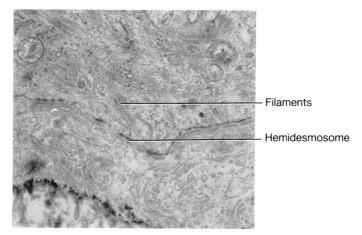

Figure 19–20. Ultrastructure of junction of oral epithelium and lamina propria. The dense-staining bars in the horizontal plane are hemidesmosomes.

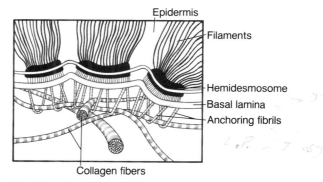

Figure 19–21. Diagram of hemidesmosome attaching oral mucosal cells to underlying lamina propria.

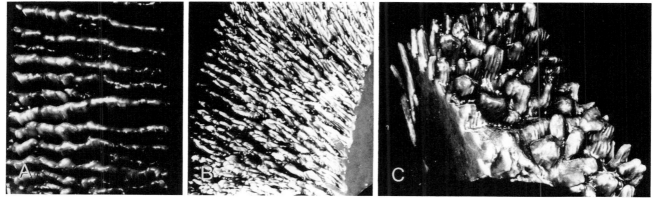

Figure 19–22. Variations in projections of connective tissue into gingival epithelium with age, as shown on wax reconstructions of sectioned papillae. (A). 20 years of age. (B). 40 years of age. (C). 60 years of age.

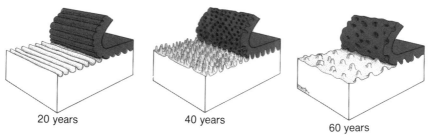

Figure 19–23. Diagram of interface of connective tissue papillae and epithelium at same age intervals as in Figure 19–22.

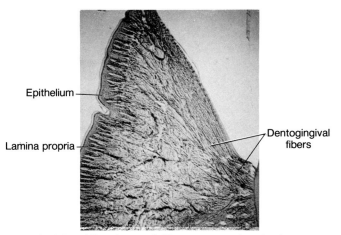

Figure 19–24. Histology of fiber groups in gingiva.

Table 19–2.
Gingival Ligaments

Group Name	Origin	Insertion
Dentogingival (free gingival)	Cervical cementum	Free and attached gingiva
Alveologingival	Alveolar crest bone	Free and attached gingiva
Circular or circumferential	Gingiva	Gingiva
Dentoperiosteal	Cervical cementum	Periosteum of outer cortical plates and cementum adjacent tooth

Clinical Application

Junctional epithelium has a higher rate of cell division than other areas of the oral mucosa. These cells have a higher rate of turnover by approximately six times more than other areas of the oral mucosa.

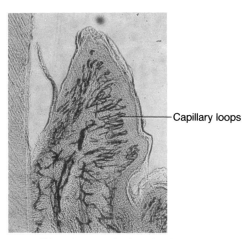

Figure 19–25. Blood vessels in gingiva (injected with India ink). Observe the vascular loops in connective tissue papillae.

Lamina Propria

The lamina propria of the gingiva is made up of the papillary and reticular zones and of dense bundles of collagen fibers that support the free and the attached gingiva (Fig. 19–24). The gingiva has no submucosa. Because the gingiva functions in mastication, its fibrous connective tissue is organized to withstand masticating forces. The fibers of the free and the attached gingiva are called gingival fibers. They arise from the periosteal surface of the alveolar crest and the cervical area of the cementum and are interspersed with fibers that course around the teeth and extend from the surface of one tooth to that of the next. The arrangement of these fibers are summarized in Table 19–2.

The lamina propria of the gingiva contains few elastic fibers except those associated with the walls of the larger gingival blood vessels. This is in contrast to the lamina propria of the alveolar mucosa, which contains numerous elastic fiber bundles.

Vascularity

Gingival connective tissue is highly vascular. The vessels have their origins in the periodontium and extend into the lamina propria of the gingiva. After perfusion with India ink, the well-organized capillary loops can be seen in the connective tissue papillae (Fig. 19–25). In the adjacent specimen that is of clinically healthy gingiva, the superficial boundary of free interdental arteries arising from the alveolar arteries is shown. Histologically, the connective tissue of the papilla of the lamina propria shows loops arising from the larger vessels of the free and attached gingiva (Fig. 19–25).

Classification of the Nervous System Relative to the Oral Region

The initial contents of this section includes a basic description of the nervous system. These paragraphs are intended as a review and for general background information.

The nervous system is divided into two main parts, the central nervous system (CNS) and the peripheral nervous system. The CNS is the brain and spinal cord. The peripheral nervous system includes the peripheral nerves that enter and leave the CNS, and the associated peripheral ganglion associated with the nerves. Nerve impulses from the CNS to the periphery travel on efferent nerves, and nerve impulses from the periphery to the CNS are carried by afferent nerves. The afferent nerves are the sensory nerves (Fig. 20–1).

Efferent nerves in the oral area can be divided into two large groups: (1) nerves to the skeletal muscle (facial and mastication), and (2) nerves to smooth muscles and glands (autonomics). The peripheral nerves are classified by alphabetic characters modified by Greek letters (see Table 20–1). The nerves to skeletal muscle are Aα fibers, which are the largest in diameter and also the fastest in the velocity of impulse conduction. Nerves to skeletal muscle end in a motor end plate that is in close relation to the cell membrane (sarcolemma) of the skeletal muscle cell (fiber). At this neuromuscular junction, acetylcholine is released from the end plate and initiates contraction of the skeletal muscle. Contraction of skeletal muscle is rapid and under the voluntary control of the individual.

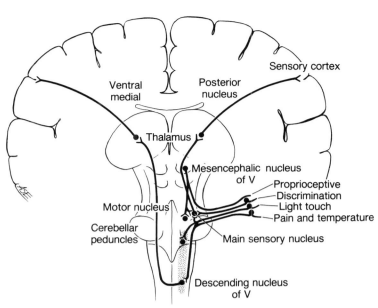

Figure 20–1. Nuclei of cranial nerves innervating oral region.

Table 20–1.
Cutaneous Receptor Organs

Class	Functional Category	Morphological Category	Size of Axon	Probable Sensory Role	Type of Skin
Mechanoreceptor position (and velocity) dectors	Type I	Merkel's cell ending; touch corpuscle	Aα	Touch-pressure	Hairy; glabrous (hairless)
	Type II	Ruffini's corpuscle	Aα	Touch-pressure	Hairy; glabrous
Velocity detector	RA (rapidly adapting)	Meissner's corpuscle	Aα	Flutter	Glabrous
Transient detector	Pacinian (phasic, tap)	Pacinial corpuscle	Aα	Vibration, tap	Subcutaneous
Thermoreceptor	Warm	?Free endings	C	Warmth	Hairy; presumably glabrous
	Cold	Free endings	Aδ or C	Cooling	Hairy; glabrous
Nociceptor	Aδ or C high-threshold mechanoreceptor	?Free	Aδ or C	Pain from mechanical stimulation	Hairy; glabrous
	Aδ thermal	?Free	Aδ	Pain from thermal or mechanical stimulation	Hairy; glabrous
	C polymodal	?Free	C	Pain from mechanical, thermal, or chemical stimulation	Hairy; glabrous

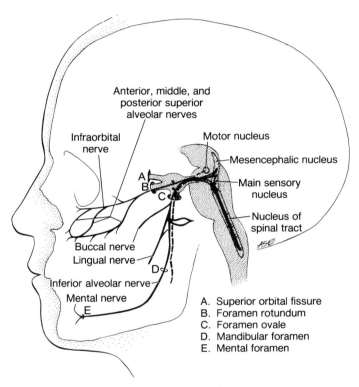

Anterior, middle, and posterior superior alveolar nerves

Infraorbital nerve

Motor nucleus

Mesencephalic nucleus

Main sensory nucleus

Nucleus of spinal tract

Buccal nerve
Lingual nerve

Inferior alveolar nerve
Mental nerve

A. Superior orbital fissure
B. Foramen rotundum
C. Foramen ovale
D. Mandibular foramen
E. Mental foramen

Figure 20–2. Trigeminal nerve: central nuclei and peripheral terminal branches to the oral region.

The second group of efferent nerves is distributed to smooth muscles and glands. This group represents the autonomic nervous system. The name "autonomic" signifies that it is autonomous or independent from voluntary control. Smooth muscles of the oral area are primarily associated with blood vessels. The nerves to these muscles are vasomotor nerves. Smooth muscle is arranged circumferentially around the vessel, and when the muscles contract the amount of blood flowing through the vessel is diminished. Vasocontriction in smaller arteries and arterioles play an important role in this control of blood flow. Efferent nerves to glands, also part of the autonomic nervous system, cause secretion. The term *secretomotor* is frequently used to describe these nerves. Autonomic nerve fibers are classified as B and C fibers and are smaller in diameter and slower in the velocity of impulse conduction (Table 20–1).

Efferent nerves (from the periphery to the CNS) of the oral cavity can be divided into three main categories: (1) sensory nerves that correspond to the afferent nerves of the autonomic nervous system. These visceral sensory nerves are not considered to be "the autonomic nervous system." However, they do provide regulatory feedback and sensory information for vasomotor and secretomotor control; (2) afferent nerves for taste, olfaction, vision, and hearing. These are termed *special* afferent nerves. The nerves for taste are discussed in the last section of this chapter; (3) general afferent nerves for mechanoreception, nociception, and thermoreception (Fig. 20–2).

Structure and Function of Peripheral Sensory Receptors Found in Oral Mucosa

What is known about the function of somatic sensory receptors in the oral mucosa has largely been extrapolated from physiological studies of hairy and non-hairy (glabrous) skin. To this date, only a partial correlation between structure and function has been achieved (Table 20–1).

The mechanoreceptors include receptors for touch, pressure, position, flutter, and vibration. They are classified as rapidly acting (RA) and slowly acting. The RA nerves conduct the fastest (60–120 m/s), are myelinated, and are the largest in diameter (10–20 μm). They are classified as Aα fibers, similar to the myelinated nerve fibers of skeletal muscle. Merkel's and Ruffini's corpuscles are nerve endings associated with the RA nerves. Other mechanoreceptors (Meissner's and Pacinian corpuscles) are associated with afferent nerves that are slowly adapting and have smaller diameter (5 to 15 μm) and slower conduction velocities (30 to 80 m/s). The nerves of the thermoreceptors and nociceptors are smaller in diameter (0.2 to 8 μm) and conduct more slowly (0.5 to 30 m/s).

Pain receptors and nociceptors are terms that require definition. The term *nociceptors* is more appropriately used for these neuroreceptors, as the term *pain* generally has a broader interpretation relating to the overall subjective response of the individual. Nociceptors respond to intense mechanical stimulation, intense thermal stimuli, and noxious chemical stimulation. Nociceptors are primarily associated with unmyelinated and lightly myelinated nerve fibers.

Complete uniformity in the classification of sensory receptors has not been achieved, but with the use of ultrastructural morphology the receptors can be divided into two general categories: (1) corpuscular receptors and (2) free nerve endings.

Corpuscular Sensory Receptors

Corpuscular sensory receptors are characterized as having specialized cell types associated with their axon terminals: (1) *Meissner's corpuscles* are located high in the connective tissue papillae; (2) *Merkel's corpuscles* are located at the base of epithelial rete ridges; and (3) *simple coiled corpuscles* are located at the base of connective tissue papillae or in the subpapillary lamina propria.

Meissner's Corpuscles

Meissner's tactile corpuscles are located within the lamina propria, at the apex of the connective tissue papillae, in close proximity to the overlying oral epithelium (Figs. 20–3 through 20–5). The corpuscle is surrounded by an incomplete capsule composed of flattened fibroblasts that lack a basal lamina, and of elastic fibers that are continuous with the general

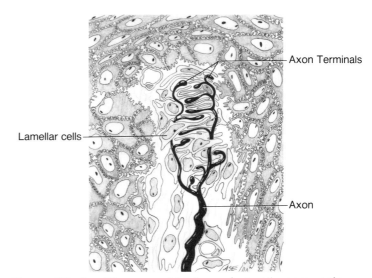

Figure 20–4. Diagram of Meissner's tactile corpuscle.

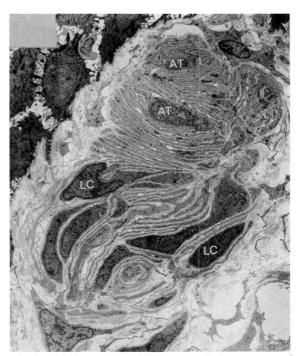

Figure 20–5. Meissner's tactile corpuscle is composed of flattened lamellar cells (LC) surrounding axon terminals (AT).

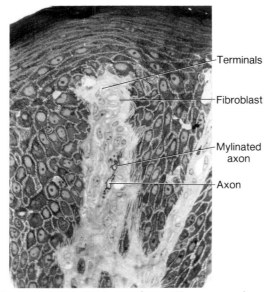

Figure 20–3. Meissner's tactile corpuscle.

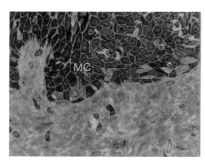

Figure 20–6. Merkel (mechanoreceptor) cells (MC).

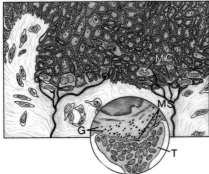

Figure 20–7. Merkel cell (MC) with axon terminal. MS, membrane specialization; T, terminal; G, secretory granules.

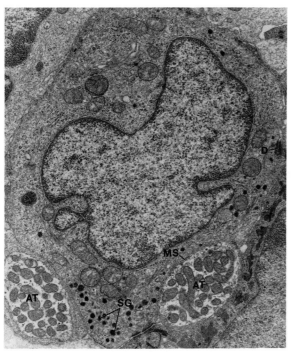

Figure 20–8. Merkel cell with associated axon terminal (AT) and secretory granules (SG). Note the lobulated nucleus. MS, membrane specialization; D, desmosome.

elastic network of the adjacent dermis. Most Meissner's corpuscles are innervated by two or more myelinated axons that, upon penetration of the capsule, lose their myelin sheaths and become positioned between stacks of cytoplasmic lamellae, which arose from specialized lamellar cells. the lamellar cells are separated from each other by considerable amounts of amorphous, filamentous material containing a small number of collagen fibrils. A basal lamina surrounds each lamellar cell and its cytoplasmic extensions. numerous pinocytotic vesicles are present along the cell membranes and appear to be most abundant adjacent to the axolemma of the axon terminal. The axon terminal contains many mitochondria. Neurofilaments and neurotubules are found but lack the uniform organization seen in the proximal parts of peripheral nerves. Meissner's corpuscles are characterized electrophysiologically as rapidly adapting mechanoreceptors functioning in tactile two-point discrimination.

Merkel's Corpuscles

Merkel cells and their associated axon terminals are specialized intraepithelial complexes found individually, or in clusters, at the base of epithelial rete ridges. In semithin (1 μm) sections, clusters of Merkel cells can be readily identified under the light microscope (Fig. 20–6). Merkel cells (MC) appear to be less intensely stained than the surrounding keratinocytes (Fig. 20–7). The nucleus of the Merkel cell is lobulated and often eccentrically placed, occupying proportionately less of the total cell volume than do the nuclei of neighboring keratinocytes (Fig. 20–7). Most Merkel cells are located at the periphery of the rete ridge, with their plasma membranes in contact with the basal lamina. A vacuolated area is often observed adjacent to the cell. This pale area corresponds to the axon terminal, seen in greater detail with the electron microscope (Fig. 20–8).

In the electron microscope, Merkel cells appear to be larger and less electron-opaque than surrounding keratinocytes. They are characterized by the presence of electron-dense, membrane-bound secretory granules, cytoplasmic spikes extending between epithelial cells and into the lamina propria, and desmosomes joining the cell to the adjacent keratinocytes. The secretory granules are polarized in the cytoplasm between the nucleus and an associated intraepithelial axon terminal (Fig. 20–8). Membrane specializations such as thickenings are often present between the Merkel cell and the associated axon.

Myelinated fibers 2 to 4 μm in diameter supply the Merkel corpuscle. As these fibers approach the base of the rete ridge, they lose their myelin sheath and continue as unmyelinated fibers, 0.5 to 1 μm in diameter. Merkel corpuscles have been characterized electrophysiologically as a type I slowly adapting mechanoreceptor, functioning as a position detector. The osmophilic granules in the cytoplasm of the Merkel cell are thought to contain a neurotransmitter; however, this neurotransmitter has not yet been identified.

Simple Coiled Corpuscles

Simple coiled corpuscles are organized similar to Meissner's corpuscles. They are found at the base of connective tissue papillae (Fig. 20–9), but are not limited to this location, often being located deeper in the lamina propria (Fig. 20–10). Since their initial discovery, they have been known by a variety of names, such as *Dogiel corpuscle, Krause end-bulb, lingual corpuscle, genital corpuscle,* or *mucocutaneous end-organ.* In contrast to Meissner's corpuscles, the simple coiled corpuscle is usually smaller and more oval in shape (Fig. 20–11). The corpuscle lacks a true capsule and the axon terminal forms a loose coil as it winds through the lamellar cells. This results in a greater number of axon profiles when the corpuscle is sectioned for electron microscopy. The precise function of this receptor has not been determined.

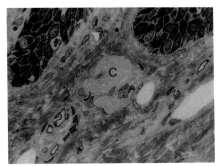

Figure 20–9. Simple coiled corpuscle (C) adjacent to oral epithelium.

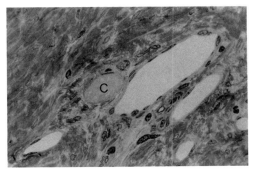

Figure 20–10. Simple coiled corpuscle (C) adjacent to small blood vessels in lamina propria.

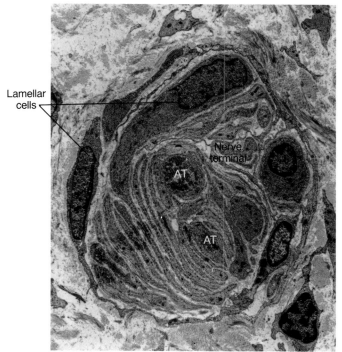

Figure 20–11. Simple coiled corpuscle with axon (AT) wound among lamellar cells.

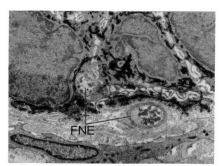

Figure 20–12. Free nerve ending (FNE) adjacent to basal lamina.

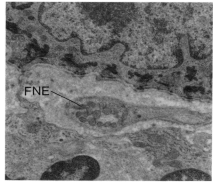

Figure 20–13. Free nerve ending (FNE) in connective tissue papilla adjacent to oral epithelium.

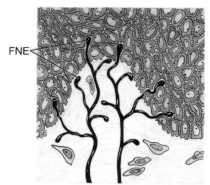

Figure 20–14. Diagram of intraepithelial free nerve ending. Terminals are found in the zone of stratum germinativum and connective tissue papillae.

Free Nerve Endings

Free nerve endings are found in abundance throughout the entire body. They may be the terminal arborization of thick or fine myelinated axons, but most often have their origin from nonmyelinated fibers. In the oral cavity free nerve endings are either intraepithelial or located in nonmyelinated fibers. In the oral cavity free nerve endings are either intraepithelial or located in the lamina propria, just beneath the basal lamina (Figs. 20–12 through 20–14). Within the epithelium, the free nerve endings are found within folds of epithelial cells in the basal and prickel-cell (Fig. 20–14). Free nerve endings within the lamina propria are characterized by abundant mitochondria in their axoplasms and partial or incomplete investment of Schwann cell cytoplasm (Fig. 20–13).

Free nerve ending are generally believed to respond to more than one sensory modality. They exist in all tissues that respond to painful stimuli, and are the only type of ending found in the tooth pulp, the classic model of pure nociception. In addition, they have been implicated as thermoreceptors.

Nerve Plexus

The oral mucosa contains a superficial nerve plexus just beneath the epidermis in the lamina propria, and a deep plexus within the submucosa. The deep plexus contains large nerve fibers that send smaller terminal branches toward the surface. The superficial plexus contains large and medium-size fibers, along with an abundance of sympathetic fibers.

The superficial nerve plexus allows nerve impulses from various receptors to reach a major nerve trunk via different collateral routes. Because of this arrangement, minor nerve injury does not result in sensory loss in the superficial tissues. It is also believed that this arrangement allows for more accurate localization of stimuli and discrimination between their intensities.

Modality Distribution

Figures 20–15 through 20–18 illustrate the distribution of pain, heat, cold, and touch endings in the oral cavity. Pain endings are concentrated in the lips and posterior oral region. The distribution of heat and cold endings indicates that the lips are the most highly innervated. Heat receptors are concentrated in the lips. The greatest concentration of cold receptors is found in the posterior palate, tongue tip, lips, and ventral surface of the tongue. The tip of the tongue and the lips are most highly innervated by touch receptors. Table 20–2 provides a summary of the distribution of these endings in the oral cavity.

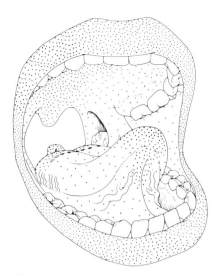

Figure 20–17.   Location of cold receptors in oral cavity.

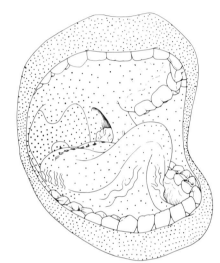

Figure 20–15.   Location of pain receptors in oral cavity.

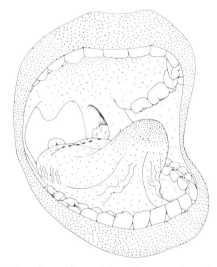

Figure 20–18.   Location of touch receptors in oral cavity.

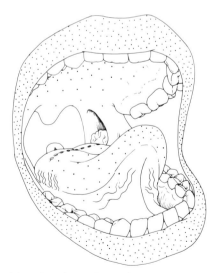

Figure 20–16.   Location of heat receptors in oral cavity.

Table 20–2.
Levels of Sensitivity of Oral Region

| | Sensitivity of Lips and Oral Mucosa | | |
Sensation	Greatest	Moderate	Least
Pain	Lips, pharynx, base of tongue, teeth	Anterior tongue, gingiva	Buccal mucosa
Heat	Lips	Anterior teeth	Ventral tongue, palate
Cold	Lips, posterior palate	Base and ventral tongue	Dorsum tongue, buccal mucusa
Touch	Lips, tip of tongue, anterior palate	Gingiva	Base tongue, buccal mucosa

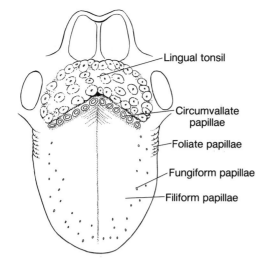

Figure 20–19. Tongue with site of taste buds.

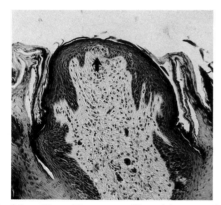

Figure 20–20. Fungiform papilla with taste bud (arrow).

Taste and Taste Receptors

Specialized sensory receptors within the oral mucosa are primarily responsible for taste. Taste reception is caused by a large number of taste receptors located on the tongue, pharynx, epiglottis, and soft palate. For a long time, it was thought that taste modalities had a corresponding location in the mouth and that these taste buds were especially sensitive to a particular taste stimulus. More recently, these differences have been shown not to be pronounced. A combination of differing taste modalities cannot explain the wide variety of taste sensations experienced by humans. Modified epithelial cells are the receptors of taste and conduct this stimulus to nerves that are in contact with these cells. The nerves then conduct impulses to the brain.

Taste-bearing Papillae

The sense of taste is a chemical sense that is associated with specific, discrete receptor organs, the taste buds. Taste buds were recognized over 100 years ago and have been a subject of continued interest. In the human adult, taste buds number about 10,000 on the tongue, approximately 2500 on the soft palate, over 900 on the epiglottis, over 600 on the larynx and pharynx, and 250 or more on the oropharynx. Taste buds are located on the dorsum and edges of the tongue and are associated with the fungiform, circumvallate, and foliate papillae (Fig. 20–19). The filiform papillae bear no taste buds, although they are the most numerous of the dorsal lingual papillae.

Taste buds begin to develop and mature early in human fetal life. They appear at 7 weeks after conception and are differentiated by 14 weeks. By this time, the tongue is well developed. The fifth, seventh, and ninth cranial nerves are also located in this area underlying the mucosa. This relationship is important to the development of taste buds because an unknown neurotrophic substance is probably responsible for differentiation and maintenance of taste buds.

Fungiform Papillae

Fungiform papillae are mushroom-shaped papillae, about 0.5 to 1 mm in diameter, and are larger at their free surface than at their base. They project slightly above the surface of the tongue (Fig. 20–20). In 40% of these rounded papillae, taste buds are located on the epithelium of the convex dorsal surface (Figs. 20–19 and 20–20). In approximately half of the 40%, one to three taste buds are found, and in the remainder four or more are found. Because the fungiform papillae project slightly above the surrounding filiform papillae, tasteable substances have easy access to these receptors. Taste buds of the fungiform papillae appear to be somewhat different from the circumvallate and foliate. The three cell types present in the other papilla are not clearly recognizable in the fungiform. This may be because the innervation is from the seventh nerve and the others are from the ninth. (Remember this when you read the description of the taste buds later in this chapter.) Fungiform papillae are located mainly on the tip and along the sides of the tongue. The threshold for sweet, salty, and sour modalities is least in these areas.

Circumvallate Papillae

As described earlier, the circumvallate papillae are named for their shape, as each round papilla is surrounded by a trench and a wall (vallum): thus the term *circumvallate* (Figs. 20–21 and 20–22). In humans, a row of 8 to 12 circumvallate papillae, each 2 to 4 mm in diameter, is located at the junction of the body (anterior two thirds) and base (posterior one third) of the tongue. Approximately 250 taste buds are contained in the wall of each papillae (Fig. 20–23). Therefore, approximately 2500 taste buds occur in this location. No taste buds appear on the dorsal aspect of the papilla: only in the walls facing the trench. Beneath these papillae are located the *serous glands* (of von Ebner), which produce a serous fluid. This fluid functions to flush out the trenches around the papillae so that new tastes may be perceived. In Figures 20–22 and 20–23, observe the ducts that open from these glands into the floor of the trenches. A variety of taste sensations, such as salty, sour, bitter, and sweet, are perceived by these taste cells.

Foliate Papillae

Foliate papillae are leaflike, consist of eight to 12 clefts, and are located along the lateral posterior borders of the tongue (Fig. 20–19). The taste buds of these papillae are similar to those of the circumvallate papillae, as both walls of the clefts (Fig. 20–24) and number approximately 1280 taste buds per cleft or 2560 per papilla (Figs. 20–21 and 20–24). They are most sensitive to the sour, salty, and bitter modalities. Like the trenches of the circumvallate papilla, the trenches of the foliate papilla have ducts of underlying serous glands opening into them.

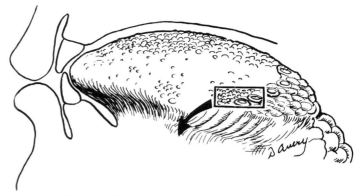

Figure 20–21. Circumvallate papilla.

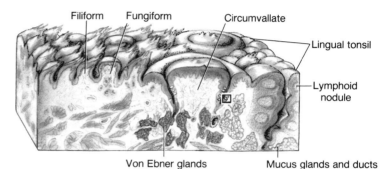

Filiform Fungiform Circumvallate

Lingual tonsil

Lymphoid nodule

Von Ebner glands Mucus glands and ducts

Figure 20–22. Circumvallate papilla with taste buds and serious glands (von Ebner).

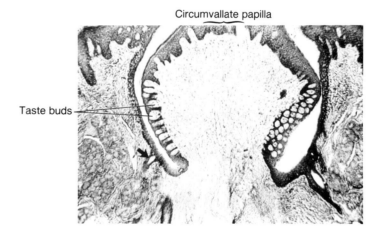

Circumvallate papilla

Taste buds

Figure 20–23. Circumvallate papilla with ducts of serious glands (arrow).

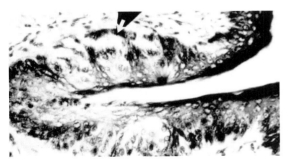

Figure 20–24. Foliate papilla with taste buds (arrow).

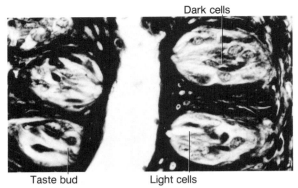

Figure 20–25. Taste buds.

Table 20–3.
Number of Taste Buds in Human Circumvallate Papilla from Birth to Old Age

Age	Mean No. of Taste Buds per Papilla and Trench Wall
0–11 m	251
1–3 y	260
4–20 y	326
30–45 y	242
50–70 y	268
74–85 y	101

Taste Bud Structure

Taste buds are goblet-shaped clusters of cells that are oriented at right angles to the surface of the epithelium (Fig. 20–25). Each barrel-shaped taste bud has a small pore that opens into the oral cavity, through which the tasteable substances may contact the taste bud cells (Fig. 20–24). Taste buds are relatively constant in size, measuring between 60 to 80 μm in length and 35 to 45 μm at their maximum diameter. Taste cells extend from the basal lamina in contact with the connective tissue to the free surface of the epithelium, where the taste pore is surrounded by as few flattened epithelial cells. The cells of the taste bud are *modified epithelial cells* that function as taste receptors. Because they transmit to nerve endings, these receptors are considered to be *neuroepithelial* cells. Under the light microscope, taste buds appear to contain two types of cells: thick, light-staining cells and thin, dark-staining cells (Fig. 20–25). Some investigators believe one cell type comprises the functional receptor cells whereas accompanying cell types are support cells. Taste cells have been found not to divide, and each type is renewed by differentiation from the more peripheral or basal cells in the taste bud or the surrounding epithelium. Thus, each cell type is a distinct line of cells with no transition between lines. In regenerating, early forms of each type appear at about the same time. The approximate numbers of taste buds in human circumvallate papillae have been determined from birth to old age (Table 20–3). The number of taste buds in each circumvallate papilla appears to be relatively constant throughout life. There may be a slight decrease in number in old age, although other investigators note negligible loss in older, healthy individuals. Therefore, even in older individuals, taste loss may be minimal.

When taste buds are examined under the electron microscope, taste bud structure is seen to consist of several types of stave-shaped cells (Figs. 20–26 and 20–27). *Type 1 dark cells* represent 60% of all cells in the bud. They appear to have an electron-dense cytoplasm and their apical cytoplasm contains dark granules.

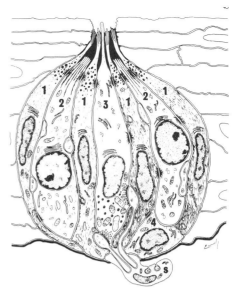

Figure 20–27. Diagram of taste bud. Type 1 dark cells represent 60% of cells; type 2 light cells, 30%; type 3, 7%; and type 4, basal cell.

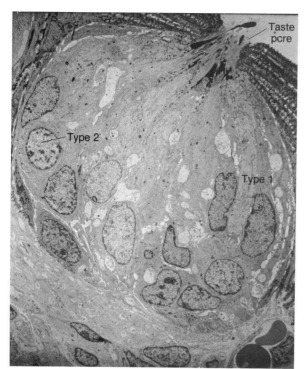

Figure 20–26. Transmission electron micrograph of taste bud.

Clinical Application

Trigeminal neuralgia or tic douloureux is one of the most painful conditions associated with the head and neck. Although the cause of this disease is not totally understood, it is thought to be due to vasospasms or compromises to the blood supply of the trigeminal ganglion. Another hypothesis is that following abnormal nerve healing, trigger zones are created at tooth extraction sites. The severe pain associated with this disease usually originates along the distribution of the specific sensory nerve to the area.

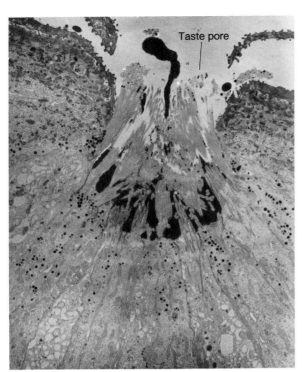

Taste pore

Figure 20-28. Taste pore. Epithelial cells surround pore. Note microvilli of type 1 and 2 cells and dense substance (below) in type 1 cell and between cells (above).

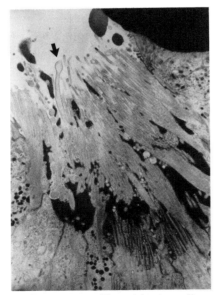

Figure 20-29. Taste pore. Note blunt ending of type 3 cell (arrow). Observe microvilli of type 1 and 2 cells surrounding it.

These cells terminate in microvilli consisting of 30 to 40 slender processes that enter the outer taste pore (Fig. 20-27). *Type 2 cells* have a lighter cytoplasm, with clear apical ends and with shorter less-numerous microvilli that terminate in the inner pore (Figs. 20-27 and 20-28). The latter type cells represent about 30% of the total cells in the bud. *Type 3 cells* represent approximately 7% of the taste cells and are similar to type 2 cells in appearance. Type 3 cells do not terminate in microvilli, as do types 1 and 2, but have a blunt rounded tip that ends into the outer taste pore (Figs. 20-27 and 20-28). Type 4 cells are the basal cell located in the base of the bud (Fig. 20-27). Cell types 1, 2, and 3 reach from the base of the bud to the pore. Type 1 cells separate the other two types and are extensively in contact with each other (Fig. 20-27).

Taste cells or *gemma cells* are generally lighter than the surrounding perigemmal epithelial cells, which are notable for their content of dense fibrils (Fig. 20-28). The nuclei of the taste cells are confined to the lower third or middle of the type 1, 2, and 3 cells. At the base, the taste bud is in contact with a basement lamina, which is in contact with the connective tissue. The taste bud opens centrally to the underlying tissue by a basal pore (Fig. 20-27).

The outer pore on the oral surface is an opening in the flattened keratinized cells. The details of a taste pore and its inner pit are seen in Figures 20-27 and 20-28. The epithelial cells surround and form the outer pore, (Fig. 20-28) into the surface of which the microvilli of the dark cells (type 1) extend. The inner taste pore is a ring. Its walls are formed by the apices of the type 1 cells and the floor by the apices of the type 2 cells (Figs. 20-27 through 20-29). Type 3 blunt-ending cells extend through the inner pore to a position close to the surface of the outer pore (Fig. 20-29). The pit and inner pore are filled with a dense substance that appears to be similar to the granules seen in the apical parts of the type 1 cells. Junctional complexes between the adjacent cells effectively seal the floor of the inner pit, from entrance of oral fluids and tasteable substances into the interior of the taste bud. Tasteable substances therefore absorb onto the surface of microvilli membranes, which causes depolarization of the taste bud cells. The depolarization causes generation of an action potential in the afferent nerve fibers.

Taste Receptor Nerve Supply

Taste reception for the anterior two thirds of the tongue (fungiform papillae) is carried by the facial nerve (chorda tympani fibers). The circumvallate and foliate papillae and the posterior third of the tongue receive innervation from the ninth cranial nerve (glossopharyngeal). Taste buds in the soft palate are innervated by the greater petrosal nerve, a branch of the seventh cranial nerve. Those in the walls of the pharynx and epitglottis relay their taste impulses by way of the 10th cranial nerve (vagus) (Fig. 20–30). All taste fibers from these three cranial nerves converges into the *tractus solitarius* in the brainstem (Fig. 20–30). Gustatory nerves are responsive to the four basic taste modalities, to some degree but there are basic differences in levels of sensitivity. The lateral parts of the body of the tongue comprise a receptive zone of the seventh nerve. The more anterior part of this zone is sensitive to sweetness and saltiness, and the posterior portion, to sourness.

Nerve fibers to the taste cells arise from nerve plexus in the underlying connective tissue and enter the taste bud through the basal pore, as shown in Figure 20–31. One nerve fiber may supply four or five papillae, or many nerve fibers may supply a single papillae (Fig. 20–31). This may explain some of the overlap in levels of sensitivity to various tastes.

The total number of nerve fibers found in a taste bud far exceeds the number of nerves entering a taste bud. This means that there is a high degree of branching of the terminal portion of the taste receptor fibers (Fig. 20–32). Some axons are noted to contact type 1 cells in the basal region whereas others spiral around the taste cells into the apical regions of the bud. No typical synapses are seen with the nerves and types 1 and 2 cells, and this is called a diffuse relationship (Fig. 20–33). A chemical synapse is seen with

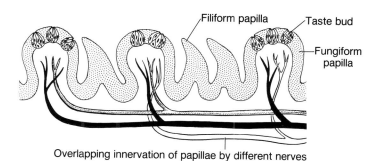

Figure 20–31. Innervation of taste buds. One nerve supplies several papillae. A second nerve may supply the same papillae.

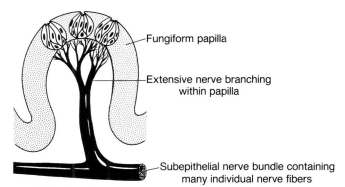

Figure 20–32. Branching of nerve fibers in fungiform papilla.

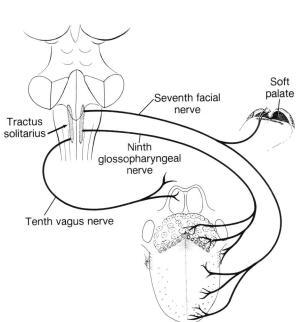

Figure 20–30. Nerves from anterior and posterior tongue, epiglottis, and soft palate lead to the tractus solitarius in the brainstem.

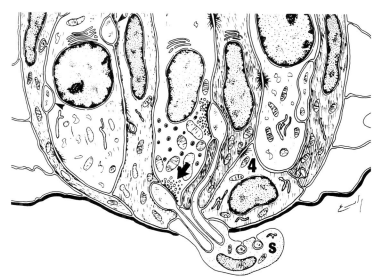

Figure 20–33. Nerve and taste cell relation. Large arrow, chemical synapse; small arrow, diffuse relations; 4, vasal cell; S, Schwann cell.

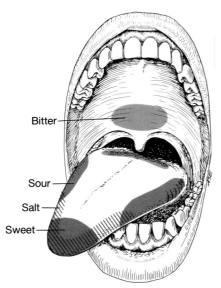

Figure 20–34. Location of taste perception in oral cavity.

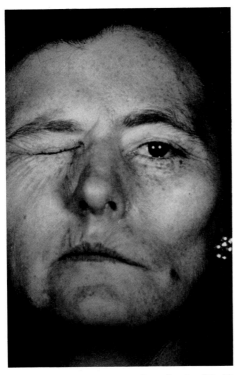

Figure 20–35. Appearance of patient with Bell's palsy.

type 3 cells, however, and this is known as a direct relationship (Fig. 20–33). Observe that adjacent to the nerve endings shown in Figure 20–33 (arrow) are light or dark vesicles that indicate the presence of neurotransmitter substance. Thus, the type 3 cell may be the taste receptor cell, or there may be two types of pathways, one that relates to type 1 and 2 (diffuse) cells and one that is a direct chemical pathway in type 3 cells.

Although there is evidence of taste cell turnover, the nerve fibers in the taste bud are permanent. It is unlikely that there is a continual shifting of the taste cells during which their relation with the nerves is maintained.

Nerves are important to the maintenance of the taste cells. Resection of nerves to the taste buds in experimental animals results in degeneration and loss of taste cells. This occurs rapidly, with disorganization of cells seen after 2 days, and with the disappearance of most taste buds by 7 days. A few taste cells persist for longer periods, up to 14 days. After the nerve supply is re-established to the area, taste cells reappear and function returns. The pattern of cell renewal suggested by these studies is that new epithelial cells originate from the lateral boundaries of the bud. As differentiation occurs, the three main cell types form in the central regions.

Taste Receptor Function

Classically, four taste modalities have been recorded: sweet, salty, sour, and bitter. They are perceived to some extent in different localities on the tongue and oropharynx (Fig. 20–34). Concentrations are a factor, as at low levels bitter taste has a slightly lower threshold on the front of the tongue. At higher concentrations, a bitter stimulus is more notable at the posterior of the tongue. Perception of water taste is believed to be due to a process of adaptation, and electric taste is recognized when one touches two dissimilar metals to the tongue. No separate receptors have been located for any of the four basic taste modalities, or water or electric.

Clinical Application

Patients with Bell's palsy, which results in paralysis of the seventh cranial nerve, are sometimes encountered in the dental office (Fig. 20–35). Various causes of this condition include an injection, trauma and iatrogenically induced lesions, and anesthesia, all of which can be disconcerting to the patient. Slurred speech, drooping facial musculature, and reduced ability to eat or drink are some of the signs of this disease. Fortunately for the patient, the effects of Bell's palsy is usually limited from a few weeks to 2 months.

Mixing the four basic modalities cannot account for every flavor we are capable of experiencing. Factors such as temperature, texture, and odor also contribute to flavor determination. All taste buds appear to be able to detect subtleties in taste, such as the difference between citric and acetic acid or between lactose and fructose. This illustrates a discriminatory ability within taste cells, as they can identify substances even when they are mixed. Investigations have shown that taste buds possess a wide spectrum of enzymes. As tasteable substances absorb on the microvilli membranes, they may function in depolarization of the taste cell, which, in turn, generates the action potential in the close-lying nerves.

Clinical Application

Trigeminal neuralgia or tic douloureux is one of the most painful conditions associated with the head and neck. Although the cause of this disease is not totally understood, it is thought to be due to a relatively poor blood supply to the trigeminal ganglion. Another hypothesis is that following abnormal nerve healing, trigger zones are created at tooth extraction sites. The severe pain associated with this disease usually originates along the distribution of the specific sensory nerve to the area.

Herpes simplex 1 and herpes zoster (varicella zoster) are two diseases that may be manifested in the oral mucous membranes (Fig. 20–36). These viruses enter the body either through direct sexual contact or by abrasions of the skin or mucous membrane. The virus then migrates, via a sensory nerve, to the sensory ganglion and eventually resides in the trigeminal ganglion. During times of stress or debilitation, the virus travels anterogradely to the nerve terminal to infect adjacent epithelial cells, with resultant formation of multiple painful vesicles which rupture and then heal, usually in 9 to 14 days. Both viruses are found over part or all of the distribution of the sensory divisions of the trigeminal nerve.

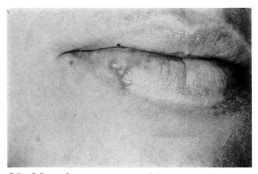

Figure 20–36. Appearance of herpes simplex 1 lesion.

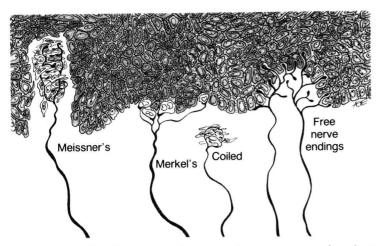

Figure 20–37. Summary diagram of appearance of various nerve endings located in oral mucosa.

Summary

The oral mucosa is richly innervated with sensory nerve endings and receptors that provide a significant role in the perception of pain (nociceptors), temperature (thermoreceptors), and touch (mechanoreceptors) (Fig. 20–37). A substantial number of sympathetic nerves also contribute to vascular tone and possibly to the perception of pain. The cranial nerves supplying the oral cavity originate from the trigeminal, facial, glossopharyngeal, and vagus nerves. Mechanoreceptors for touch and pressure include Meissner's corpuscles, Merkel's corpuscles, and simple coiled corpuscles. Meissner's corpuscles adapt rapidly whereas Merkel's corpuscles adapt slowly. Free nerve endings are characterized as thermoreceptors and nociceptors. Superficial and deep nerve plexuses also are located in the oral mucosa. They provide collateral pathways for the innervation of sensory receptors. Table 20–2 provides a summary for various sensation types in the oral cavity.

Taste buds are small ovoid neuroepithelial structures located primarily on the dorsal and lateral surfaces of the tongue and oropharynx. They are located in fungiform, circumvallate, and foliate papillae, and function in tasting sweet, salt, sour, and bitter. Taste buds are goblet-shaped clusters of four types of cells. Type 1 (dark) cells are long and thin and represent the majority of the taste cells. Type 2 cells contain no dark granules and represent about 30% of the cells, and type 3 cells represent about 7% of the taste cells and exhibit chemical synapses with the nerve endings. Type 4 are basal cells whose function is not understood. Type 3 cells show evidence of neural reception of taste. There are about 14,000 taste buds in the human oral pharynx. It is believed that the sense of smell makes an important contribution to taste.

Self-Evaluation Review

1. List the types of nerve endings found in the oral mucosa. Where are they located?
2. Describe the general somatic afferent (GSA) innervation of the oral mucosa.
3. What functions are assigned to free nerve endings?
4. Briefly characterize corpuscular receptors.
5. What plexus has an abundance of autonomic fibers?
6. Discuss the location and number of taste buds in the adult. Do these change in number during life?
7. Describe the several kinds of cells of the taste bud.
8. What nerves carry taste impulses from the oral cavity?
9. What happens if you resect a nerve to a taste bud?
10. Locate the greatest number of pain, heat, cold, and touch receptors in the oral cavity.

Acknowledgments

I wish to acknowledge the contribution of Professor Raymond G. Murray, Department of Anatomy, University of Indiana, School of Medicine, who read and assisted with the section of taste for the first edition, and contributed Figures 20–26 through 20–29 and Figure 20–33. I further wish to recognize the contributions of Professor Robert M. Bradley, DDS, who reviewed the first editing of the text concerning taste, and contributed Figures 20–31 and 20–32.

Suggested Readings

Barr ML, Kierman JA. *The Human Nervous System, An Anatomical Viewpoint*. 6th ed. Philadelphia, Pa: Lippincott; 1993:35–45.

Bradley RM. *Basic Oral Physiology*. Chicago, Ill: Yearbook; 1981.

Dubner R, Sessle BJ, Storey AT. *The Neural Basis of Oral and Facial Function*. New York, NY: Plenum Press; 1978.

Kruger L, Mantyh P. Gustatory and related chemosensory systems. In: Bjorklund A, Hokfelt T, Swanson LW, eds. *Handbook of Chemical Neuroanatomy*. Vol. 7. *Integrated Systems of the C.N.S., Part II*. Amsterdam: Elsevier; 1989.

Oakley B. Neuronal-epithelial interactions in mammalian gustatory epithelium. In: *Regeneration of Vertebrate Sensory Receptor Cells*. Chichester: Wiley; 1991:277–287.

Palay SL. The general architecture of sensory neuroepithelia. In: *Regeneration of Vertebrate Sensory Receptor Cells*. Chichester: Wiley; 1991:3–24.

Rustioni A, Weinberg RJ. The somotosensory system. In: Bjorklund A, Hokfelt T, Swanson LW, eds. *Handbook of Chemical Neuroanatomy*. Vol. 7. *Integrated Systems of the C.N.S., Part II*. Amsterdam, Elsevier; 1989.

Development, Structure, and Function of Salivary Glands

Robert M. Klein

Introduction

The human salivary glands are important organs of the oral cavity that produce saliva, an essential fluid required for normal speech, taste, mastication, swallowing, and digestion. Saliva functions in the maintenance of oral health through its antimicrobial, cleansing, lubricating, and buffering functions as well as its role in digestion. While the functions of saliva will be discussed in Chapter 22, the purpose of this chapter is to discuss the development, structure, and function of the major and minor salivary glands and the role of these organs in health and disease.

Objectives

After reading this chapter, you should be able to describe the embryological development of the salivary glands and the role of the extracellular matrix in the developmental processes of morphogenesis and cytodifferentiation; classify the salivary glands following morphological and functional criteria; describe the histology (including ultrastructure) and innervation of the salivary glands; describe the general functions of these glands and the cell biologic concepts involved in regulation of secretion including the cyclic AMP and calcium-mediated pathways in salivary gland secretion; and give examples of the pathologic alterations and aging changes that occur in these glands of the oral cavity.

Development of the Salivary Glands
General

The development of glandular tissue in mammals involves interactions of the epithelium with the underlying *mesenchyme* to form the functional part of the gland. These *epithelial–mesenchymal interactions* are defined by developmental biologists as proximate tissue interactions, also known as *secondary induction*, in which the presence of mesenchyme, in close proximity to the epithelium, is required for the normal development of the epithelium. For example, epithelial–mesenchymal interactions regulate both the initiation and growth of the glandular tissue and the eventual *cytodifferentiation* of cells within the salivary glands. Mesenchyme therefore has an essential role in development as well as in forming the supporting part of the adult gland.

Mesenchyme is composed of undifferentiated pluripotential connective tissue cells (e.g., fibroblasts, mast cells, and macrophages) and *extracellular matrix*. The extracellular matrix can be classified as: (1) *basal lamina* and (2) surrounding extracellular matrix. The basal lamina is composed of *type IV collagen*, *heparan sulfate* and other *proteoglycans*, as well as *laminin* and *entactin*, two glycoproteins that interact with each other and with other components of the extracellular matrix. The basal lamina is secreted by the epithelium and serves supportive and filtering functions as well as regulating migration, polarity, and differentiation of epithelial cells. The surrounding extracellular matrix is synthesized by connective tissue cells and contains extracellular matrix molecules such as *collagen types I and III*, the glycoproteins *fibronectin* and *tenascin*, and proteoglycans such as *chondroitin sulfate*. The components of the basal lamina and surrounding extracellular matrix therefore differ in the types of glycoproteins and proteoglycans present in each location.

The extracellular matrix provides regulatory cues for *cell proliferation*, *cell differentiation*, and *morphogenesis*, the major developmental processes required for the formation of adult structures. Cell proliferation is the increase in number of cells that occurs throughout development as organs enlarge, and also in cell replacement systems (e.g., gastrointestinal epithelium) throughout life. Proliferating cells enter the cell cycle, replicate their DNA, and subsequently undergo cytokinesis to form two progeny (i.e., daughter cells). These cells may either undergo specialization or remain as part of a dividing or stem cell population that continues to proliferate. Differentiation describes those processes responsible for the development of cell specificity and diversity as observed at the morphological or molecular level. Differentiated cells express a specific portion of the genome that is characteristic of that particular cell type. Morphogenesis describes those developmental processes that are responsible for the formation of the shape and form of an organ. Glandular branching as occurs in the developing salivary glands is one of the best examples of a morphogenetic process. Morphogenesis and differentiation are independent, but concurrent processes required for the development of adult architecture and specificity of cell types, respectively.

All salivary glands follow a similar development pattern. The functional glandular tissue (*parenchyma*) develops as an epithelial outgrowth (glandular bud) of the buccal epithelium that invades the underlying mesenchyme. The connective tissue *stroma* (capsule and septa) and blood vessels form from the mesenchyme. The mesenchyme is composed of cells derived from both mesoderm and neural crest and has therefore been called ectomesenchyme or mesectoderm. Ectomesenchyme is essential for the normal differentiation of the salivary glands. However, as mentioned previously, it is

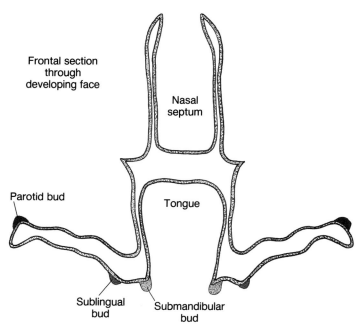

Figure 21–1. Composite schematic diagram of the origin of salivary glands (frontal view).

Frontal section through developing face

Nasal septum

Parotid bud

Tongue

Sublingual bud

Submandibular bud

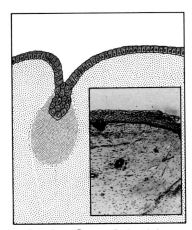

Figure 21–2. Stage I, bud formation.

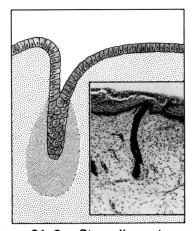

Figure 21–3. Stage II, cord growth.

the extracellular matrix components, synthesized by mesenchymal connective tissue cells, that provide important signals that direct the morphogenesis and differentiation of the glandular bud.

As the epithelial bud forms during development, those portions of the bud closest to the *stomodeum* (primitive oral cavity) eventually differentiate into the main excretory duct of the gland whereas the most distal portions arborize to form the terminal portions of the duct system, the secretory end pieces or acini. The origin of the epithelial buds is believed to be ectodermal in the parotid and minor salivary glands and endodermal in the submandibular and sublingual glands. The breakdown of the oropharyngeal (buccopharyngeal) membrane during the 4th week of development, however, permits the intermingling of stomodeal ectoderm and cranial foregut endoderm, which complicates the identification of specific germ layer origin of the salivary glands.

The parotid glands originate near the corners of the stomodeum by the 6th week of prenatal life. The submandibular glands arise from the floor of the mouth at the end of the 6th or the beginning of the 7th week in utero. The sublingual gland forms lateral to the submandibular primordium at about the 8th week. The sites of origin of the major salivary glands are shown in Figure 21–1, which is a composite diagram representing multiple serial sections. All minor salivary glands form from the epithelium overlying a specific area of the oral cavity, but do not begin to develop until the 12th prenatal week.

Stages of Development

Salivary gland development may be divided into six stages.

Stage I. Formation: Induction of Oral Epithelium by Underlying Mesenchyme. The mesenchyme underlying the buccal epithelium induces proliferation in the epithelium, which results in tissue thickening and formation of the epithelial bud (Fig. 21–2). The growing bud is separated from the condensation of mesenchyme by a basal lamina secreted by the epithelium. Although the site and the time of development differ slightly for the three major salivary glands, the processes involved in development are similar.

Stage II. Formation and Growth of Epithelial Cord. A solid cord of cells forms the epithelial bud by cell proliferation (Fig. 21–3). Condensation and proliferation occur in the surrounding mesenchyme, which is closely associated with the epithelial cord. The basal lamina, although not visible at the magnification used for Figure 21–3, is found between the cord and the mesenchyme. It is composed of glycosaminoglycans, collagen, and glycoproteins. The basal lamina as well as the surrounding mesenchyme play a role in influencing morphogenesis and differentiation of the salivary glands throughout their development. The role of the basal lamina and extracellular matrix will be discussed in more detail in the sections of this chapter dealing with the developmental processes involved in the ontogeny of the salivary glands (pp. 356–360).

Stage III. Initiation of Branching in Terminal parts of Epithelial Cord and Continuation of Glandular Differentiation. The epithelial cord proliferates rapidly and branches into terminal bulbs (presumptive acini). The growth in length of the solid epithelial cords and the differentiation of the berrylike terminal bulbs are shown in Figure 21–4.

Stage IV. Repetitive Branching of Epithelial Cord and Lobule Formation. The branching continues at the terminal portions of the cord, forming an extensive treelike system of bulbs. This branching process is evident in Figure 21–5, which shows a section from a developing human salivary gland. As branching occurs, connective tissue differentiates around the branches, eventually producing extensive lobulation. The glandular capsule forms from mesenchyme and surrounds the entire glandular parenchyma.

Stage V. Canalization of Presumptive Ducts. Canalization of the epithelial cord, with formation of a hollow tube or duct, usually occurs by the 6th month in all three major salivary glands (Fig. 21–6). Experimental studies have led to the proposition of two main theories to explain the mechanism of canalization: (1) different rates of cell proliferation between the outer and inner layers of the epithelial cord; and (2) fluid secretion by the duct cells, which increases the hydrostatic pressure and produces a lumen within the cord. Further branching of the duct structure and growth of connective tissue septa continue at this stage of development (Fig. 21–6).

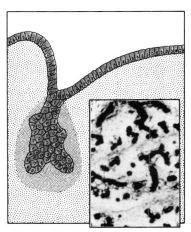

Figure 21–4. Stage III, branching of cords.

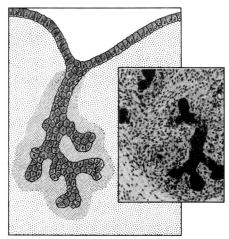

Figure 21–5. Stage IV, lobule formation.

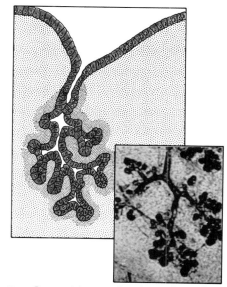

Figure 21–6. Stage V, canalization of cords to form ducts.

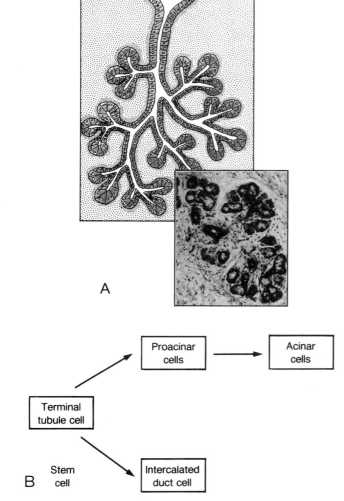

Stage VI. Cytodifferentiation. The final morphological stage of salivary gland development is the cytodifferentiation of the functional acini and intercalated ducts. During this period, mitotic activity shifts from the entire epithelial cord to the terminal bulb portions. Cells of the bulb region differentiate into terminal tubule and proacinar cells (Fig. 21–7A). The terminal tubule cells are believed to be stem cells for the proacinar cells that undergo cell division and subsequent differentiation to form adult acinar cells (Fig. 21–7B). *Myoepithelial* cells probably arise from epithelial stem cells in the terminal tubules and develop in concert with acinar cytodifferentiation. Maturation of the acinar cells occurs in specific stages classified according to the morphology of secretory granules and cellular organelles. Acinar development differs for serous and mucous cells. Therefore, the parotid, submandibular, and sublingual salivary glands show variation in cytodifferentiation patterns. Terminal tubule cells eventually differentiate into the intercalated duct cells of the adult glands. Secretagogue stimulus–secretion coupling mechanisms and innervation of the gland continue to mature following cytodifferentiation.

Processes Involved in Salivary Gland Development

General

Development of the salivary glands is influenced by intrinsic and extrinsic factors that regulate the processes of cell proliferation, differentiation, and morphogenesis. The intrinsic factors are defined as the preprogrammed pattern of gene expression specific for each cell type. Following this preprogrammed script with genes turned on and off at appropriate times leads to the normal development, growth, and differentiation of cells. Extrinsic factors are signals provided by cell–cell and cell–matrix interactions as well as by cytokines and growth factors in the extracellular milieu.

Figure 21–7. (A). Stage VI, cytodifferentiation. (B). Schematic of differentiation of terminal tubule cells.

Branching of the Epithelial Cord

Branching is the primary morphogenetic process in salivary gland development, and it has been studied extensively by analysis of salivary gland rudiments grown in vitro. Cleft formation in distal buds initiates the branching process, which is followed by epithelial proliferation (Fig. 21–8). Collagen type III accumulates at cleft points and appears to be a key substance in the morphogenetic process of branching (Fig. 21–8B). Types I and IV collagen appear to be more important for maintenance and support of established branches (Fig. 21–8C). The independence of epithelial expansion and branching has been demonstrated by use of tunicamycin with salivary gland rudiments in vitro. Tunicamycin inhibits N-linked glycosylation, resulting in dramatically decreased protein accumulation, and cell proliferation (i.e., epithelial expansion), but epithelial branching is unaffected. Control

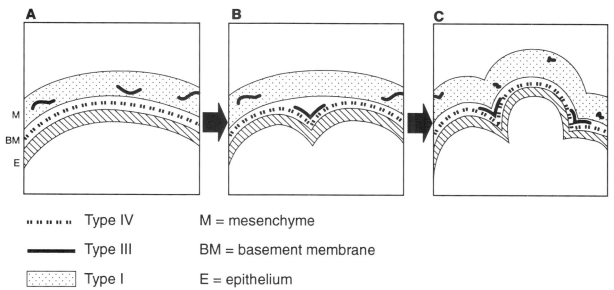

······· Type IV   M = mesenchyme

——— Type III   BM = basement membrane

▓ Type I   E = epithelium

Figure 21–8. Schematic of cleft formation during salivary gland branching. A, B, and C are sequential steps during branching morphogenesis. The interaction of the mesenchyme, epithelium, and basement membrane as well as the location of the collagen subtypes during development are illustrated.

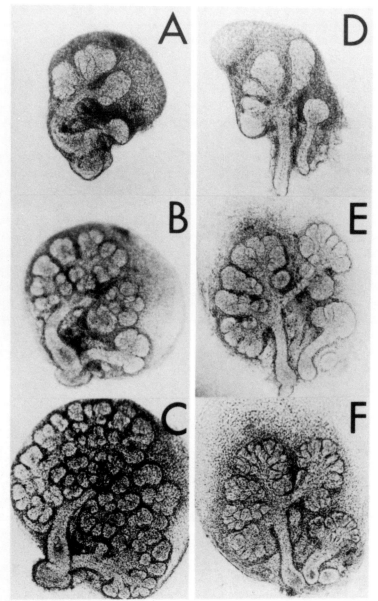

Figure 21–9. Living salivary gland rudiments in organ culture. (A) through (C). Control rudiments after 0, 24, and 48 h of culture. (D) through (F). Tunicamycin-treated rudiment after 0, 24, and 48 h of culture.

cultures are shown in Figures 21–9A through C and tunicamycin cultures are shown in Figures 21–9D through F. After tunicamycin treatment, branching occurs and lobules form normally, with inhibited cell proliferation, resulting in a smaller rudiment with miniature lobes. In contrast, both the size and number of lobules increase in control cultures.

Branching and proliferation must be coordinated processes for normal development of the salivary glands to occur. Mitotic activity is normally localized in the most peripheral regions of the bud (Fig. 21–10A). Treatment with *hyaluronidase* disrupts the basal lamina, interfering with the signal required for cleft formation. Destabilization of the basal lamina therefore inhibits cleft development, but also affects subsequent events such as cell proliferation. For example, in the absence of a normal basal lamina there is an absence of branching, and uniform cell proliferation replaces localized mitotic activity (Fig. 21–10B). The basal lamina is therefore implicated in the stabilization of the epithelium and the initiation and maintenance of lobular morphology.

The basal lamina may regulate morphogenetic changes directly or by selective filtration or channeling of materials to the epithelium. For example, the regulation of the flow of ions such as Ca^{++} (Fig. 21–10C) to the epithelium may alter the function of microtubules and microfilaments in cellular proliferation, migration, and differentiation. Collagenogenic and collagenolytic activity is also instrumental

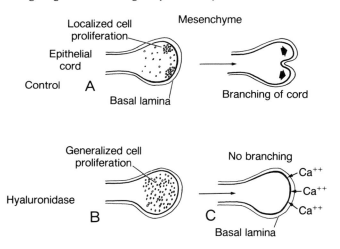

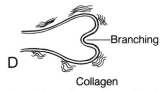

Figure 21–10. (A). Branching of salivary gland cell cords (control). (B). Hylauronidase treatment altering basal lamina and resulting in lack of branching. (C). Alteration of Ca^{++} flow affecting cell proliferation and other developmental processes. (D). Importance of collagen and collagenolytic activity during morphogenesis.

in salivary gland development. For example, collagen synthesis by the mesenchyme provides structural stabilization after branching has occurred (Fig. 21–10D). The stabilization appears to be provided by types I and IV collagen, which are associated with maintenance and support of the branched organization of the adult gland (Fig. 21–8B and C). In addition, collagenolytic activity in the epithelium and mesenchyme may allow for selective breakdown of the basal lamina (type IV collagen in Fig. 21–8) and communication between the epithelium, basal lamina, and surrounding mesenchyme at key stages of development.

The role of the extracellular matrix in morphogenesis is highlighted by studies in which salivary gland rudiments branch in vitro in the absence of mesenchymal cells, but in the presence of other factors. A 13-day mouse submandibular gland rudiment is shown in Figure 21–11A; when the epithelium is recombined with mesenchyme, three-dimensional branching occurs in a similar fashion to that in vivo (Fig. 21–11B). Use of an artificial matrix such as Matrigel, composed primarily of laminin, type IV collagen, heparan sulfate, entactin, and nidogen, results in only two-dimensional branching of the gland (Fig. 21–11C). When rudiments are grown in vitro with epidermal growth factor (EGF, an important growth-stimulatory peptide), there is extensive branching (Fig. 21–11D). Omission of EGF or Matrigel results in an absence of morphogenesis (Fig. 21–11E and F). The extracellular matrix in concert with growth factors appears to regulate the morphogenesis occurring during salivary gland development.

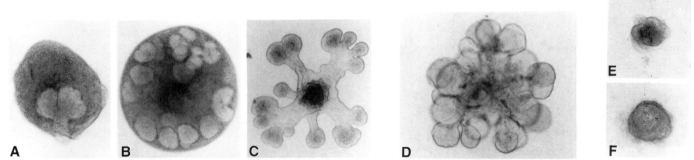

Figure 21–11. Submandibular gland rudiments in cluture. (A). Freshly isolated gland. (B). An epithelium separated from the mesenchyme, and then recombined with it and cultured. (C). An epithelium covered with Matrigel, separated from the mesenchyme by a filter, and then cultured. Branching morphogenesis occurred two-dimensionally. The epithelium was photographed after the mesenchyme below the filter was removed. (D). An epithelium covered with Matrigel and cultured in medium containing EGF. The epithelium underwent extensive branching and each lobule formed a spherical swelling. (E). Rudiment grown under the same conditions as (D) except in the absence of EGF, the outline of the epithelium was uneven. (F). An epithelium grown without Matrigel, but in the presence of EGF. No branching morphogenesis occurred.

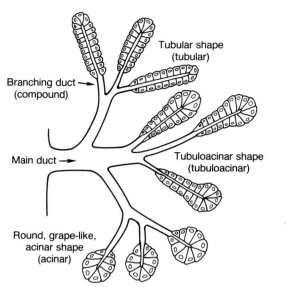

Figure 21–12. Diagram of a tubuloacinar-type gland.

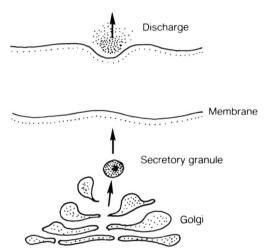

Figure 21–13. Diagram of the merocrine-type secretory process.

Clinical Application

Mucoceles are retention cysts of the minor salivary gland ducts and contain mucus. They may be found throughout the oral cavity wherever minor salivary gland ducts open, but are most common on the lower lip. Mucoceles probably arise following irritation or mechanical trauma to the salivary gland ducts, which results in rupture or, sometimes, the obstruction of the duct. The seepage of mucus into the surrounding connective tissue (lamina propria and submucosa) leads to inflammation and the formation of granulation tissue.

Cytodifferentiation

The initiation of cytodifferentiation of salivary gland acinar cells is believed to be dependent on preprogrammed development occurring in early stages of morphogenesis. There is evidence, however, that secretory cell differentiation may proceed independently of mesenchymal factors. A period of in situ epithelial–mesenchymal contact is required for cytodifferentiation, and once this contact has taken place, exocrine cell differentiation occurs without continued presence of mesenchyme. Therefore, it appears that there is a "partial coupling" of the independently controlled processes of gland morphogenesis and cytodifferentiation. Full differentiation of functional secretory components is apparent at birth but is not complete until the onset of a solid diet and the presence of masticatory stimuli.

This postnatal development process includes: (1) the maturation of stimulus–secretion coupling, which links secretagogue-membrane receptors to signal transduction pathways within the cell and controls acinar cell secretion; and (2) the establishment of neural connections from the autonomic nervous system, the primary regulator of salivary gland function.

Classification of the Salivary Glands

The glands of the body may be classified into two general types: (1) *exocrine*—that is, those glands with a duct system to transport secretion from the glands; and (2) *endocrine*—that is, those ductless glands dependent on blood supply for delivery of their secretory product(s). Salivary glands are classified as exocrine glands, but recent research has associated these glands with a number of biologically active substances (e.g., nerve growth factor and epidermal growth factor) that may be secreted by an endocrine mechanism. The salivary glands are classified as compound tubuloacinar glands, which indicates the presence of a branched duct system and secretory units with both tubular and acinar portions (Fig. 21–12).

The glands of the body are also classified according to the method of secretory production. The salivary glands are *merocrine* glands. The term merocrine is derived from the Greek words *meros*, meaning part, and *krino*, meaning to separate. The classification of these glands as "partially secreting" is not completely correct, however. Salivary glands are repeatedly functional, as secretory release occurs through a process of fusion of membranous secretory vesicles (granules) with the apical plasmalemma (cell membrane) known as *exocytosis* (*ex* = out of; *osis* = process). The process of storage of secretory product in membrane-bound vesicles coupled with the insertion of vesicular membrane into the apical membrane of the cell preserves the vesicular contents and conserves cell membrane. The vesicular membrane that is added to the apical membrane is later recycled through *endocytosis* for reutilization in the formation of new secretory vesicles (Fig. 21–13).

The salivary glands of mammalian species may be divided into *major and minor salivary glands*. The major salivary glands produce most of the 0.5 to 0.75 L of saliva produced daily. These three glands are located apart from the oral cavity with which they communicate by large excretory ducts. There are three pairs of major salivary glands: the *parotid*, the *submandibular* (formerly submaxillary), and the *sublingual* glands. The minor salivary glands are found in the oral cavity and are named according to their location: buccal, labial, lingual, palatine, and glossopalatine. In addition, the salivary glands may be classified by types of secretion: serous, mucous, and mixed. Mucous secretion produces mucin, which acts as a lubricant to aid in mastication, deglutition, and digestion. Serous secretion contains water, enzymes (primarily salivary amylase and some maltase), a variety of salts, and organic ions. Although the serous secretion aids in mastication and the removal of debris from the oral cavity, its digestive potential in the breakdown of carbohydrates is probably minimal, as a result of the short period of time between chewing and the entrance of foods into the esophagus and stomach. The parotid gland is an example of a purely serous secreting gland, the palatine glands are purely mucous, and the submandibular and sublingual glands are mixed-type glands (Tables 21-1 and 21-2).

Table 21-1.
Minor Salivary Glands*

Name	Location	Type of Secretion
Labial (superior and inferior)	Lips	Mixed (predominantly mucous)
Buccal	Cheek	Mixed (predominantly mucous)
Glossopalatine	Anterior faucial pillar Glossopalatine fold	Pure mucous
Palatine	Hard palate Soft palate Uvula	Pure mucous
Lingual (tongue)	Anterior	Mixed (predominantly mucous)
	Circumvallate papillae (von Ebner's glands)	Pure serous
	Posterior	Pure mucous

*Contribution to saliva—5–10%.

Table 21–2.
Major Salivary Glands

Gland	Size	Location	Type of Secretion	Capsule	Approximate Contribution to Saliva (%)	Striated Ducts	Intercalated Ducts	Sympathetic Innervation Vasomotor	Parasympathetic Innervation (Secretomotor)		Blood Supply	
									Preganglionic	Postganglionic	Arterial	Venous
Parotid	Largest	Anterior to ear	Purely serous in adult, predominantly serous in newborn	Extensive	25	Long	Long and narrow	Postganglionics via superior cervical ganglion (SCG)	Inferior salivatory nucleus→ninth nerve	Otic ganglion→auriculotemporal nerve→gland	Branches of external carotid artery	Veins generally follow the course of the arteries
Submandibular	Intermediate	Beneath the mandible near the angle	Predominantly serous	Extensive	60	Longer than in parotid	Shorter than in parotid	Postganglionics via SCG	Superior salivatory nucleus→chorda tympani of seventh nerve	Submandibular ganglion → gland	Branches of facial and lingual artery	Same as for parotid gland
Sublingual	Smallest	Anterior floor of the mouth	Predominantly mucous	Minimal	5	Very short	Inconspicuous	Postganglionics via SCG	Superior salivatory nucleus→chorda tympani of seventh nerve	Submandibular ganglion → gland	Sublingual and submental artery	Same as for parotid gland

Major Salivary Glands

The locations of the major salivary glands in an adult human are shown in Figure 21–14. The parotid, which is the largest gland, is located anterior to the external acoustic meatus and mastoid process, inferior to the zygomatic arch, lateral and posterior to the ramus of the mandible, and on the surface of the masseter muscle. Anatomically, the parotid gland is closely associated with the facial nerve, external carotid artery, superficial temporal and maxillary veins, and numerous cervical lymph nodes. The close anatomic relation of the parotid gland to the facial nerve renders complete or partial parotidectomy (i.e., in the case of a parotid tumor) a difficult surgical procedure. The relationship of the gland to the facial nerve begins early in fetal development (Fig. 21–15 shows anatomic relation at about 10 weeks of prenatal age). The anatomic position of the parotid gland, close to the mandible, has clinical relevance in glandular inflammatory diseases (such as mumps), which are characterized by masticatory pain. The parotid (Stensen's) duct extends from the lateral surface of the gland, anteriorly, across the masseter muscle and the buccal fat pad. At the anterior border of the masseter, it bends medially at a sharp angle, piercing the fat pad and buccinator muscle to open into the oral cavity in a papilla opposite the crown of the second maxillary molar tooth. The epithelium of the duct becomes continuous with the mucous membrane of the mouth.

The submandibular gland is located medial to, and under partial cover of, the mandible. It is closely associated with the mylohyoid and medial pterygoid muscles, submandibular lymph nodes and facial arteries and veins. The submandibular (Wharton's) duct extends anteriorly, in the floor of the mouth, to open into the oral cavity at the sublingual papilla at the side of the frenulum of the tongue.

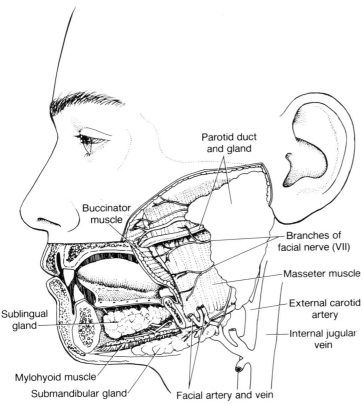

Figure 21–14. Diagram of anatomic structures of glands and associated structures.

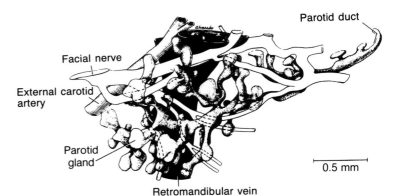

Figure 21–15. Relation of facial nerves to developing fetal parotid gland.

The sublingual is the smallest of the major salivary glands and is located beneath the mucous membrane of the floor of the mouth. Although the parotid and submandibular are encased in an extensive connective tissue capsule, the sublingual gland lacks a distinct capsule. Compared with the parotid and the submandibular, the sublingual consists of a large portion and a collection of small glands rather than a single, clearly delineated gland. The main excretory duct of the sublingual gland (Bartholin's), may join the submandibular duct or open into the oral cavity with a separate sublingual papilla. Numerous smaller sublingual ducts (ducts of Rivinus) may join the submandibular duct or open separately into the floor of the mouth.

General Structural Plan of Salivary Glands

The general arrangement of the glands is similar to the arrangement of grapes on a vine, with the stems representing the branching duct system of the compound glands and the grapes representing acini composed of five to seven secretory acinar cells. Figure 21–16 illustrates the general structural plan of a compound tubuloacinar gland. There are three types of secretory endpieces: serous, mucous, and mixed (both serous and mucous). There also are several types of ducts: intercalated and striated (intralobular) ducts and excretory (interlobular) ducts. Surrounding and supporting the duct and secretory system is a capsule of connective tissue (more extensive in the parotid and submandibular glands) which extends into the glands as septa dividing the *parenchyma* into lobes and lobules. The connective tissue is essential both as a framework for support of the glands and as

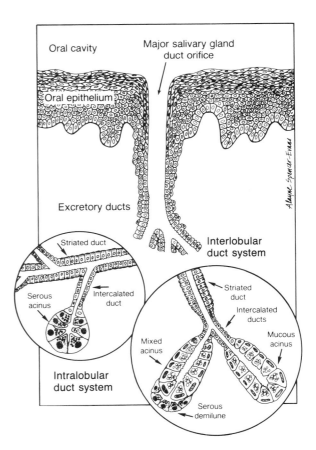

Figure 21–16. Histological plan of compound tubuloacinar gland and duct system.

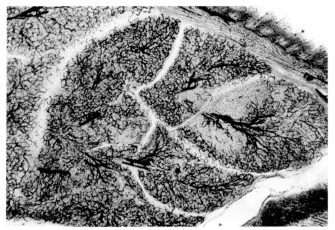

Figure 21–17. Histology of microvascular injection of dye to demonstrate the distribution of blood vessels within a salivary gland lobule.

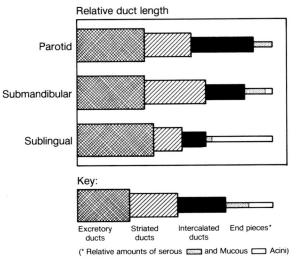

Figure 21–18. Diagram comparing salivary gland duct system in parotid, submandibular, and sublingual glands.

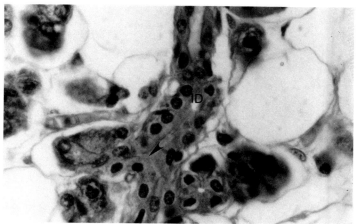

Figure 21–19. Histology of intercalated duct (ID).

a conduit for nerves (primarily autonomic), blood vessels, and lymphatics. The pattern and extent of the vascular supply of the salivary glands is demonstrated in Figure 21–17, which shows the rat parotid gland injected with India ink. The injection reveals how the larger vessels enter each lobe at one point and branch to supply each lobule. The duct system of the salivary glands drains the lobules and lobes in a similar manner.

Duct System

The duct system differs in each of the major salivary glands (see Table 21–1). Figure 21–18 illustrates the differences in the ductal distribution between the parotid, submandibular, and sublingual glands. The duct system has two main structural parts: the *intralobular* and the *interlobular* portions. Intralobular ducts are of two types: *intercalated* and *striated (secretory)*. The other portion of the duct system is termed the *excretory* ducts. In Figure 21–18, the excretory ducts are indicated by cross-hatched areas; striated ducts, by the striped areas; and intercalated ducts, by darkly shaded areas. The secretory portions or end pieces are either mucous (unshaded), serous (spotted), or mixed. The intercalated ducts are longest in the parotid, intermediate in the submandibular, and shortest in the sublingual glands. The sublingual glands have the fewest number of intralobular ducts, as both striated and intercalated ducts are very short.

Histology of Duct System

Intercalated ducts (ID) are the first (most distal) element of the intralobular duct system, are lined by a low cuboidal epithelium (Fig. 21–19), and drain the secretory end pieces (acini). The intercalated duct cells contain a few secretory granules, some rough endoplasmic reticulum (RER), mitochondria, and a round or oval centrally placed nucleus (Fig. 21–20). *Striated ducts* are the next largest introlobular type and are located between the intercalated and the excretory ducts. The striated ducts (also known as the secretory or salivary ducts) are lined by tall columnar epithelial

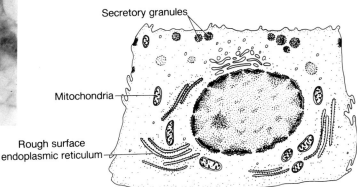

Figure 21–20. Diagram of intercalated duct cell.

(G). Autoradiographic grains are present over immature granules present in the Golgi regions. These granules often possess coated membrane evaginations that have been associated with secretory sorting processes. For example, proteins may be sorted into vesicles for constitutive release from the cell. The inset in Figure 21–28C shows the coat (arrowhead) of the granule located in the center of the field.

Specific processes occur in each intracellular compartment during the maturation of secretory proteins. Several processes occur within the RER including initiation of: (1) folding, (2) glycosylation, and (3) processing of sugar molecules on the maturing secretory proteins. Membranous *transport vesicles* (Fig. 21–27) provide the mechanism for RER to Golgi transport. These vesicles move to the Golgi apparatus, where the protein synthesized by the RER is further modified (e.g., glycosylation) and where packaging of secretory granules is completed (Fig. 21–27). The secretory vesicle or granule is the vehicle for movement of secretory proteins from the Golgi to the cell membrane. The majority of salivary secretory proteins are released by fusion of the granule with the cell membrane—that is, *exocytosis* under the regulation of acinar cell secretagogues. This process is known as *regulated secretion* in contrast to the secretagogue-independent mechanism of continual vesicular shuttling known as *constitutive secretion* (Fig. 21–29). Vesicles in acinar cells are responsible for transport of membrane proteins to the apical or basolateral surfaces of these highly polarized cells. Vesicles also contain secretory proteins destined for release in the absence of secretagogue (Fig. 21–29). Some of these vesicles may bud from immature secretory granules, as shown in Figure 21–28C.

Lysosomal activity also plays an important role in the secretory process. *Mannose-6-phosphate* is attached to lysosomal enzymes during maturation and becomes the signal that directs these enzymes from the Golgi to lysosomes. Lysosomes contain *acid hydrolases*, which are required for intracellular degradation. For example, after response to a *secretagogue*, the acinar cell produces an abundance of protein that must be degraded. A similar process, called crinophagy, occurs after prolonged absence of secretagogue. In the absence of secretagogue lysosomal vesicles fuse with secretory granules causing breakdown of excess granules. In addition to crinophagy, lysosomes are required for processing of endocytosed material and for autophagy of intracellular organelles.

The ultrastructural features of a serous acinus are shown in Figure 21–30. Granules ready for release are observed near the lumen. Serous cells in the salivary glands are responsible for the production of salivary amylase. This enzyme catalyzes the hydrolytic breakdown of α-1,4-glucosidic bonds typical of complex carbohydrates. Some authors have classified these cells as seromucous because periodic-acid-Schiff (PAS) stains the cells positively for glycoprotein. The traditional nomenclature of serous acinar cells is used in this chapter, however.

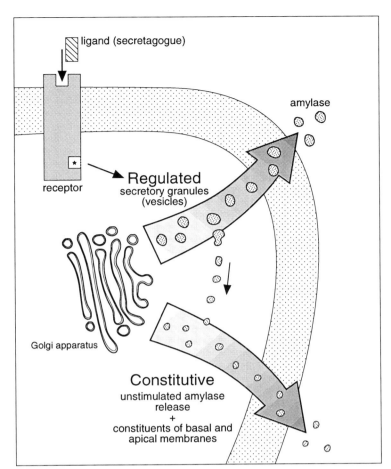

Figure 21–29. Regulated versus constitutive secretion in a salivary gland acinar cell. *Indicates conformational change that occurs after ligand binding.

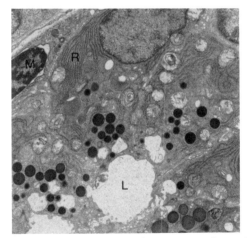

Figure 21–30. Ultrastructure of serous acinus lumen (L), rough endoplasmic reticulum (R), and myoepithelial cell (m).

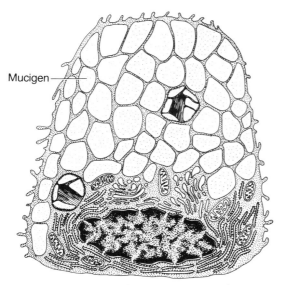

Figure 21-31. Diagram of ultrastructure of mucous cell.

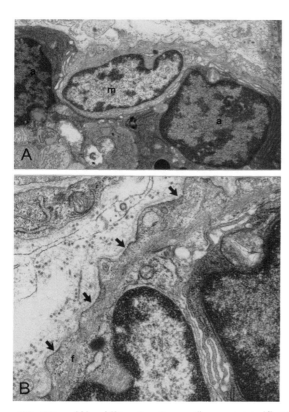

Figure 21-32. (A). Ultrastructure (low magnification) of myoepithelial cell (m) encompassing an acinar cell (a). (B). Ultrastructure (higher magnification) of myoepithelial cell with parallel microfilaments (f). Arrowheads indicate the extent of the basal lamina surrounding the myoepithelial cell and acinus.

Mucous Cells

Mucous cells are triangular or pyramidal and contain numerous granules containing mucins. The appearance of mucous cells depends on the secretory phase of the cells (Fig. 21-31). They are reduced in size after release of mucin. Mucous cells require special stains, such as PAS or mucicarmine, to demonstrate the presence of mucin granules. In normal hematoxylin and eosin (H & E) preparations, these cells generally have a washed-out cytoplasm because organic solvents remove mucin. These cells typically are observed to possess a flattened basal nucleus (Fig. 21-33).

Myoepithelial Cells

Basket or basal myoepithelial cells are branched stellate cells that lie between the basal lamina and the acinar cells (Figs. 21-32A and B and 21-33). The myoepithelial (*m*) cells have long processes that encompass the acinus and intercalated duct. In light microscopy, only the nuclei of the cells usually are visible, but ultrastructurally these cells have parallel microfilamentous (*f*) arrangements similar to those demonstrated in smooth muscle cells (Figs. 21-32A and B).

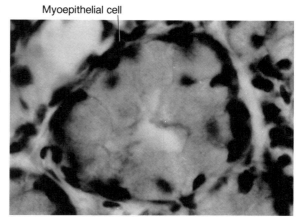

Figure 21-33. Histology of mucous acinus with myoepithelial cell on the periphery.

Scanning electron micrographs of myoepithelial cells are shown in Figure 21–34, with cell processes surrounding the terminal portions of the acini of the sublingual gland (Fig. 21–34A) and submandibular gland (Fig. 21–34B). There are morphological differences in myoepithelial cells between the salivary glands. Note the absence of myoepithelial cells around terminal acini in the parotid gland where the myoepithelial cells surround the intercalated ducts (Fig. 21–34C). Myoepithelial cell processes wrap around portions of the duct system and serve to squeeze secretion from the acinus and the associated duct system. Contraction of the myoepithelial cells facilitates the movement of secretory products from the acinus toward the oral cavity.

Histological Structure of the Acinus

The acinus or secretory portion (end piece) of the gland varies form a purely serous or a purely mucous type to a mixed type that contains both serous and mucous cells (Fig. 21–35). Serous and mucous acini differ in shape and size, with mucous acini having a more tubular shape. Mixed acini have mucous and serous cells in different positions within the secretory end piece. The mucous cells are closest to the intercalated ducts, with the serous cells forming *demilunes* (*sd*) capping over the blind ends of the mucous acini (Fig. 21–35). The serous cells are not separated from the lumen of the acinus but are connected to it by *secretory* (*intercellular*) *canaliculi* that pass between the mucous cells. All acini are surrounded by a *basal lamina* that structurally supports them. Myoepithelial cells are located between the acinar cells and the basal lamina (Figs. 21–32 and 21–36).

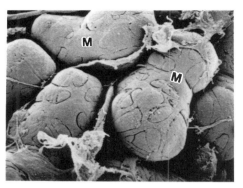

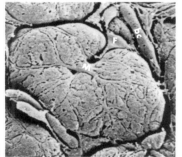
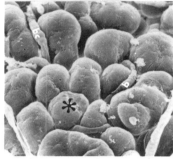

Figure 21–34. Scanning electron microscopy of myoepithelial cells. (A). The terminal portion of a sublingual acinus. The myoepithelial cells (m) cover a large part of the acinus (f, fibroblastlike cells). (B). The terminal portion of a submandibular acinus. Myoepithelial cells (m); blood capillary (bc). (C). The terminal portions (*) of the parotid gland are shown; note the absence of myoepithelial cells.

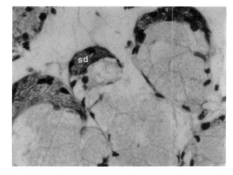

Figure 21–35. Serous demilune (sd) in mixed acinus.

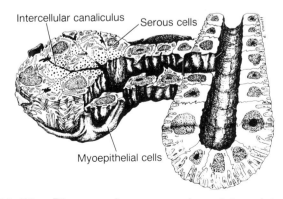

Figure 21–36. Diagram of a serous acinus, intercalated, and striated duct.

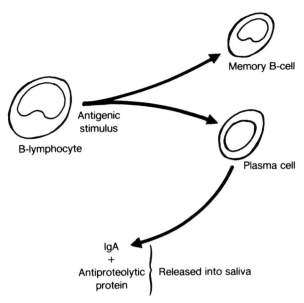

Figure 21–37. Diagram illustrating formation of immunoglobulin by plasma cells derived from B-lymphocytes.

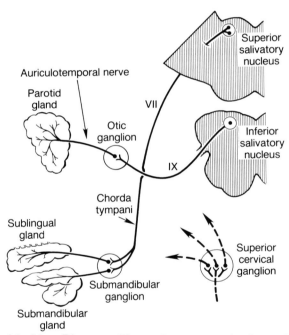

Figure 21–38. Diagram illustrating sympathetic and parasympathetic innervation of salivary glands.

Connective Tissue Cells

The connective tissue that forms the capsule and septa of the salivary glands and surrounds ducts and acini contains plasma cells, fibroblasts, macrophages, and lymphocytes. B-lymphocyte-derived *plasma cells* secrete *immunoglobulins* (primarily IgA) (Fig. 21–37). IgAs are bound to proteins that prevent proteolysis, and the complex is released into the oral cavity for defense against bacterial, viral, and other pathogens.

Innervation of Salivary Glands

Salivary gland secretion is regulated primarily by sympathetic and parasympathetic autonomic nerves (Fig. 21–38). Sympathetic fibers arise from the thoracolumbar region of the spinal cord, synapse primarily in the superior cervical ganglia, and travel with blood vessels to reach the salivary glands. These fibers are of two kinds: (1) vascular (primary vasoconstrictive) and (2) secretory-type sympathetics. Parasympathetic fibers originate in the superior and inferior salivatory nuclei of the brainstem and synapse in a ganglion in close proximity to the gland (Table 21–1 and Fig. 21–38). In the parotid gland, preganglionic fibers travel with the glossopharyngeal (ninth cranial) nerve to the otic ganglion; from the ganglion, postganglionic fibers travel with the auriculotemporal nerve to the gland. The parasympathetic innervation of the sublingual and submandibular glands originates in the superior salivatory nucleus. The pathway involves the facial nerve (VII) via the chorda tympani (preganglionic) to the submandibular ganglion. After synapsing, the postganglionic fibers innervate the glands. There is some evidence that individual acinar, myoepithelial, and duct cells may receive a dual autonomic innervation. Parasympathetic nerve stimulation produces a profuse watery secretion whereas sympathetic stimulation produces a less voluminous, thick, mucous saliva. The parasympathetic nervous system appears to be the primary neural regulator of salivary gland function. Species and gland differences, difficulty in isolationg or including all sympathetic fibers in stimulation experiments, and the diversity of sympathetic neurotransmitters have hindered delineation of the precise role of sympathetic fibers in the secretory process.

Pharmacology of Salivary Glands

The extensive autonomic innervation of the salivary glands establishes a sensitivity to autonomic pharmacological agents. Postganglionic sympathetic nerves release the neurotransmitter norepinephrine. Preganglionic sympathetic and preganglionic and postganglionic parasympathetic nerves release acetylcholine. Sympathetic noradrenergic endings are influenced by pharmacological adrenergic agonists and antagonists which may be classified into two subclasses of receptors: α and β (Fig. 21–39). Isoproterenol is a β-adrenergic agonist that stimulates secretion in the salivary glands by binding to receptors on acinar cell plasma membranes. β-receptors function through the intracellular second messenger, *cyclic AMP*. Stimulation of α-receptors induces the release of K^+ ions across the plasmalemma at both apical and basal surfaces. Parasympathetic cholinergic agents such as pilocarpine stimulate both preganglionic sympathetic fibers and parasympathetics. These drugs function through cholinergic receptors that are also located on acinar cells. Pilocarpine stimulates salivary gland secretion and alters the tonicity of the saliva. Atropine, a parasympatholytic drug, inhibits the watery parasympathetic-mediated secretion of the salivary glands. Extreme dryness of the mouth (*xerostomia*) and difficulty in swallowing and talking may result from atropine administration. Diminished salivary gland secretion is a side effect of drugs such as antihistamines, opiates, and barbiturates. Dryness of the mouth is associated with stress and adrenaline secretion. It is often assumed that this reaction is part of the flight, fight, or fright sympathetic response. However, the mechanism for stress-related dryness of the mouth is central inhibition from higher centers, which influence the salivatory nuclei, rather than direct peripheral inhibition by the sympathetic nervous system.

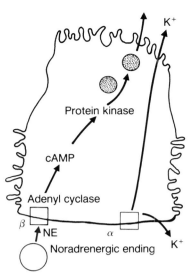

Figure 21–39. Diagram illustrating pharmacological effects on cell metabolism.

Clinical Application

Endocrine diseases such as diabetes mellitus, neurological disorders (especially those affecting the autonomic nervous system), and alcoholism result in sialadenosis, a noninflammatory and non-neoplastic disease of the salivary glands. Sialadenosis is characterized by acinar cell hypertrophy, acinar hyperplasia, and alteration of the quantity and content of the saliva. Sialadenitis (also known as sialoadenitis) is inflammation of the salivary glands caused by infection or by obstruction of a salivary gland duct (see Clinical Application on duct stones, page 379). The parotid gland is the most often affected salivary gland in both sialadenosis and sialadenitis. The result in both diseases is a decrease in salivary gland flow rate.

Regulation of Secretion

The secretory process can be separated into two parts: (1) secretion of fluid and electrolytes and (2) secretion of proteins by exocytosis. Exocytotic processes appear to be regulated through the action of β-receptors whereas α- and muscarinic receptors may affect exocytosis in addition to their role in regulation of fluid and ion secretion. β-receptors act through a cyclic AMP pathway; α-, muscarinic, and other neurotransmitter receptors function primarily through calcium-mediated pathways involving the phosphoinositide cycle.

β-Adrenergic Receptors and Cyclic AMP

Isoproterenol as well as naturally occurring catecholamines bind to β-receptors. These receptors are single polypeptide chain transmembrane glycoproteins that transverse the lipid bilayer of the plasma membrane more than once (i.e., multipass structure). In fact, they have a precise orientation with a distinct seven-pass structure characteristic of receptor proteins linked to GTP-binding regulatory proteins (i.e., G-proteins). There is a large family of receptor proteins that facilitate guanosine-triphosphate (GTP)-binding required for the activation of the receptor–G-protein complex. One of these G-proteins is stimulatory (i.e., G_s) and in the inactive state is bound to GDP (Fig. 21–40). When isoproterenol binds to the β-receptor a G_s-binding site is exposed and the G_s-protein binds to the β-receptor (Fig. 21–40). The resulting complex is capable of binding GTP in exchange for GDP activating the G-protein. A subunit of the activated G_s-protein activates adenylate cyclase. The G-protein system allows for amplification of the receptor-signal transduction response at two levels during ligand–receptor binding: (1) the production of numerous activated G_s-molecules, and (2) prolongation of the activation of adenylate cyclase. Activation ends when the G-protein hydrolyzes GTP to GDP, and another cycle can begin. Adenylate cyclase is the enzyme that catalyzes the conversion of adenosine triphosphate (ATP) to the intracellular second messenger, cyclic AMP. This messenger regulates many aspects of intracellular metabolism and function, including secretion, through the phosphorylating action of cyclic AMP-dependent protein kinase (A-kinase). The resulting protein phosphorylation stimulates exocytosis (e.g., to release amylase-containing secretory granules), but also leads to activation of nuclear regulatory factors and induction of gene expression (e.g., increased transcription of the amylase gene) (Fig. 21–40).

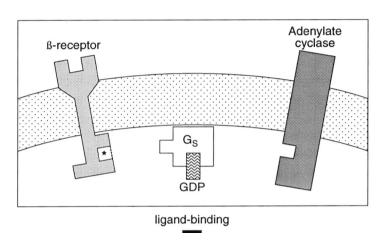

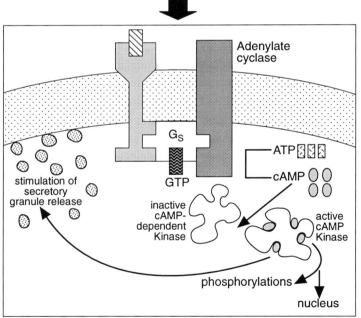

Figure 21–40. Diagram of the β-receptor-activated cyclic AMP-dependent regulatory process. *Indicates conformational change that occurs after ligand binding, exposing the G_s binding site.

Calcium and the Phosphoinositide Cycle

Stimulation of acinar cells by muscarinic cholinergic, a-adrenergic (specifically the α_1-subtype), and some peptide neurotransmitters results in an elevation of intracellular calcium. Binding of ligands to these specific receptors activates another G-protein known as G_p, which serves to activate phospholipase C (Fig. 21–41). Activation of phospholipase C is the key step in the phosphoinositide pathway and catalyzes the formation of diacylglycerol (DAG) and inositol triphosphate (IP$_3$) from the substrate phosphatidylinositol 4,5-*bis*-phosphate (PIP$_2$). DAG activates protein kinase C, which in turn phosphorylates cytosolic proteins, but may also increase specific gene transcription (Fig. 21–41). IP$_3$ binds to receptors on intracellular membranes, resulting in mobilization of intracellular calcium by opening of gated-Ca^{++} channels.

Other Pathways and Interactions of Pathways

Muscarinic and a specific subtype of α-receptor (α_2) also inactivate adenylate cyclase through the inhibitory G-protein known as G_i. These receptors are linked to adenylate cyclase by an inhibitory G-protein that subsequently binds GTP rather than the GDP that is bound in the inactive state. In addition, there is interaction between the cyclic AMP and the calcium pathways. For example, the A-kinase that is dependent on cyclic AMP elevation may phosphorylate Ca^{++}-channel proteins in intracellular membranes, or the plasma membrane, changing calcium fluxes within the cell or between the cell and its environment.

Growth Factors and Peptides Secreted by the Salivary Glands

Two major growth factors have been isolated from the rodent salivary glands. Nerve growth factor stimulates the growth of sympathetic ganglion cells whereas epidermal growth factor influences tooth eruption, epidermal keratinization, and cell proliferation and differentiation throughout the body. These growth factors are localized in specialized duct cells known as the granular convoluted tubules of the submandibular gland in rodents. Epidermal growth factor is found in human salivary glands, but predominantly in the intercalated ducts of the parotid gland. Granular convoluted tubule cells do not exist in the human submandibular glands. Nerve growth factor and its transcripts have not been identified in human salivary glands. Atrial natriuretic peptide, renin, and other factors have been found in several species whereas glucagonlike protein has been found in the human submandibular gland. Atrial natriuretic peptide is a protein first identified in the atria of the heart, which plays an important role in electrolyte balance. Because ANP has been localized in the salivary glands it may have a function in fluid balance in these organs, which produce fluid equal to 20% of the plasma volume.

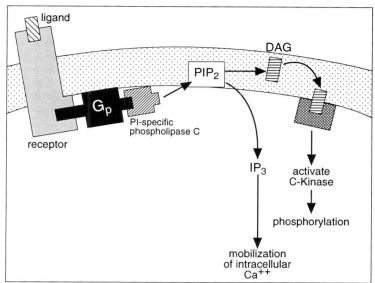

Figure 21–41. Diagram of the phosphoinositide cycle and calcium regulatory process.

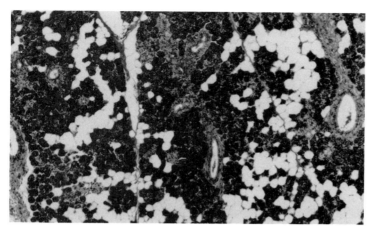

Figure 21-42. Histology of the parotid gland.

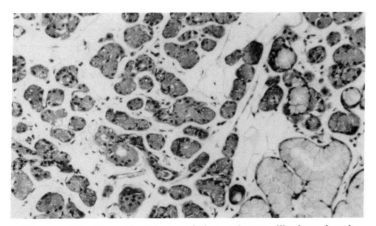

Figure 21-43. Histology of the submandibular gland.

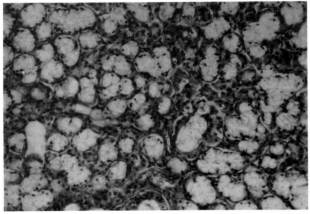

Figure 21-44. Histology of the sublingual gland.

Distinguishing Histological Characteristics of the Major Salivary Glands

Parotid Gland

The parotid gland is a purely serous gland in humans. The interlobular connective tissue contains a large number of fat cells that increase with age (Fig. 21-42). Fat cells may be distinguished from mucous cells by their totally vacuolated appearance and lack of mucigen. In the parotid gland, serous cells stain deeply with H & E, and intralobular ducts are prominent (Fig. 21-42).

Submandibular Gland

The submandibular gland is a mixed type of gland (in humans the majority of acini are serous). The histological structure of this gland is similar to that of the parotid gland, but with more striated ducts and fewer intercalated ducts. Acini are either purely serous or mixed tubules of smaller serous and larger mucous cells (Fig. 21-43). Serous demilunes are evident. In some species, striated duct cells are modified in structure and are called granular convoluted tubule cells. In rodents, these specialized ducts store and secrete hormones and other pharmacologically active substances, such as nerve growth factor, renin, and epidermal growth factor. Granular convoluted tubule cells do not exist in the human salivary glands.

Sublingual Gland

Most of the acini in this gland are mucous-secreting. There are few purely serous acini in humans (Fig. 21-44). There are, however, a few mixed acini with serous demilunes. Both segments of the intralobular duct system are poorly developed, and intercalated ducts are virtually absent. There is an absence of striations in the columnar cells lining the intralobular ducts that resorb sodium from the saliva. The absence of striations would imply that the resorption machinery is absent from the sublingual gland duct system. In fact, sublingual saliva has a much higher concentration of sodium than the other major salivary glands.

Distinguishing Histological Characteristics of the Minor Salivary Glands

The minor salivary glands are located throughout the oral cavity in the lips, cheeks, hard and soft palates, tongue, and sublingual sulcus or floor of the mouth. They are unencapsulated and are named by their location (i.e., labial, buccal, glossopalatine, and lingual). There are serous, mucous, and mixed-type minor salivary glands, as indicated in Figure 21–45 and Table 21–2. These glands produce enzymatic and mucous secretions that are similar to those of the major salivary glands. Their secretory activity appears to be continuous rather than in response to specific stimuli. The secretory products of the minor salivary glands empty into the oral cavity through numerous small ducts. Figure 21–46 shows an excretory duct surrounded by mucous acini (*m*) from a human labial salivary gland.

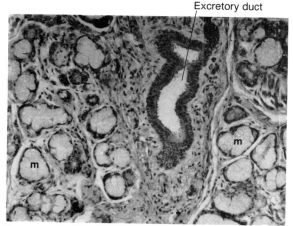

Excretory duct

Figure 21–46. Histology of labial salivary gland.

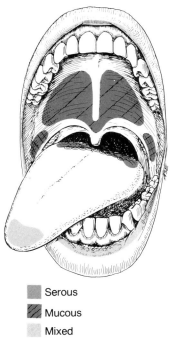

Serous

Mucous

Mixed

Figure 21–45. Diagram illustrating the location of the minor salivary glands.

Clinical Application

A few diseases that alter the structure and function of the salivary glands are diagnosed by the use of an important x-ray technique, sialography. In sialography, a radio-opaque substance is injected into the main salivary duct system before an x-ray is taken. Figure 21–47 shows a normal sialogram with the duct (arrow) and mandible (m) labeled. Sialography is useful in the diagnosis of patients with tumors, Sjögren's syndrome, and salivary calculi.

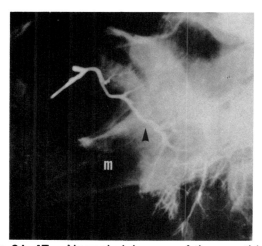

Figure 21–47. Normal sialogram of the parotid gland.

Clinical Application

Sjögren's syndrome is an autoimmune disease resulting in exocrine dysfunction and characterized by the absence or diminution of saliva and/or tears. This syndrome is often associated with rheumatoid arthritis. The submandibular, parotid, palatal, and labial glands are the most frequently affected by the disease, which is manifested by extensive lymphoid infiltration and atrophy of the ductal, acinar, and myoepithelial cells. Proliferation of lymphoepithelial elements results in narrowing of the duct, with localized dilations proximal to the zones of narrowing. Sacculation of the parotid duct and the excretory ducts is shown in Figure 21–48, a lateral sialogram from a patient with Sjögren's syndrome.

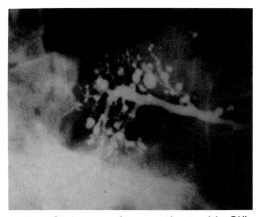

Figure 21–48. Sialogram from patient with Sjögren's syndrome (sacculation of the parotid duct) should be noted on the X-ray.

Summary

The human salivary glands are important organs of the oral cavity that produce saliva, an essential fluid required for normal speech, taste, mastication, swallowing, and digestion. In addition to its role in digestion, saliva maintains oral health through its antimicrobial, cleansing, lubricating, and buffering functions.

The three major salivary glands are the parotid, submandibular, and sublingual. In addition, there are numerous minor salivary glands in the cheeks, tongue, palate, lips, and other sites in the oral cavity that contribute to the production of the saliva.

The salivary glands develop following a pattern of epithelial–mesenchymal interactions between the outgrowths of the oral (buccal) epithelium and the underlying mesenchyme. Salivary gland development requires the processes of differentiation, proliferation, and morphogenesis. The growth (proliferation of cells), cytodifferentiation (development of specific cellular phenotypes), and morphogenesis (development of shape and form) of the gland depend on both intrinsic and extrinsic factors. The programmed pattern of cell specific gene expression is the genetic script established early in development whereas extrinsic factors include cell–cell and cell–matrix interactions and growth factors.

Interactions between cells, as well as between cells and the extracellular matrix, influence each of the steps in salivary gland development. The glands develop in six stages: (1) induction of bud formation from the oral epithelium by the underlying mesenchyme, (2) formation and growth of the epithelial cord, (3) initiation of branching in terminal parts of the cord, (4) lobule formation through repetitive branching of the epithelial cord, (5) canalization of the cords to form ducts, and (6) cytodifferentiation.

Branching is the primary morphogenetic process during salivary gland development. Branching begins with cleft formation followed by coordinated cell proliferation; however, branching and growth remain independent events. An intact basal lamina and the presence of mesenchyme are required for normal branching. Collagen synthesis stabilizes and maintains the branch points.

The salivary glands are classified as: (1) exocrine (having a duct system), (2) compound tubuloacinar (a branched duct system with both tubular and acinar end pieces), (3) merocrine (repeatedly functional) because cytoplasmic contents and cell membrane are conserved during secretion.

The salivary glands are classified as major and minor with serous, mucous, and mixed types of secretion. Three pairs of major salivary glands secrete into the oral cavity: parotid, submandibular, and sublingual glands. The major salivary glands produce most of saliva, although the minor glands contribute their secretions to the 0.5 to 0.75 L of saliva produced daily. The parotid glands are the largest salivary glands, located anterior to the ear, and in humans secrete primarily an enzyme-rich serous secretion. The submandibular glands are mixed glands, mostly serous, which are located beneath the angle of the mandible. The sublingual glands are located beneath the floor of the oral cavity and are of the mixed type, albeit primarily mucous secretion.

The duct system of the salivary glands consists of intralobular and interlobular portions and is responsible for modifying the primary salivary secretion produced by the acinar cells. The intralobular portions include the intercalated ducts draining the acini and the striated (or secretory) ducts. Striated ducts are responsible for sodium and potassium exchange and are believed to function in a manner similar to that of cells of the distal renal tubule. The intercalated ducts are longest in the parotid gland, and the striated ducts are longest in the submandibular gland. The secretory ducts empty into the interlobular (excretory) ducts, which ultimately unite to form the main excretory duct, which subsequently opens into the oral cavity.

The secretory portions of the glands are called acini and contain serous, mucous, or both serous and mucous cells. Serous cells primarily secrete salivary amylase. The mucous cells secrete mucin. Myoepithelial cells, which appear to be of epithelial origin, wrap around the acinus and serve a contractile function, squeezing secretory material from the acinar cells.

Secretion has been studied extensively in the serous cells of the salivary glands. Release of amylase occurs primarily by a regulated secretory pathway in response to the binding of a secretagogue to cell surface receptors. Constitutive secretion uses vesicular shuttling to maintain basal (unstimulated) amylase secretion and to transport membrane components to the apical and basolateral membranes. Specific processes occur in each intracellular compartment. The rough endoplasmic reticulum is the site of synthesis and initiation of folding, glycosylation, and processing of the sugars attached to proteins. In the Golgi apparatus further glycosylation as well as packaging and concentration of secretory products occurs. Secretory granules (vesicles) carry amylase to the cell surface, where exocytosis occurs as the secretory granule fuses with the cell membrane.

Secretion is regulated by several intracellular systems. β-Adrenergic drugs bind to β-receptors, stimulating a cascade of events involving stimulatory G-protein (G_s) and cyclic AMP. For example, when

Clinical Application

Salivary duct stones occur most commonly in the submandibular duct and less commonly in the parotid duct. When such stones are small, they may have only a minor influence on gland function; larger stones, however, may obstruct the duct and produce large back-pressure on the gland, which induces destruction of the parenchyma in severe cases. Calcium phosphate in the form of hydroxyapatite is the primary mineral component. Microorganisms are found within the calculi and are probably involved in the formation and growth of these structures. Figure 21–49 demonstrates a large laminated stone at the orifice of Wharton's duct.

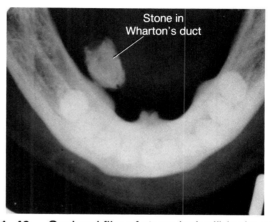

Figure 21–49. Occlusal film of stone (calculi) in the submandibular (Wharton's) duct.

isoproterenol binds to the β-receptor a G_s-binding site is exposed intracellularly and G_s-protein binds to the β-receptor. This complex binds GTP and activates cAMP, the well-defined second messenger that regulates metabolic events through phosphorylation and more indirectly through nuclear events. Intracellular calcium also regulates secretion through interaction with another G-protein called G_p. This G-protein activates the phospholipase C, which catalyzes the formation of diacylglycerol (DAG) and inositol triphosphate (IP_3). Diacylglycerol increases cytosolic protein phosphorylation and gene transcription; inositol triphosphate opens intracellular calcium channels. Another G-protein (G_i) plays an important role in muscarinic and α_2-receptor stimulation. This inhibitory G-protein inactivates adenylate cyclase. These intracellular systems do not exist independently, but interact to regulate secretory events.

The salivary glands receive an elaborate autonomic innervation from both sympathetic and parasympathetic nerves, and they are sensitive to autonomic pharmacological agents. The salivary glands provide an important role in digestion, immune responses, and other normal functions. These important organs of the oral cavity are affected in a number of pathologic conditions, such as Sjögren's syndrome, salivary calculi, mucoceles, and cystic fibrosis, and are significantly altered during the normal aging process.

Self-Evaluation Review

1. Describe the six stages in the development of the salivary glands. What are the roles of mesenchyme and the basal lamina in salivary gland morphogenesis and cytodifferentiation?
2. Which developmental processes are involved in salivary gland development? What is the mechanism of ductal branching in the developing salivary glands?
3. How are the salivary glands classified on the basis of secretion or structure?
4. What is the location of the major and minor salivary glands? Which of these glands are serous, mucous, or mixed type? How do the three major salivary glands differ in histological appearance?
5. Define the following terms: parenchyma, stroma, exocytosis, demilunes, intercellular (secretory) canaliculi, xerostomia, sialography, salivary calculi, Sjögren's syndrome, and mucoceles.
6. Describe the order of ducts from the acinus to the oral cavity in the parotid gland. Which ducts are intralobular in location? How does the duct system modify the primary secretion produced by the acinar cells? How do the three major salivary glands differ in the length of the various ductal types?
7. Describe the appearance of the intercalated, striated, and excretory ducts and of serous, mucous, and mixed acinar cells at the light-microscopic and ultrastructural level. Which acinar cell organelles are involved in serous secretion?
8. Describe the role of cyclic AMP, G-proteins, the phosphoinositide cycle, and calcium in the regulation of salivary secretion.
9. What is meant by regulated and constitutive secretion? How do these secretory pathways relate to acinar cell function in the salivary glands?
10. What is the function of myoepithelial cells? Where are they found?
11. What substances are produced by the connective tissue in the salivary glands?
12. Describe the parasympathetic and sympathetic innervation of the salivary glands.

Acknowledgments

Figure 21–9 is reproduced with permission of the author and publisher from: Spooner, BS, Bassett KE, Spooner BS Jr. Embryonic salivary gland epithelial branching activity is experimentally independent of epithelial expansion activity. *Devel Biol.* 133: 569–575, 1989 (Academic Press Inc).

Figure 21–11 is reproduced with permission of the author and publisher from: Nogawa H, Takahashi Y. Substitution for mesenchyme by basement-membrane-like substratum and epidermal growth factor in inducing branching morphogenesis of mouse salivary epithelium. *Development* 112:855–861, 1991 (The Company of Biologists, Ltd.).

Figure 21–15 is reproduced with permission the author and publisher from: Gasser R. The early development of the parotid gland around the facial nerve and its branches in man. *Anatomical Record* 167:63–78, 1970 (Alan R. Liss Inc).

Figure 21–28 is reproduced with the permission of Zastrow MV, Castle JD. Protein sorting among two distinct export pathways occur from the content of maturing exocrine storage granules. *J Cell Biol.* 105:2675–2684, 1987 (The Rockefeller University Press).

Figure 21–33 is reproduced with permission of the author and publisher from: Nagato T, Yoshida H, Yoshida A, Uehara Y. A scanning electron microscope study of myoepithelial cells in exocrine glands. *Cell Tissue Res.* 209:1–10, 1980 (Springer-Verlag).

Figure 21–36 is reproduced with permission of the author and publisher from: Tandler B. 1978. Salivary glands and the secretory process. In: Shaw JH et al. eds. *Textbook of Oral Biology,* Philadelphia (WB Saunders Co), pp. 547–592.

Figures 21–47 through 21–49, two sialograms and one X-ray, are copied (with permission) from the Diagnostic Radiological Health Sciences Learning Laboratory, as developed by the Radiological Health Sciences Education Project, University of California–San Francisco, under contract with the Bureau of Radiological Health, the Food and Drug Administration, and in cooperation with the American College of Radiology. (Additional information is available from the American College of Radiology, 560 Lennon Lane, Walnut Creek, Ca 94598.)

The author thanks the late Karl A. Youngstrom, MD, PhD, for his assistance with the reproduction of the sialograms and X-rays, and Mrs. Barbara Fegley and Mr. William Bopp for electron microscopic technical assistance. I am grateful to Doctors Bernard Tandler, Raymond F. Gasser, J. David Castle, Toshikazu Nagato, Brian Spooner, and Hiroyuki Nogawa, and the American College of Radiology for their contribution of figures. Drs. James C. McKenzie and Robert C. De Lisle and Beth E. Klein are acknowledged for their painstaking care in proofreading the manuscript. Electron microscopy was provided by the University of Kansas Medical Center Electron Microscopy Research Service Laboratory. The electron microscopy was funded in part by grants from the National Institute of Dental Research.

Suggested Readings

Alberts B, Bray D, Lewis J, Raff M, Roberts K, Watson JD. *Molecular Biology of the Cell*, 3rd ed. New York, NY: Garland Publishing Inc; 1994.

Banerjee SD, Cohn RH, Bernfield MR. Basal lamina of embryonic salivary epithelia. Production by the epithelium and role in maintaining lobular morphology. *J Cell Biol.* 1977;73:445–463.

Baum BJ, Ambudkar IS, Horn VJ. Neurotransmitter control of calcium mobilization. In: Dobrosielski-Vergona K, ed. *Biology of the Salivary Glands*, Boca Raton, Fla: CRC Press; 1993: 105–127.

Bradley RM. Salivary secretion. In: Getchell TV et al., eds., *Smell and Taste in Health and Disease.* New York, NY: Raven Press; 1991:127–144.

Castle D. Cell biology of salivary protein secretion. In: Dobrosielski-Vergona K, ed. *Biology of the Salivary Glands*, Boca Raton, Fla: CRC Press; 1993:81–104.

Cutler LS. The dependent and independent relationships between cytodifferentiation and morphogenesis in developing salivary gland secretory cells. *Anat Rec.* 1980;196:341–347.

Field A, Scott J. Changes in the structure of salivary glands with age. In: Dobrosielski-Vergona K, ed. *Biology of the Salivary Glands.* Boca Raton, Fla: CRC Press; 1993:397–439.

Garrett JR. The proper role of nerves in salivary secretion: A review. *J Dent Res.* 1987;66:387–397.

Gasser RF. The early development of the parotid gland around the facial nerve and its branches in man. *Anat Rec.* 1970;167:63–78.

Lawson KA. The role of mesenchyme in the morphogenesis and functional differentiation of rat salivary epithelium. *J Embryol Exp Morphol.* 1972;27:497–513.

Nakanishi Y, Nogawa H, Hashimoto Y, Kishi J-I, Hayakawa T. Acculumation of collagen III at the cleft points of developing mouse submandibular epithelium. *Development* 1988;104:51–59.

Palade GE. Intracellular aspects of the process of protein synthesis. *Science* 1975;189:347–358.

Quissell DO. Stimulus-exocytosis coupling mechanism in salivary gland cells. In: Dobrosielski-Vergona K, ed. *Biology of the Salivary Glands.* Boca Raton, Fla: CRC Press; 1993:105–127.

Rice DH, Becker TS. *The Salivary Glands.* New York, NY: Thieme Medical Publishers; 1994.

Schramm M, Selinger Z. The function of α- β-adrenergic receptors and a cholingergic receptor in the secretory cell of rat parotid gland. In: Ceccarelli B, Cleminti, F Meldolesi, J. eds. *Advances in Cytopharmacology.* New York, NY: Raven Press; 1974:29–32.

Shear M. The structure and function of myoepithelial cells in salivary glands. *Arch Oral Biol.* 1966;11:769–780.

Spooner BS, Wessells NK. An analysis of salivary gland morphogenesis: role of cytoplasmic microfilaments and microtubules. *Dev Biol.* 1972;27:38–54.

Tandler B. Ultrastructure of the human submaxillary gland. I. Architecture and histological relationships of the secretory cells. *Am J Anat.* 1962;111:287.

Tandler B. Salivary glands and the secretory process. In: Shaw JH, Sweeney EA, Cappuccino CC, Meller, SM, eds. *Textbook of Oral Biology.* Philadelphia, Pa: WB Saunders; 1978:547–592.

Turner RJ. Mechanisms of fluid secretion by salivary glands. *Ann NY Acad Sci.* 1993;694:24–35.

Work WO, Johns ME. Symposium on salivary gland diseases. *Otolaryngol Clin North Am.* 1977;10:259–463.

Young JA, Van Lennep EW. *The Morphology of Salivary Glands.* New York, NY: Academic Press; 1978.

22

Histology of Saliva, Pellicle, Plaque, and Calculus

James K. Avery

Introduction

Salivary glands daily secrete approximately 7500 cc of saliva. It is a complex secretion and has two major functions: to keep the oral tissues moist and to provide protection from caries. The latter function is accomplished by constant deposition of salivary mucoprotein and sialoprotein onto the tooth surface. This will result in the gradual formation of the acquired tooth covering termed the pellicle (also termed the cuticle). The *acquired pellicle* is a structureless, nonmineralized layer, initially less than 1 μm thick, that forms rapidly on the polished tooth surface when it is contacted by saliva. Soon microorganisms may appear on or within the pellicle and begin proliferating. Within 24 h, in a protected site and without cleansing, a soft, observable deposit termed *plaque* appears. Plaque may lead to either mineralized calculus or caries, which are important in the consideration of oral histology. These structures are on or in the teeth of most individuals, and can cause pathology. Thus in the absence of adequate oral hygiene, saliva may transcend its protective function and serve as a medium for microorganisms that contribute to caries or periodontal disease. Saliva is 90% water; the other 10% is composed of small amounts of numerous other substances. Amylase, which acts on carbohydrates and produces glucose and maltose, is found in saliva. A lipolytic enzyme produced by the lingual glands hydrolyzes triglycerides to diglycerides and fatty acids. Digestion, to a limited extent, thus begins in the oral cavity. In addition, at least four salivary proteins inhibit the growth and the secretion of peroxidase by oral bacteria. Thiocyanate and iodine in saliva are bactericidal, and lysozyme hydrolyzes bacterial cell walls. Salivary IgA inhibits adherence of microorganisms to oral tissues.

Objectives

After reading this chapter, you should be able to describe the composition and histology of saliva. You should also be prepared to discuss the formation and histology of the pellicle, plaque, and calculus.

Saliva

Desquamated epithelial cells are the most common cellular elements other than bacteria found in saliva. These cells are sloughed into the saliva and can be found in any salivary smear (Fig. 22–1). They are large, flat, and polygonal, can be found floating free in the saliva and, on swabbing of the mucosa, are found in large numbers. Because most of the oral mucosa is nonkeratinized, the majority of observed epithelial cells are nucleated. The nucleated cells, when viewed microscopically, reveal sex differences. The presence of a large chromatin granule adjacent to the nuclear membrane indicates the nucleus of a female. A view of an epithelial cell at a higher magnification than that seen in Figure 22–1 reveals the centrally located nucleus and numerous bacteria adhering to the surface of the cell (Fig. 22–2).

Saliva also contains lymphocytes and polymorphonuclear leukocytes. When these are in the oral cavity, they are termed *salivary corpuscles*. The number of salivary corpuscles in saliva is dependent on the state of oral health. Elevated levels of lymphocytes in saliva are observed, if the tonsils are infected. Higher levels of leukocytes and lymphocytes originate from the gingival crevice as a result of infected pockets around the teeth. Figure 22–3 is a view of inflamed gingiva with numerous leukocytes, lymphocytes, and plasma cells. A gingival pocket with plaque, bacteria, and inflammatory cells is seen in Figure 22–4, with the epithelium on the left and root cementum and dentin on the extreme right. Leukocytes, as well as densely stained plaque, are seen on the right.

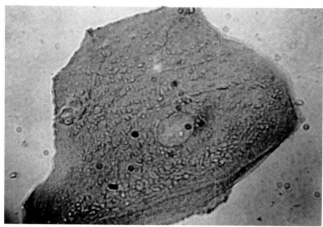

Figure 22–2. Bacteria on surface of epithelial cell.

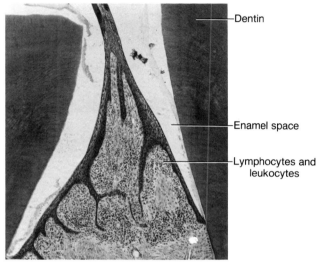

Dentin

Enamel space

Lymphocytes and leukocytes

Figure 22–3. Gingivitis resulting in leukocytes and lymphocytes in saliva.

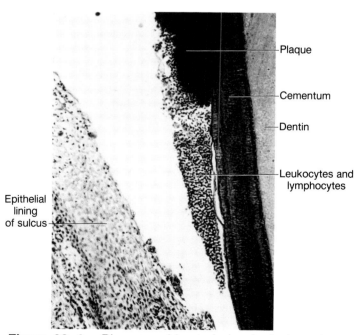

Plaque

Cementum

Dentin

Leukocytes and lymphocytes

Epithelial lining of sulcus

Figure 22–4. Plaque and bacteria in gingival crevice.

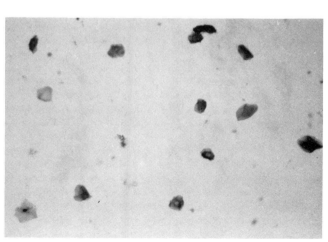

Figure 22–1. Salivary smear showing epithelial cells.

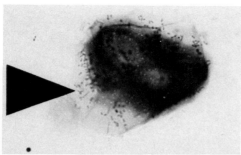

Figure 22–5. Salivary corpuscle: lymphocyte with bacteria on its surface (arrow).

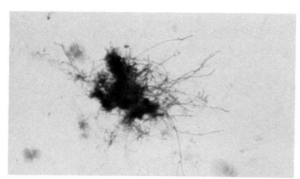

Figure 22–6. Clumps of mucin in saliva.

Clinical Application

The destructive events occurring on the tooth's surface lead from deposition of bacteria that form a plaque to the condition of caries or periodontal disease. If acidic, enamel dissolution may occur; if basic, calculus may form in plaque remnants that irritate the gingiva and lead to inflammation and tissue necrosis.

Some lymphocytes wander away from the germinal centers of the tonsils, especially if the tonsils are infected. They migrate out of the tonsillar crypts into the pharyngeal and oral cavities to become *salivary corpuscles.* Lymphocytes may function in antibody–antigen relationship and may also function as macrophages, as is seen in Figure 22–5. Note the engulfed coccal bacteria in this salivary lymphocyte.

Analysis of a slivary smear will likely yield, in addition to desquamated epithelial cells and salivary corpuscles, clumps of mucin to which bacteria are attached (Fig. 22–6). Secretory glycoproteins or mucins represent the main organic substance of saliva and may be readily seen if the salivary smear is stained.

Pellicle

The structures that cover the tooth surface may be either *developmental* or *acquired.* The *developmental cuticles* include the *primary acellular cuticle* or dental cuticle, formed as the final secretory product of ameloblasts, and the *secondary cellular cuticle,* formed from remnants of the reduced enamel epithelium. The term "cellular" is misleading in that as the secondary cuticle becomes keratinized, cellular outlines are lost. Both developmental cuticles are lost, or worn away almost entirely, because of mastication. Some reduced enamel epithelium initially remains in the depths of the gingival crevice and is eventually "turned over" as the basal epithelium cells proliferate throughout life. A third developmental tooth covering is the *coronal cementum* found as thin patches of acellular cementum in the cervical area of the crown.

The *acquired coverings* of the tooth surface include the cuticle, preferably termed the *pellicle*, which is thin, structureless membrane that forms as a result of salivary mucoproteins and sialoproteins bathing the tooth surface (Fig. 22–7). The presence of a deep, narrow central fissure in the occlusal surface allows the salivary proteins to accumulate in its depth. The inability of a toothbrush to clean such a fissure properly results in an area such as is seen in Figure 22–8. Although an acquired pellicle covers the tooth surface, it will penetrate in any convenient discrepancy on the tooth surface, such as a crack, an overhanging filling, or a lamella.

At an ultrastructure level, the acquired pellicle has a fine granular appearance and is approximately 500 Å in thickness. It may be devoid of microorganisms. The tooth surface seen in Figure 22–9A and B, happens to be bacteria-free. The thin pellicle is seen overlying the densely packed crystals of enamel apatite, which have their long axes perpendicular to the enamel surface. This area is described as the prismless zone of enamel.

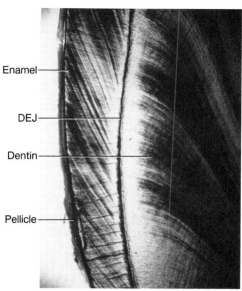

Figure 22–7. Pellicle on surface of enamel. DEJ, dentinoenamel junction.

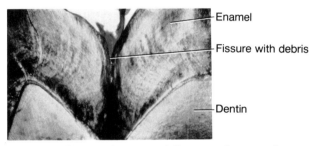

Figure 22–8. Plaque in central fissure of enamel.

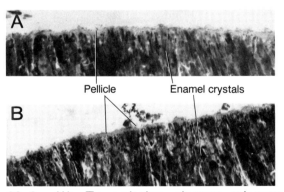

Figure 22–9. (A). Transmission electron micrograph of bacteria-free acquired pellicle on surface of enamel. (B). Ultrastructure of bacteria-free acquired pellicle on enamel surface.

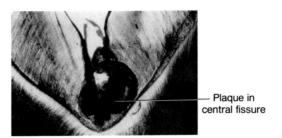

Figure 22–10. Plaque and early caries in central fissure of human molar.

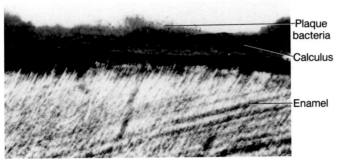

Figure 22–11. Plaque bacteria on surface of thin layer of calculus on cervical enamel.

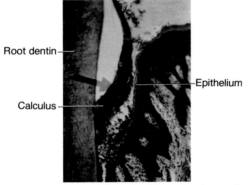

Figure 22–12. Gingival sulcus with calculus, plaque, and bacteria (arrow). Enamel was removed in tissue preparation, producing enamel space.

Plaque

The central fissure in a premolar or molar is a site for accumulation of oral microoganisms that readily colonize this fissure. They attach to any convenient mucins and take advantage of any food debris. These microorganisms rapidly form into a thick plaque and attack the enamel surface (Fig. 22–10). In Figure 22–10, the developing cavity is limited to the enamel but will probably soon expand along the dentinoenamel junction to penetrate the dentinal tubules.

The cervical area of the tooth is another region susceptible to plaque development and subsequent destruction of the tooth surface. In Figure 22–11, the filamentous bacteria of the plaque are seen on the cervical enamel surface. Beneath the plaque is a thin deposit of calculus. Instead of caries destroying the surface of the tooth shown in Figure 22–11, the pH was sufficiently alkaline to result in the deposit of minerals on the cytoskeleton of bacteria and calculus was formed. Mineralization rather than demineralization has occurred.

When plaque development takes place in a gingival sulcus, the bacteria increase in number, and with the addition of the calculus as an irritant, inflammation of the gingiva occurs (Fig. 22–12). In Figure 22–12, calculus is seen overlying the enamel space (enamel dissolved in tissue preparation), and cells and organisms are seen in the plaque at the depth of the pocket. Observe that the epithelial attachment is on the surface of the cementum, not the enamel. Inflammatory cells are also seen in the lamina propria underlying the epithelium.

The plaque or microbial flora is not static and is closely related to the state of periodontal health. The flora in the supragingival and subgingival zones is different, with the kind of difference depending on the extent of disease. The following brief description summarizes some of these differences. In patients with *normal* tissues, a thin layer of coccoid bacteria may appear on the pellicle. In patients with *gingivitis*, more filamentous bacteria with a corncob appearance have been reported supragingivally, and greater numbers of Gram-negative bacteria, flagellated cells, nd spirochetes can be found in the sulcus. In patients with periodontitis, as in patients with the gingivitis, more filamentous bacteria with a corncob appearance have been reported supragingivally, and a greater number of Gram-negative bacteria, flagellated cells, and spirochetes adhere to the root surface subgingivally. Periodontosis patients exhibit predominantly (although sparsely) Gram-negative bacteria. These patients also exhibit a unique lobulated cuticular deposit that appears electron dense.

A transmission electron micrograph (Fig. 22–13) reveals the appearance of 7-day-old dental plaque. At the bottom of the field is the surface of the enamel covered with a thin, dark-staining pellicle. Above this line is the feltwork of plaque microorganisms. Filamentous bacteria are seen at the top of the micrograph. When the deeper portion of the 7-day-old plaque is studied at higher magnification with transmission electron microscopy, the identity of the bacteria on the enamel surface can be seen (Fig. 22–14). The clear space at the bottom of the field represents the demineralized surface enamel. overlying it is a thin, electron-dense pellicle. The deepest part of the plaque consists of a condensed microbial layer that appears as a darkly stained band resting on the pellicle. Above this layer is a superficial layer of coccoid and filamentous microorganisms. The light areas in the plaque contain cell remnants, mucopolysaccharide substances, and glycoproteins. In this zone, active acid production by the cocci occurs, resulting in surface etching and dental caries.

A higher magnification of the condensed microbial layer of plaque, on an enamel surface, is seen in Figure 22–15. Below is enamel with the thin black pellicle on its surface. At this high magnification, a pellicle is seen to be discontinuous. The remainder of the field shows the condensed microbial layer consisting of coccoid microorganisms, which appear to be dividing in a plane perpendicular to the enamel surface. Polysaccharides are located between the bacteria. Ribosomes can also be observed in a few bacteria.

Clinical Application

Plaque bacteria ferment sugars to lactic acid, which will then destroy the mineralized enamel. Destruction of the protective pellicle and the enamel surface is a progressive process. A disclosing agent can expose plaque bacteria to facilitate its removal but plaque will re-form unless appropriate oral hygiene is practiced.

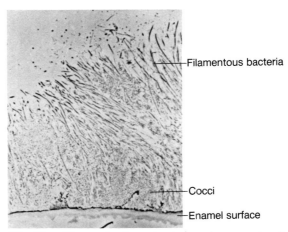

Figure 22–13. Transmission electron micrograph of plaque bacteria on enamel surface after 7 days.

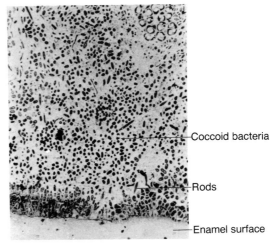

Figure 22–14. Electron micrograph of bacteria on enamel surface seen in Figure 22–13, with coccoid and rods noted.

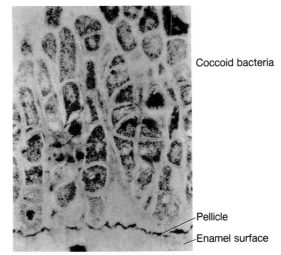

Figure 22–15. Ultrastructure of condensed bacterial layer on enamel surface denotes the region of active cell division.

22: Histology of Saliva, Pellicle, Plaque, and Calculus **387**

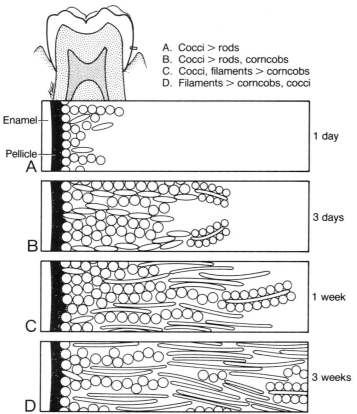

Figure 22-16. Changes in composition of plaque with time. On day 1, cocci and rods can be seen; after 1 week, filamentous bacteria appear.

A. Cocci > rods
B. Cocci > rods, corncobs
C. Cocci, filaments > corncobs
D. Filaments > corncobs, cocci

Enamel
Pellicle

A — 1 day
B — 3 days
C — 1 week
D — 3 weeks

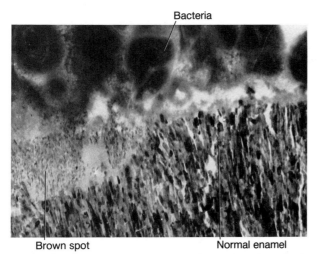

Figure 22-17. Electron micrograph of initial carious lesion on enamel surface, with enamel crystal dissolution (left) under bacteria.

Bacteria
Brown spot
Normal enamel

Numerous dental investigators have shown that the composition of plaque changes with time (Fig. 22-16). Initially, cocci and rods appear, and after a week, filamentous organisms are seen. The composition of the plaque is dependent on the extent of gingival disease and its location supragingivally or subgingivally.

As noted in Figure 22-9A and B, the outermost area of enamel in the teeth of most patients is composed of a prismless zone about 30 μm thick. In this zone, the c-axis or long axis of the apatite crystals is situated almost perpendicular to the tooth surface (Fig. 22-9). The initial carious lesion involves this zone, as plaque bacteria cause dissolution of some of these crystals. This dissolution is illustrated in Figure 22-17; a brown spot is seen on the left, and normal tooth structure is seen on the right. Situated between the overlying bacteria of the plaque and the enamel surface is an amorphous-appearing pellicle. Enamel crystal dissolution is seen in the superficial zone on the left. Another case of a superficial lesion in the enamel of an adult human is seen in Figure 22-18. In this figure, a small penetrating defect filled with organic materials is observed. A surface zone of altered enamel that is overlayed by remains of an organic pellicle can also be seen.

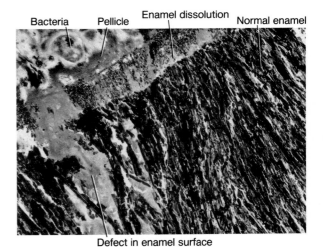

Bacteria   Pellicle   Enamel dissolution   Normal enamel

Defect in enamel surface

Figure 22-18. Electron micrograph of penetrating defect in enamel filled with organic material and of enamel dissolution under pellicle and bacteria.

Calculus

The formation of calculus begins by a process opposite to that of tooth surface dissolution. The beginning of inorganic crystallization on the tooth surface occurs in the inner organic layer of the pellicle and the overlying bacteria of the dental plaque (Fig. 22–19). Dense granular particles that appear smaller than enamel apatite crystals are around and in the bacterial matrix. Calcification then spreads between the bacteria into the adjacent plaque. Calcification first takes place in the cell walls and then the cores of the bacteria calcify to produce calculus. The surface of the tooth then becomes covered with a continuous layer of apatite crystals. This layer gradually thickens as further deposition occurs.

Figure 22–20 illustrates the appearance of calculus formed in root dentin. Dentinal tubules containing large atypical mineral crystals can be seen (lower left). This indicates that demineralization related to the carious process was reversed and precipitation of mineral had occurred. At the top of the electron micrograph, calcified bacteria and matrix can be seen.

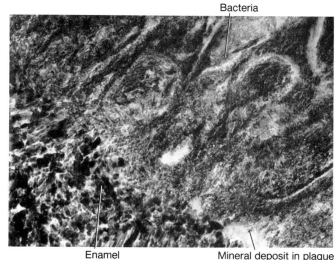

Figure 22–19. Electron micrograph of minute crystals on the surface of enamel denotes calculus formation. A calcified bacterial matrix is seen.

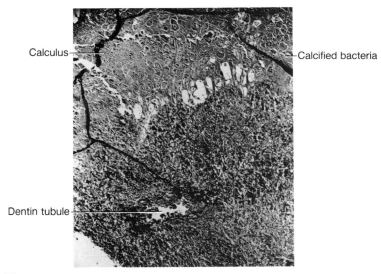

Figure 22–20. Electron micrograph of calculus on root dentin. Dissolution of mineral in dentinal tubule indicates reversal of caries process.

Clinical Application

Saliva bathes the tooth's surface and assists in the formation of the protective organic membrane, the pellicle. Microorganisms collect in protected sites forming a deposit. Thus, saliva, which usually serves as a protective function in bathing the tooth, then serves as a medium for growth of organisms on the tooth.

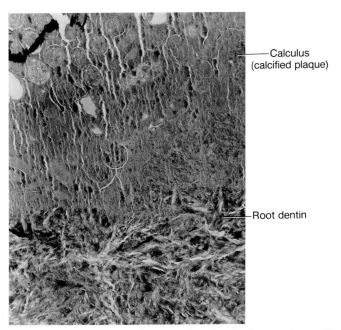

Figure 22-21. Electron micrograph of calculus on irregular surface of dentin after root scaling. Note the minute size of the crystals in the calculus compared with those in the dentin.

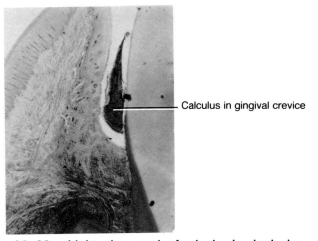

Figure 22-22. Light micrograph of calculus in gingival crevice. Enamel was lost in tissue preparation.

As is seen in Figure 22–21, there is close adaption of calculus to the irregular surface of root dentin. The adaption seen in this figure was a result of scaling of the root surface. The calcified bacteria appear as circular profiles. Observe how much smaller the hydroxyapatite crystals are in the calculus compared with the underlying dentin. Calculus forms in a calcospheric manner as the calcium salts derived from saliva are deposited within the organic matter. The glycoprotein matrix and the bacterial become mineralized, if the oral environment maintains an alkaline pH. As the plaque mineralizes, it loses its ability to produce an acid environment. Calculus varies in composition and in hardness. Very hard calculus contains a higher percentage of inorganic salts. Softer calculus has a higher percentage of protein. Calculus most often is found near the opening of the parotid excretory ducts, on the buccal surfaces of the mandibular incisors, near the opening of the submandibular and sublingual gland ducts.

Calculus can be categorized clinically into two types: supragingival or salivary appearing, above the gingival crest and subgingival or *serumal*, within the gingival crevice. Subgingival calculus is much harder and forms more slowly than salivary caclulus.

A typical picture of calculus appearing in a gingival crevice is shown in Figure 22–22. This deposit has caused gingival inflammation, and inflammatory cells can be seen in the lamina propria of the gingiva. Observe the location of the gingival attachment on the dark-staining cementum rather than on the enamel. Where there is calculus, inflammatory cells usually can be found in the underlying gingival epithelium.

The mouth is said to be a micro-universe of organisms. The acquired pellicle is an amorphouse organic deposition on enamel, on which plaque may form. Plaque is derived from desquamated epithelial cells and is composed of mucin, dextrans, sugars, and bacteria. The composition of the plaque changes with time, location, and extent of the disease process. The composition of supragingival and subgingival plaque varies, as does the bacterial composition in the periodontal pocket. These variables are expressed in Figure 22–23. If the pH of the saliva is alkaline, calculus may develop from mineralization of the plaque, and this may be salivary or serumnal.

Figure 22–24 is an example of a mouth that requires extensive care and patience. This patient is dependent on your knowledge of oral hygiene.

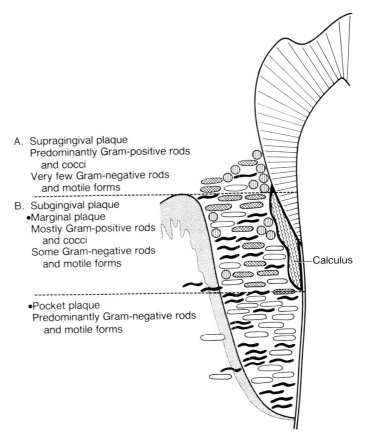

Figure 22–23. Summary of presence and identification of bacteria in supragingival, subgingival, and periodontal pocket.

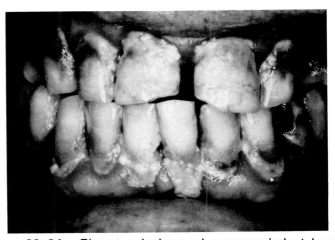

Figure 22–24. Plaque, calculus, and severe periodontal problems can be seen in this patient's mouth.

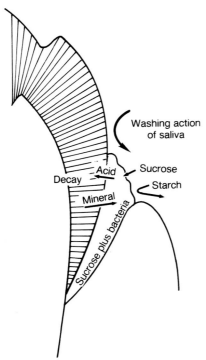

Figure 22–25. Summary of plaque activity and enamel dissolution.

Summary

Figure 22–25 is a diagram summarizing the activity occurring within plaque. This diagram illustrates the typical location of development of plaque at the interdental gingival margin. Above the gingiva is seen the washing action of saliva, which assures the self-cleansing of enamel areas. Plaque accumulates at the gingival margin, and the presence of sucrose gives rise to a synthesis of slimy extracellular oligosaccharides and glucose, which diffuse into the deeper layers of the plaque. There they may be fermented to lactic acid, which penetrates into the enamel and causes mineral diffusion into the plaque. The large polysaccharide molecules of starches do not diffuse into the plaque.

Clinical Application

Cells of the saliva include, most commonly, epithelial cells shed from the mucosa, lymphocytes, and leukocytes. The two latter cells are termed salivary corpuscles and are prevalent when either of these sites of origin is infected. Lymphocytes arise from the tonsils and leukocytes from gingival crevices.

Self-Evaluation Review

1. Name and characterize the outermost layer of enamel.
2. Describe the changes that occur in the plaque from 1 day to 3 weeks.
3. On what matrix does calculus form?
4. What changes occur in the pellicle underlying the plaque?
5. Describe some histological characteristics of the plaque.
6. Where does plaque usually form?
7. Describe the cells and their origin that are found in saliva.
8. What is the composition of a pellicle?
9. What organisms are deep in the plaque supragingivally? Subgingivally?
10. How long does it take for an acquired pellicle to form?

Acknowledgments

Photomicrographs for Figures 22.9 A and B, 22.17, 22.18, and 22.19 are provided by Dr. R. F. Frank, Professor and Dean, and by Dr. M. Brendel, Faculty de Chirurgie Dentaire, Strasburg, France.

Photomicrographs for Figures 22.20 and 22.21 are provided by Knut A. Selvig, Professor and Head, Department of Dental Research, School of Dentistry, University of Bergen, Bergen, Norway.

Photomicrographs for Figures 22.13, 22.14 and 22.15 are provided by scientists at the National Institute for Dental Research, Bethesda, Maryland.

Data for Figure 22.24 are provided by Dr. Walter Loesche, University of Michigan School of Dentistry, Ann Arbor, Michigan.

Suggested Readings

Frank RM, Brendel A. Ultrastructure of the approximal dental plaque and the underlying normal and carious enamel. *Arch Oral Biol.* 1966;11:883–912.

Hand AR. Salivary glands. In: *Orban's Oral Histology and Embryology*, 11th ed. Bhaskar SN, ed. St. Louis, MO: CV Mosby; 1990.

Koulourides T, Feagin F, Pigman W. Remineralization of dental enamel by saliva. *Ann NY Acad Sci.* 1965;131:751–757.

Lie T. Early dental plaque morphogenesis. *J Periodont Res.* 1977;12:73–89.

Listgarten MA. Structure of the microbial flora associated with periodontal health and disease in man. *J Periodontol,* 1976;47:1–18.

McHugh WD. *Dental Plaque.* Edinburgh; E. & S Livingstone; 1970.

Meckel AH. The formation and properties of organic films on teeth. *Arch Oral Biol.* 1965;10:585–598.

Newman HN. Update on plaque and periodontal disease. *J Clin Periodontol.* 1980;7:251–258.

Saxton CA. Scanning electron microscope study of the formation of dental plaque. *Caries Res.* 1973;7:102–119.

Selvig KA. Attachment of plaque and calculus to tooth surfaces. *J Periodont Res.* 1970;5:8–18.

Shannon JL, Suddick RP, Dowd FJ. Saliva composition and secretion. *Monogr Oral Sci.,* 1974;2:1–103.

Silverstone LM, Johnson NW, Hardie JM, Williams RAD. The formation, structure and microbial composition of dental plaque. In: Silverstone LM, Johnson NW, Hardie JM, Williams RAD, eds. *Dental Caries Aetiology, Pathology and Prevention.* New York, NY: Macmillan; 1981:103–132.

Histology of Nasal Mucosa, Paranasal Sinuses, and Olfaction

Donald S. Strachan

Introduction

This chapter discusses the nasal cavity, the paranasal sinuses, and olfaction. Initially, the anatomic relation of the nasal cavity will be described. The nasal septum divides the cavity into two parts. The lateral wall contains projections that vastly increase the area exposed to respiratory air. The mucosa of the nasal cavity aids in humidification and warming or cooling of the air during respiration. Epithelium lining the nasal cavity is respiratory epithelium (ciliated pseudostratified columnar epithelium with goblet cells), and the lamina propria contains numerous glands and a rich venous sinusoidal network.

The paranasal sinuses will be described. They are a group of air containing spaces around the nasal cavity. In the adult, the frontal, sphenoid, and maxillary sinuses are large paired sinuses. There are numerous ethmoid sinuses in the superior parts of the nasal cavity. The mucosa of these sinuses is similar to the nasal cavity, but the epithelium and lamina propria are thinner.

Olfactory mucosa is found in the superior parts of the nasal cavity. Neuroreceptor cells for the sense of smell are located within the epithelium of this mucosa. The neuroreceptor cells are first-order neurons and are considered to be part of the central nervous system. These cells have the ability to regenerate and re-establish connections with the central nervous system.

Objectives

After reading this chapter, you should become familiar with the microscopic structure of the nasal tissues and paranasal sinuses. Included in this knowledge should be an understanding of the function of these tissues. You should be able to describe the histological detail of the olfactory mucosa and the basic neuroanatomical connections for olfaction. Also, you should be able to discuss the regeneration capacity of the olfactory epithelium, and to describe the anatomic basis for the sense of smell (olfaction).

Frontal, Ethmoid, and Sphenoid Sinuses

These three sinuses have a thinner mucosa than the maxillary sinuses. They have only a moderate number of seromucous glands, and have a reduced number of goblet cells in their epithelium. The columnar epithelial cells lining their surfaces contain cilia. All of these sinuses have openings (ostia) to the lateral walls of the nasal cavity (Figs. 23–8 and 23–9). Ciliary beating moves the mucous coating over the epithelium toward the ostium of each sinus. In addition to the ciliary action, negative air pressure created during breathing can help in the clearance of mucous from the system.

The connective tissue fibers of the lamina propria in the paranasal sinuses generally are not organized into a distinct periosteal covering. The epithelium and lamina propria together form a thin membrane that lines these sinuses. With exceptions of the medial walls of the maxillary sinuses and areas close to the ostia, the lamina propria of the paranasal sinuses does not contain many seromucous glands.

Ostia of the Paranasal Sinuses

The ostia of the sphenoid sinuses are found above the superior concha (Fig. 23–9). Most of the numerous ethmoid sinuses and the maxillary sinus open into the middle meatus, beneath the middle concha. The ostia for the frontal sinuses are found in the anterior part of the middle meatus. The frontonasal duct of the frontal sinus communicates with the nasal cavity. In most sinuses, the ostium is a short pathway. Also opening into the nasal cavity in the inferior meatus is the nasolacrimal duct. Excess lacrimal secretions (tears) that reach the medial aspect of the eye are transported to the nasal cavity by this duct (Fig. 23–9).

At birth, the ostium for the maxillary sinus is situated at the same level as the floor of the nasal cavity. With development and growth of the maxillary dentition and with increases in height of the maxillae and palate, the ostium becomes located more superiorly and, as already stated, empties into the middle meatus. Frequently, there is an accessory ostium for the maxillary sinus located posteriorly to the main ostium.

Clinical Application

Clinical Application

It is usually difficult to place osseointegrated type implants into the posterior parts of the maxillary as there is not enough bone present and because of the proximity of the maxillary sinus. However, surgical procedures have been designed to place bone from the patient or bone substitutes into an enlarged space between the sinus mucosa and the bony floor. The purpose is to create newly organized osseous tissue to support the implant. More investigation is required to analyze the success of this technique.

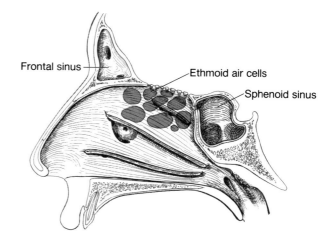

Figure 23–8. Diagram of location of frontal ethmoid and sphenoid sinuses, sagittal view.

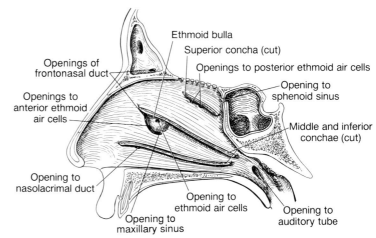

Figure 23–9. Diagram of location of ostia of sinuses shown in Figure 23–8.

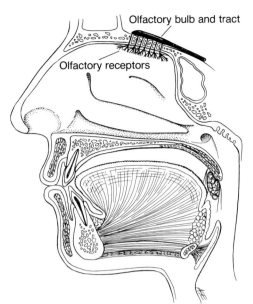

Figure 23–10. Taste receptors are located on the dorsum on the tongue, and olfactory receptors are located in the superior aspect of the nasal cavity.

Clinical Application

Orthognathic surgery for moving the maxillary arch sometimes requires the separation of the maxillary alveolar process and teeth as a block (La Fort I). Ostia of the nasolacrimal ducts should be superior to the surgical cuts that free the maxillary segment. Scarring or closure of the duct results in tears flowing over the face from the inner corners of the eye.

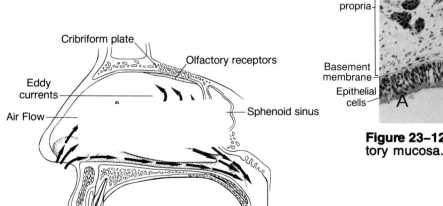

Figure 23–11. Nasal chamber with olfactory receptors. Eddy currents contact olfactory area.

Olfaction

Olfaction occurs as airborne substances contact cilia of sensory cells that are located in the superior region of the nasal mucosa. There are direct neural pathways between olfactory stimuli and the central nervous system. How the olfactory receptors sense and discriminate between various odors is not fully understood (Fig. 23–10).

Olfactory Mucosa Structure

The zone of olfactory mucosa is located in the superior aspects of the nasal cavity. This area is above the superior nasal conchae and includes the roof of the nose and the upper part of the nasal septum (Fig. 23–11). This area is out of the main air flow. Thus, the receptors in this area are activated by eddy currents carrying the smellable substances to them. In histological sections the junction between the olfactory mucosa and the nasal mucosa is abrupt. A comparison of the thickness of the nasal olfactory mucosa is seen in Figure 23–12. With increasing age the amount of olfactory mucosa diminishes, and there is an uneven border between the two types of mucosae. However, when viewed microscopically, the boundary is clearly seen. In some areas, islands of olfactory mucosa are surrounded by nasal mucosa.

The olfactory receptors arise embryologically from neuroblasts that differentiate directly from cells of the paired olfactory placodes. The placodes are thickenings in the superficial ectoderm of the face and they invaginate to form the olfactory pits. Primary receptor (sensory) cells develop from this ectoderm, and then form axons that join with the olfactory nerve that is part of the brain.

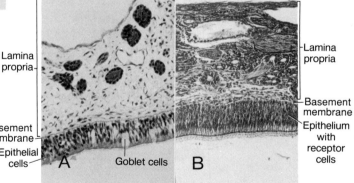

Figure 23–12. (A). Respiratory mucosa. (B). Olfactory mucosa.

The olfactory mucosa consists of an epithelial cell layer and a lamina propria that is adjacent to the underlying bone (Fig. 23–12). In the lamina propria are serous glands (Bowman's) whose ducts drain onto the surface of the epithelium. In Figure 23–12, the respiratory epithelium (A) and the olfactory epithelium (B) can be seen side by side. However, there are several basic differences. Both are pseudostratified columnar-type epithelium, but the olfactory epithelium is taller (approximately 70 μm) than the respiratory epithelium (45 μm). Both types of epithelium have cilia. The respiratory epithelium contains goblet cells, whereas the olfactory epithelium contains olfactory receptor cells. Both have basal cells. Respiratory epithelium has a distinct basement membrane visible with the light microscope; the olfactory epithelium has a basement membrane, but it is less distinct and is best visualized at the ultrastructural level. Beneath the olfactory mucosa is the periosteum of the ethmoid bone (Fig. 23–13). There is no submucosa underlying the olfactory epithelium. In contrast, there is a significant submucosa found under respiratory epithelium and this submucosa contains numerous venous sinusoids and glands.

Olfactory epithelium consists primarily of three cell types: tall ciliated columnar receptor cells, supporting cells with microvillar cells, and basal cells that lie adjacent to the basement membrane. When olfactory epithelium is viewed with the electron microscope, distinct layers are seen (Fig. 23–13). The nuclei of supporting cells lie close to the surface of the epithelium. The nuclei of the neural cells form a band midway from the free surface to the deep lying basal cells. On the free surface of the mucosa is a mucous layer some 10 to 40 μm thick.

At higher magnification (Fig. 23–14), the cilia of the neural receptor cells and the microvilli of the supporting cells can be seen. The tall slender olfactory receptor cells end at the epithelial surface with a bulb shaped olfactory vesicle from which the cilia extend onto the surface of this epithelium (Figs. 23–14 through 23–16). Cilia of the epithelial cells of nasal mucosa (respiratory epithelium) move or beat constantly whereas cilia of olfactory epithelium do not.

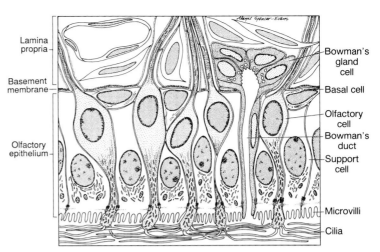

Figure 23–14. Diagram of olfactory epithelium denotes olfactory neural receptor and supporting cells. Serous glands underlie the olfactory epithelium.

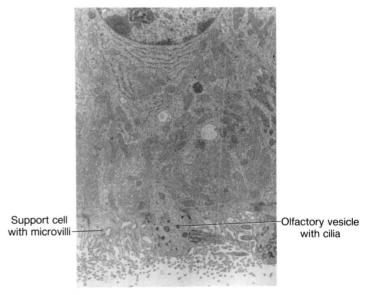

Figure 23–15. Ultrastructure of olfactory vesicle and cilia and microvilli of support cells.

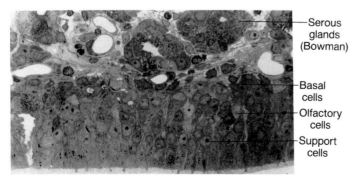

Figure 23–13. Olfactory mucosa with three layers of nucleated cells (bottom to top); superficial (light-stained) support cells; wide band of olfactory cell nuclei (dark nuclei); and basal cell nuclei at junction with basal lamina.

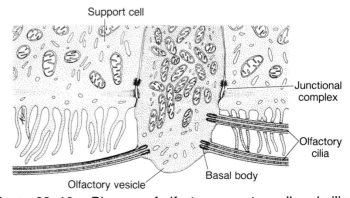

Figure 23–16. Diagram of olfactory receptor cell and cilia.

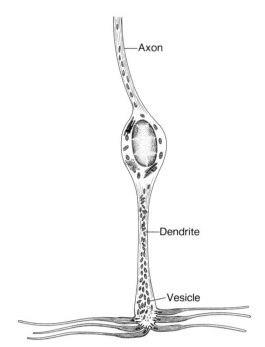

Figure 23–17. Diagram of olfactory cell and axon.

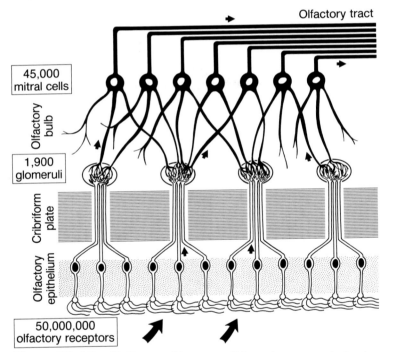

Figure 23–18. Pathway of how smell impulses pass to brain.

Clinical Application

Patients with defects between the oral and nasal cavities (cleft palate or surgical defects) require a physical separation of these cavities so that breathing can occur when ingesting food or for normal sounding speech to occur. An oral prosthesis (obturator) can be constructed to help close the defect.

The olfactory receptor cell is a primary neuron. This slender, flask-shaped columnar cell with its cylindrical dendrite terminates as an olfactory vesicle at the epithelium–mucous interface (Fig. 23–17). This vesicle may appear flat or dome-shaped. It contains neurotubules indicating its neural function in olfaction, and contains the ciliary basal bodies of numerous cilia (10 to 60) per cell (Figs. 23–16 and 23–17). The cilia vary in length from 50 to 200 μm and exhibit the usual pattern of "9 + 2" microtubules in each cilium. The cilia probably provide a role in olfactory transduction. Adjacent to the olfactory vesicle is a constricted zone and junctional complex. This junctional complex has characteristic zonular occludens, zonular adherens, and macula adherens (desmosome), with adjacent supporting cells. This junctional complex seals the intercellular space from the external environment. The receptor cells vary from 5 to 8 μm in diameter, with a nucleus almost as large, so that most of the cell cytoplasm is at the distal pole, where it is continuous with the cylindrical dendrite (olfactory rod) (Fig. 23–17). Figure 23–18 is a diagram of the pathway of smell impulses to the brain. The olfactory sensory cell is a first-order neuron. The process that extends from the proximal pole of the olfactory cell is actually an unmyelinated axon. This axon joins with other axons to form small Schwann cell-wrapped bundles. These bundles then join with other similar bundles and pass through the cribriform plate of the ethmoid bone to terminate in the glomeruli of the bilateral olfactory bulbs. The glomeruli are areas where axons of the olfactory sensory cells intermingle with dendrites of the mitral cells.

The basal cells shown in Figure 23–14 are shaped like a pyramid, and are in direct contact with the basement membrane. Basal cells are the site of numerous mitotic figures, and thus produce cells that replace the supporting and receptor cells (Fig. 23–14). New cells are required to replace the cells that normally turn over because of age, injury, or exposure to noxious chemicals. The new neural receptor cells re-establish their contact with the olfactory nerves of the brain and with adjacent cells. Olfactory neogenesis is unique in the body as neural cells are not replaced elsewhere and the process continues throughout life.

Observe the relationship of the adjacent olfactory support cells and basal cells seen in Figure 23–16. On their free surface, microvillae are seen extending from the support cells, and their cytoplasm is filled with secretory granules. In addition to the ciliated receptor cells, support cells, and basal cells, an additional support cell with microvillae has recently been described the literature, which may be a second type of receptor cell. Olfactory cells contain many neurotubules and mitochondria, and cilia protrude from the surface of the olfactory vesicle (Fig. 23–16). Underlying the olfactory epithelium in the lamina propria are the serous *glands of Bowman*. These glands are tubular alveolar glands with secretory cells penetrating the epithelial cell layer; their ducts open onto the surface (Fig. 23–14). Although these cells are classified as serous cells, they contain mucopolysaccharide staining granules. These glands, as well as the supporting cells, contribute to the mucous layer overlying the olfactory epithelium.

Olfactory Receptor Nerve Supply

Although the first cranial nerve is responsible for olfaction, trigeminal nerve fibers (cranial nerve V) have been found in olfactory mucosa. These fibers, arising from terminal nasal branches, terminate among the olfactory cells. Their role in olfaction is unknown, but they may provide a role in sensory function.

Olfactory Receptor Function

What part the cilia provide in olfactory reception is not known, although cilia and microvilli cause considerable increase the surface of these receptors. Findings indicate that the secretion from Bowman's glands, along with the secretory products of the supporting cells, have a role in the diffusion of odor molecules over the epithelial surface. These secretions are renewed by production of new materials within these cells. Functionally, the olfactory receptor is thought to be an independent unit. Recent information on replacement of receptor cells and their close relation to adjacent cells by junctional complexes indicates that the difference in the basal and supportive cells may relate to stages of growth.

Figure 23–18 illustrates a large number of receptor cilia in the olfactory mucosa. Considering the number of cilia per cell and the number of receptor cells in the olfactory mucosa, there are millions of these cilia. Cilia are at the luminal end of the cell, which is the dendritic end of this bipolar sensory neuron. At the opposite end is the axon of this cell. The axons from hundreds of receptor cells cluster, are wrapped by Schwann cells, and pass to the bilateral olfactory bulbs. At the bulbs, the axons synapse at sites called *glomeruli*, which are composed of the dendrites of mitral cells. The mitral cells are the second-order neurons. The dendrites of the mitral cells then carry olfactory impulses by their axons that form the olfactory tract. These axons proceed to centers in the brain. There are far fewer mitral cells (45,000) than sensory neurons (they number 50 million on one side), and there are even fewer (1900) glomeruli. Thus, large numbers of sensory axons synapse with each mitral cell. The axons of the mitral cells collectively form the olfactory tract, which travels to the higher brain centers. Not shown n Figure 23–18 are the many interconnections between right and left olfactory bulbs.

A regional organization of the olfactory bulb corresponds to that of the olfactory mucosa; fibers from the anterior part of the mucosa extend to the anterior part of the bulb, and fibers from the posterior portion of the mucosa extend to the posterior part of the bulb. Smells can therefore be discriminated by both detailed signal pattern and area of signal origin. Attempts have been made to classify smells into a small number of groups, but have not proven successful. Of interest, the olfactory epithelium can become fatigued to one odor but not to others. Recent investigations into the mechanism of olfaction have suggested that the sensed odors affect the enzyme balance of the olfactory cell.

Summary

The nasal passages function not only in conduction of air but in the warming (and cooling) of it by numerous blood vessels, and in adjusting the moisture content with secretions from the serous and mucous glands. Each bilateral nasal cavity contains three conchae that increase the surface area of the nasal cavities. These cavities are lined with pseudostratified ciliated columnar epithelium situated on a prominent basement membrane. Beneath the basal lamina, mucous and serous glands appear in the lamina propria. The paranasal sinuses are located around the superior and lateral parts of the nasal cavity, and drain into the nasal cavity. Maxillary sinuses are the largest of the sinuses, and molar roots lie adjacent or in the sinus floor. Therefore, maxillary sinusitis may cause painful teeth. The frontal, ethmoid, and sphenoid paranasal sinuses contain ciliated stratified columnar epithelium, which is much thinner than the epithelium of the nasal cavity and contains no seromucous glands and few goblet cells.

Odors are transmitted to olfactory epithelium as airborne substances. At the epithelium odors combine with fluid covered mucosa at the receptor site. Olfactory receptors are bipolar neurons that use cilia to detect odors, and then transmit the impulse via the olfactory nerve to the olfactory bulb and the brain. The cells of the olfactory epithelium are continuously being replaced, and the receptor-neurons re-establish connections with the olfactory bulb (cranial nerve I).

Self-Evaluation Review

1. What is the relationship of the floor of the maxillary sinus to the floor of the nasal cavity early in life? In the adult?
2. Describe major differences between mucosa of the nasal cavity and mucosa of the paranasal sinuses.
3. Give three major functions of the nasal cavity.
4. What sinuses have their openings into the middle meatus?
5. What nerve carries odoriferous signals to the brain?
6. Describe an olfactory receptor.
7. What are the differences between olfactory and respiratory epithelia?
8. Describe the life cycle of the olfactory receptor cell.
9. Compare the thickness of the mucosa of the medial and lateral wall of the maxillary sinus.
10. What is the relation of the molar roots to the maxillary sinus?

Acknowledgments

I also wish to acknowledge the contributions of Professor P. P. C. Graziadei, Department of Biologic Sciences, Florida State University, who contributed suggestions on the first edition of the text, and Figures 23–13 and 23–15.

Suggested Readings

Ballenger JJ. The clinical anatomy and physiology of the nose and accessory sinuses. In: Ballenger JJ ed. *Diseases of the Nose, Throat, Ear, Head and Neck.* 14th ed. Malvern, Pa: Lee and Febiger; 1991:3–22.

Costanzo RM. Regeneration of olfactory receptor cells. In: *Regeneration of Vertebrate Sensory Receptor Cells.* Ciba Foundation Symposium 160. Chichester: Wiley; 1991:223–248.

Drake-Lee AB. Physiology of the nose and paranasal sinuses. In: Kerr AG, Groves J, Scott-Brown WG, eds. *Scott-Brown's Otolaryngology.* Vol. 1 5th ed. London: Butterworth; 1987:162–182.

Knops JL, McCaffrey TV, Kern EB. Physiology—clinical applications. In: Rice DH ed. *Inflammatory Diseases of the Sinuses.* Philadelphia, Pa: Saunders; 1993:517–531.

McBride TP. Nasal physiology. In: Bluestone CD, Stool SE, eds. *Pediatric Otolaryngology.* 2nd ed. Philadelphia, Pa: Saunders; 1990:632–642.

Moran DT, Rowley JC, Jafek BW. Electron microscopy of human olfactory epithelium reveals a new cell type: The microvillar cell. *Brain Res.* 1982;253:39–46.

Morrison EE, Costanzo RM. Morphology and plasticity of the vertebrate olfactory epithelium. In: Serby MJ, Chobor KL, eds. *Science of Olfaction.* New York, NY: Springer-Verlag; 1992:31–50.

Naessen R. The identification and topographical localization of the olfactory epithelium in man and other mammals. *Acta otolaryngol. (Stockh),* 1970;70:51–57.

Rhys-Evans PH. Anatomy of the nose and paranasal sinuses. In: Kerr AG, Groves J, Scott-Brown WG, eds. *Scott-Brown's Otolaryngology.* Vol 1. 5th ed. London: Butterworth; 1987:138–161.

Sleigh MA, Blake JR, Liron N. The propulsaion of mucous by cilia. *Am Rev Respir Dis.* 1988;137:726–741.

Tos M. Mucous elements in the airways. *Acta Otolaryngol.* 1976;82:249–251.

Trotter CM, Hall GH, Salter DM, Wilson JA. Histology of mucous membrane of human inferior nasal concha. *Clin Anat.* 1990;3:307–316.

Widdicombe J, Sant'Ambrogio G, Mathew OP. Nerve receptors in the upper airway. In: Mathew OP, Sant'Ambrogio G, eds. *Respiratory Function in the Upper Airway.* New York, NY: Dekker; 1988.

Glossary

Accessory canals. Canals leading from the radicular pulp laterally through the root dentin to the periodontal tissue. They are particularly numerous in the apical third of the root.

Accessory root canal. Subordinate chamber of the dental pulp lying within the root portion of the tooth.

Accellular cementum. That part of the cementum covering one third to one half of the root of a tooth adjacent to the cementoenamel junction. It usually is opposed by a layer of cellular cementum. It consists of collagenous fibers and a uniform ground substance but has no cellular components.

Acid hydrolases. The content of lysosomes, the enzymes specialized for intracellular degradation.

Acinus, salivary. A small terminal saclike dilation found in salivary glands.

Acquired cuticle. Acellular organic film that is deposited on the surface of teeth after eruption. Microscopically, it is made up of several layers.

Adrenergic. Nerve fibers that secrete norepinepherine at a synapse usually associated with sympathetic nerve fibers.

Agonist. A substance that produces an effect similar to the naturally occurring substance.

Allantois. Fetal tubular diverticulum developing from the hindgut. In humans, it is vestigial and contributes to the formation of the umbilical cord and placenta.

Alloplastic material. Material suitable for implantation that is not from the human body, such as metal, plastic, or mineral.

Alveolar bone. The ridge of bone on the surface of the body of the maxilla and mandible. This term is applied to the tooth-bearing part of the mandible and maxilla, as it contains the tooth sockets.

Alveolar bone proper. A thin lamina of bone that surrounds and supports the roots of the teeth and gives attachment to principal fibers of the periodontal ligament.

Alveolar crest fibers. Those principal fibers of the periodontal ligament extending between the crest of the alveolar bone and the neck of the tooth.

Alveolar fundus. Bottom or base of the alveolar bone proper, lining the tooth socket.

Ameloblast. One of the cells of the inner layer lining the cap of the enamel organ. These cells give rise to the enamel of the teeth.

Amelogenesis. The process of production and development of enamel.

Amelogenin. A hydrophobic proline-rich protein found in newly deposited enamel matrix. Its molecular weight is about 25,000 daltons. Amelogenins are lost during maturation of enamel.

Amylase. Enzyme that catalyzes the hydrolysis of starch into smaller, water-soluble carbohydrates. In mammals, there are two forms: (1) pancreatic amylase, found in the pancreatic juice, and (2) salivary amylase (ptyalin), found in the saliva.

Anastomosis. A communication or union between two structures.

Anatomical crown. That portion of the tooth that is covered by enamel; the true crown.

Angiogenesis. Refers to the process by which capillaries develop budlike structures that will form new capillary branches.

Ankyloglossia. Restricted movement of the tongue, which results in speech difficulty.

Ankylosed. Stiffened; bound by adhesions; fused; denoting a joint in a state of ankylosis; rigid fixation of a tooth to the surrounding bony alveolus as a result of periodontal membrane ossification.

Antibody. An immunoglobulin molecule that reacts with or binds to the substance (antigen) that induced its synthesis. These proteins are produced by plasma cells.

Antigen. A substance that is recognized as foreign by the body.

Aortic arches. A series of arterial channels encircling the embryonic pharynx in the mesenchyme of the branchial arches.

Apical cementum. Cementum deposited on the apical region of the tooth root.

Apical foramen. Opening at the apex of the root of a tooth that gives passage to the nerves and blood vessels.

Arches, aortic. See *Aortic arches*.

Arches, branchial. See *Branchial arches*.

Apocrine. Sweat gland, a large tubular exocrine gland that accumulates secretion in its cell apices and ruptures the surface membrane during the secretory activity.

Articular disc. Of the temporomandibular joint; the fibrous disc that separates the joint into upper and lower cavities.

Attached gingiva. That part of the oral mucosa which is firmly bound to the tooth and alveolar process.

Attached pulp stones. Mineralized tissues that are partly fused with the dentin of the coronal or root pulp.

Basal lamina. Structural scaffolding composed of glycosaminoglycans, glycoproteins, and collagen; synthesized by epithelial cells throughout the body; probably plays an important role in developing systems and in homeostasis of adult epithelia. Thickening of the basal laminae of the body occurs in diabetes mellitus and other pathologic conditions.

Bell stage. Tooth developmental stage characterized by the differentiation of inner enamel epithelial cells into ameloblasts and the formation of the crown outline by these cells.

Bifid tongue. Split or cleft; separating the tongue into two parts.

Biocompatibility. The ability of a material to perform with an appropriate host respose in a specific situation. The material may be required to trigger or elicit a biological response from the body, such as bone formation or protein adhesion, without being harmful to the tissues.

Biological age. The maturational age; not the chronological age, but the dental age/skeletal age.

Birbeck's granule. A specific granule located in Langerhan's cells.

Birth. Passage of the child from the uterus to the outside world; the act of being born.

Blastocyst. The postmorula stage of development; a blastula with a fluid-filled cavity.

Bodily movement of a tooth. When force is applied through the center of resistance the tooth moves in a bodily fashion. All parts move the same amount and in the same direction.

Bone. Mineralized animal tissue consisting of an organic matrix of cells and fibers of collagen impregnated with mineral matter, chiefly calcium phosphate and calcium carbonate.

Bradykinin. A kinin composed of nine amino acids secreted in response to the action of trypsin on a globulin of blood plasma.

Branchial. Barlike; resembling the gills of fish.

Branchial arch cartilages. One of the cartilages formed in a branchial arch of the embryo.

Branchial arches. One of a series of mesodermal thickenings between the branchial clefts, appearing in higher forms only vestigially. During embryonic stages they contribute to the formation of the face, jaws, and neck.

Buccinator muscle. Muscle forming principal substance of the cheek.

Bud stage. Initial stage of tooth development; the enamel organ develops from this structure. The dental papilla and the dental sac enclose the bud.

Bundle bone. Specialized bone lining the tooth socket into which the fibers of the periodontal ligament penetrate; synonymous with the radiographic term *lamina dura.*

Calculus. An abnormal concretion within the body, usually formed of inorganic matter and often deposited around a minute fragment of inorganic material, the nucleus.

Calculus, dental. Hard stonelike concretion formed on the teeth or prosthesis. It varies in color from creamy yellow to black and is mostly composed of calcium phosphate.

Calvarium. Skullcap; the superior, domelike portion of the cranium.

Canaliculi. Small microscopic spaces that contain cellular projections of osteocytes and cementocytes. In dentin, the spaces occupied by branches from the main dentinal tubule.

Cap stage. Tooth development, an early stage in enamel organ formation; follows the bud stage.

Caries, dental. Localized, progressively destructive disease of the teeth that starts at the external surface (enamel) with the apparent dissolution of the inorganic components by organic acids.

Cartilage. Connective tissue characterized by its non-vascularity and firm consistency. There are three kinds of cartilage: hyaline cartilage, fibrocartilage, and elastic cartilage.

Catecholamines. One of a group of similar compounds that have a sympathomimetic action.

Cell differentiation. An increase in morphologic or chemical heterogenicity.

Cell proliferation. The developmental process in which cells pass through the cell cycle, with parent cells dividing to form two daughter cells and thereby increasing the number of cells in the tissue or organ.

Cell rests (Malassz). The epithelial remnants of the root sheaths found in the periodontal ligament.

Cell-free zone. Relatively cell-free layer adjacent to odontoblasts, overlying the cell-rich zone of the dental pulp, and composed of delicate fibrils embedded in the ground substance.

Cell-rich zone. Layer of the dental pulp situated between the pulp core and the cell-free zone, which is richly supplied with cellular elements, blood vessels, and nerves.

Cellular cementum. That part of the cementum covering the apical one half to two thirds of the root of a tooth. It is usually opposed by a layer of acellular cementum. It contains cementocytes embedded in the calcified matrix.

Cementicles. Calcified spherical bodies composed of cementum either lying free within the periodontal ligament attached to the cementum or embedded within it.

Cementoblast. Connective tissue cell type responsible for the formation of cementum.

Cementocyte. A cell found in the lacuma of cellular cementum, from 8 μm to more than 15 μm in diameter, with a wide variety of shapes from round to oval to flattened. Numerous cytoplasmic processes extend from its free surface.

Cementum. Bonelike connective tissue that covers the tooth from the cementoenamel junction to and surrounding the apical foramen.

Cementum-enamel (cementoenamel) junction. It represents the boundary between enamel and cementum that lies at the cervic of the tooth. These two tissues may overlap or be slightly separated.

Cervical loop. Growing free border of the enamel organ. The outer and inner enamel epithelial layers are continuous and reflected into one another.

Cervix. The portion of the tooth that lies at the border of the anatomical crown and root of the tooth. It is often at the cementum-enamel junction.

Chemotaxis. The movement of cells following a concentration gradient (moving towards higher concentration) of a chemical substance.

Choanae. Paired openings between the nasal cavity and nasopharynx.

Cholinergic nerves. Nerve fibers that secrete acetylcholine at a synapse primarily associated with postganglionic parasympathetic fibers.

Chorda tympani. A branch of the facial nerve that joins the lingual nerve for parasympathetic supply to the sublingual and submandibular glands.

Chondrocranium. Cartilaginous skull; the embryonic skull before ossification.

Chronologic age. Record of time elapsed since birth.

Circumpulpal dentin. Inner portion of the dentin located near the pulp organ of the tooth.

Circumvallate papilla. Papilla vallata; one of eight or ten projections from the dorsum of the tongue that form a V-shaped row anterior to the sulcus terminalis. Each is surrounded by a circular trench having a slightly raised outer wall.

Cleft lip. A congenital defect of the lip, usually the upper lip. Failure of the median nasal and maxillary process to fuse.

Cleft palate. Palatum fissum; a congenital fissure in the median line of the palate or lateral to the premaxillary process or both. It usually is associated with cleft lip.

Clinical crown. That portion of the crown exposed above the gingiva and visible in the oral cavity.

Clinical eruption. Emergence of the crown of a tooth, that portion of which can be observed clinically.

Cocci. Bacteria with round, spheroidal, or ovoid form, including *Microcossus*, gonococcus, meningococcus, *Staphylococcus*, streptococcus, and pneumococcus.

Col. Valleylike depression in the facial lingual plane of the interdental gingiva. It conforms to the shape of the interproximal contact area.

Collagen. White fibers of the corium of the skin, tendon, and other connective tissue. The fiber is composed of fibrils bound together with interfibrillar cement; the fibrils are, in turn, formed of ultramicroscopic filaments. An albumoid found in connective tissue, bone, and cartilage and notable for its high content of the amino acids glycine, proline, and hydroxyproline.

Collagen fiber. High-molecular-weight protein composed of a number of structural types that vary in diameter from less than 1 μm to about 12 μm and usually are arranged in bundles.

Compact bone. Hard, external, more highly calcified than cancellous (spongy) portion of bone.

Complement. A group of proteins that react with the antibody-antigen complex producing mediators of inflammation and causing death of foreign cells.

Concha. A shell- or scroll-like bone. Anatomically it relates to the turbinate bones projecting into the nasal cavity.

Connective tissue adhesion. Protein adhesion of connective tissue to other substances such as teeth or alloplastic materials.

Connective tissue stroma of salivary glands. Capsule and septa formed from mesenchyme and the blood vessels.

Constitutive secretion. Secretion occurring continuously with molecules transported in vesicles from the Golgi apparatus to the plasma membrane in the presence or absence of secretagogue. Some transport vesicles may bud from the secretory vesicles shuttling proteins to the plasma membrane.

Cord growth of salivary glands. Solid cord of epithelial cells that characterizes an early stage of development of salivary glands.

Corpus luteum. Yellow endocrine body, 1 to 1.5 cm in diameter, formed in the ovary in the site of a ruptured ovarian follicle.

Cranial. Pertaining to the bones covering the brain on the superior end of the body in humans.

Cranial base. Lower portion of the skull constituting the floor of the cranial cavity.

Cribriform. Bone containing perforations or numerous formina.

Crypts. Pitlike depressions or tubular recesses.

Cuticle, developmental. Skin of the teeth consisting of an extremely thin layer of organic material covering the enamel of recently erupted teeth.

Cuticle, primary. A thin film on the enamel of an unerupted tooth. A product of the degenerating ameloblasts.

Cyclic AMP (cAMP). Adenosine 3′:5′-cyclic phosphate; the second or intracellular messenger of target cells. Hormones or pharmacologic agents interact and bind to a membrane-bound receptor associated with an adenyl cyclase enzyme system. Adenyl cyclase catalyzes the conversion of ATP to AMP.

Cystic fibrosis. Lethal genetic disease characterized by a generalized dysfunction of exocrine glands throughout the body and therefore resulting in digestive and pulmonary problems.

Cytodifferentiation. The process by which cells in the developing tooth evolve and gain functional and morphological differences.

Cytokines. A group of nonantibody molecules produced by cells that function to influence and signal other cells. The principal function is the induction of cell division and the regulation of differentiation.

Dead tracts. Empty tubules left after the odontoblastic processes degenerate.

Deciduous dentition. Primary teeth or first-formed set of teeth that undergo exfoliation to provide space for the permanent teeth.

Degenerating lamina. Lysis and disappearance of the dental lamina, characteristic of teeth in the bell stage of development.

Demilune (serous demilune). Half-moon or crescent-shaped serous cells of a mixed-type acinus that form a cap over the ends of the mucous acinar cells.

Dental lamina. Horseshoe-shaped epithelial bands that traverse the upper and lower jaws and give rise to the ectodermal portions of the teeth.

Dental papilla. Formative organ of the dentin and primordium of the pulp.

Dental plaque. Organic deposit on the surface of teeth. Site of growth of bacteria or nucleus for formation of dental calculus.

Dental pulp (endodontia). Soft tissue contained within the pulp cavity, consisting of connective tissue and containing blood vessels, nerves, and lymphatics.

Dental sac (follicle). Area surrounding the developing tooth that produces the alveolar bone, cementum, and periodontal ligament and consists of (ecto) mesenchymal cells and fibers that surround the dental papilla and the enamel organ.

Denticles. A calcified structure found in the pulp of a tooth.

Dentin. Body of the tooth; surrounds the pulp and underlies the enamel on the crown and the cementum on the roots of the teeth. About 20% is organic matrix, mostly collagen, and 10% is water. The inorganic fraction (70%) is mainly hydroxyapatite, with some carbonate, magensium, and fluoride. It is yellowish in color.

Dentinal tubule. The space in dentin that contains or at one time contained an odontoblastic process.

Dentinoenamel junction. Interface of the enamel and dentin of the crown of a tooth.

Dentinogenesis. Process of dentin formation in the development of teeth.

Desmosome. Macula adherens; site of adhesion between two cells, consisting of a dense plate near the cell surface, separated from a similar structure in the adjacent cell by thin layers of extracellular materials believed to have adhesive properties. Intracellular tonofilaments are associated with this structure.

Diapedesis. The migration of cells like neutrophils through gaps between endothelial cells.

Differentiation. Growth associated with or having a distinguishing character or function from the surrounding structures or from the original type; specialization.

Diphyodont. Having two sets of teeth, as in humans and most mammals.

Displacement. Change in position of a bone due to growth at its border or movement of an adjacent bone. Change in attachment when one element, radical, or molecule is removed and is replaced by another.

Drift. The change in position of a bone due to remodeling (apposition on one side and resorption on the other). Movement of a tooth to a position of greater stability.

Drug. Any substance used as a medicine in the treatment of disease; to give medicine; to narcotize.

Duct. Tube with well-defined walls for passage of excretions or secretions.

Duct, intercalated. The smallest-diameter intralobular duct of salivary glands that conducts saliva from the acinar cells to the striated ducts. These ducts modify salivary secretions.

Duct, interlobar. Channels located outside lobes of the salivary glands.

Duct, intralobar. Channels located within lobes of the salivary glands.

Duct, striated. A type of intralobular duct of the salivary glands that is composed of columnar cells with centrally placed nuclei and striations at the basal ends of cells. These cells modify salivary secretions.

Dystrophy. Any disorder arising from defective or faulty nutrition.

Eccentric growth. That process whereby one part of the developing tooth germ remains stationary, while the remainder continues to grow. This leads to a shift in its center.

Ectoderm. Outer layer of cells of the three primary germ layers; forms nervous system epidermis and derivatives.

Ectomesenchyme. Neural crest cells, mesectoderm. This term is used to describe cells derived from the neural crest and found in the mesodermal tissues. Functions in induction. Forms spinal ganglia, much of the face, and branchial arches.

Edema. The swelling that results from fluid accumulation within the tissue following a spill of blood constitutents.

Edentulous. Without teeth, having lost the natural teeth.

Eicosanoids. A group of compounds that are converted to biologically active substances that act as mediators of inflammation.

Embedded pulp stones (denticles). Small calcified masses of dentin appearing as a function of age or trauma. They may protrude from the existing dentin wall into the pulp tissue.

Enamel crystals. Hydroxyapatite crystals found in enamel rods. They are deposited during tooth mineralization.

Enamel lamellae. Thin, leaflike structures that extend from the enamel surface toward the dentinoenamel junction. They represent defects or spaces filled entirely or partly with organic material.

Enamel organ. Originates from the stratified epithelium lining the primitive oral cavity organ; consists of four distinct layers: outer enamel epithelium, stellate reticulum, stratum intermedium, and inner enamel epithelium. The latter becomes the ameloblastic layer.

Enamel pearls. Enameloma, a developmental anomaly in which a small nodule of enamel is formed near the cementoenamel junction, usually at the bifurcation zone of molar teeth.

Enamel rod. One of the structural units of enamel, extending from the dentinoenamel junction to the surface of the tooth, averaging about 5 μm in width and 9 μm in height, and normally having a translucent crystalline appearance.

Enamel spindles. Tubular spaces in enamel found at the dentinoenamel junction in which a terminal extension of the odontoblast processes may be found.

Enamel tuft. Narrow, ribbonlike structure whose inner end arises at the dentinoenamel junction, extends one third of the distance to the enamel surface, and consists of hypocalcified enamel rods; may be filled with organic substance and extend at near right angles to the dentinoenamel junction.

Enamelin. An acidic glycosylated phosphoprotein of mature enamel. It has a molecular weight of about 55,000 daltons.

Endochondral. Relating to the type of formation of bone formed within cartilage and replacing it.

Endocrine. Refers to glands of internal secretion that release their secretory product(s) (hormones) directly into the bloodstream rather than through a duct system.

Endosseous implants. Implants that are embedded in bone and fixed throughout the entire length of the implant. The various implant types are screw, blade, and cylinder.

Entactin. An extra cellular matrix glycoprotein associated with the basal lamina.

Epidermal growth factor (EGF). A small peptide (molecular weight = 6045) originally isolated from the male mouse submandibular gland and now known to have a very wide distribution in the body. EGF stimulates cell proliferation and/or differentiation in various organs and tissues through EGF receptors that activate tyrosine-specific proteins kinases.

Epimers. Dorsal form of a myotome that forms muscles innervated by the dorsal ramus of the spinal nerve.

Epiphyseal plate of condylar head. Cartilage of the head of the mandibular condyle, a growth site.

Epithelial attachment. Dentogingival junction attachment of the gingival epithelium with the tooth's surface. The basal lamina of the epitheleum is attached by means of hemidesmosomes.

Epithelial cell rests. Remains of (Hertwig's) root sheath. The epithelial cells that cover the roots during root development. Later, they are located in the periodontal ligament near the surface of the cementum as groups of cells called "rests." There are three types: proliferating, resting, and degenerating. Occasionally, they develop into the dental cysts.

Epithelial diaphragm. Formed by the root sheath at the beginning of root development; important in formation of the root. It finally serves to narrow the width of the cervial opening of the root.

Epithelial pearls. Discrete, rounded or ovoid groups of epithelial cells, frequently keratinized, found in the lamina propria. The cells are arranged in a whorled or concentrically laminated pattern, with polygonal cells centrally

flattened and with more mature cells found peripherally. Most often found in the midline of the palate and are remnants of epithelium in the line of fusion.

Epithelium. Cellular, avascular layer covering all the free surfaces of the body internal and external and the lining of vessels. Consists of cells and a small amount of intercellular substance. Includes the glands and other structures derived therefrom.

Epithelium, inner enamel. The cells that line the concavity of the enamel organ in the cap and early bell stages of tooth development and differentiate into ameloblasts.

Epithelium, outer enamel. Cuboidal peripheral cells of the cap or the bell stage of tooth development that line the convexity of the cap.

Eruption, teeth. Appearance of teeth in the oral cavity; a stage coordinated with root growth and maturation of tissues surrounding the tooth.

Esterase. The enzyme responsible for catalyzing the hydrolysis of an ester into an alcohol and acid.

Excretory duct. Pertaining to excretion; is an interlobular duct draining the intralobular ducts, possessing a pseudostratified or stratified columnar epithelium, and believed to be involved in ionic transport.

Exfoliate. To shed or eliminate something as of scales from the surface of the body or loss of teeth from the jaws.

Exocrine. Denotes glands that release their secretory product(s) into a duct system.

Exocytosis. Discharges of secretory product(s) from the cell, preserving the cell membrane through fusion of the secretory vesicle with the cell membrane.

Extracellular matrix. Macromolecular products of mesenchymal and epithelial (basement membrane components) cells that provide a role in cellular adhesion. These substrate adhesion molecules are important in induction of epithelia and regulation of cellular migration.

Extravasate. Fluid that extrudes or escapes from a vessel into the tissues.

Fenestrated. Perforated with one or more openings.

Fertilization. Rendering gametes fertile; contact and fusion of spermatozoa and ovum and formation and merging male and female pronuclei and development of zygote.

Fibroblasts. Elongated, ovoid, spindle-shaped, or flattened cells found in connective tissue that form the connective tissue fibers.

Fibronectin. An adhesive V-shaped glycoprotein present in the basement membrane that has collagen-binding domains. There is also a heparin-binding domain and a fibrin-binding site on the molecule. Fibronectin binds to integrins called fibronectin receptors on cells. One cell-binding site contains a tripeptide sequence known as the RGD sequence (Arg-Gly-Ash).

Fibrous capsule. Capsule composed chiefly of fibrous elements.

Filamentous bacteria. Long, pleomorphic, branched, rod-shaped microorganisms.

Filiform papillae. The most numerous type of papillae of the dorsum of the tongue. They are threadlike papillae pointing toward the throat.

Fissure sealant. Composite resin "bonded" directly to the enamel surface that functions to seal out bacteria that cause caries.

Fontanelles. One of several membranous intervals at the angles of the cranial bones in the infant. Normally there are six, corresponding to the pterion and asterion, on either side, and to the bregma and lambda, in the midline.

Fordyce's spots (granules). Ectopic sebaceous glands, located at angles of the mouth.

Free gingiva. That portion of the gingiva that surrounds the tooth and is not directly attached to the tooth surface; the outer wall of the gingival sulcus.

Free pulp stones (denticles). Small calcified masses of dentin that appear as a function of aging or trauma. They develop in the connective tissue of the pulp without obvious relationship to the secondary dentin of the tooth.

Frontonasal. Region of upper anterior face between the eyes. Nasal placodes arise here.

Fungiform papillae. One of numerous minute elevations on the dorsum, tip, and sides of the tongue, of a mushroom shape, with the tip being broader than the base.

Furcation. An anatomic area of a multirooted tooth where the roots divide.

G protein. Guanosine $5'$-triphosphate–binding regulatory protein that alters an intracellular messenger (eg, cyclic nucleotides or CA^{++}).

Gap junctions. Specialized intercellular junctions between cells, with pores permeable to ions and small molecules.

Genetic. Relating to genetics or ontogenesis.

Gingiva. That soft tissue surrounding the necks of erupted teeth. It is composed of two parts: the masticatory mucosa facing the oral cavity and the sulcular (crevicula) epithelium and epithelial attachment facing the tooth. The gingiva consists of fibrous tissue, enveloped by mucous membrane, which covers the alveolar processes of the upper and lower jaws.

Gingival sulcus. The shallow V-shaped trench around each tooth, bounded by the tooth surface on one surface and the epithelial-lined free margin on the other.

Glycosaminoglycan (GAG). Noncollagenous macromolecule previously referred to as mucopolysaccharide.

Gnarled enamel. The enamel located at the tips of the cusps, in which the rods or groups of rods are twisted, bent, and intertwined.

Gonial angle. Angle between the lower border and posterior ramus of the mandible.

Granular layer of Tomes. A thin layer of defective dentin adjacent to the cementum, which appears granular and located along the root surface.

Granulation tissue. The tissue that replaces the blood clot and is formed by new connective tissue and new capillaries.

Granulocytes. Blood cells that have granules in their cytoplasm. These include neutrophils, eoisinophils, and basophils.

Granuloma. A nodule of granulation tissue that contain growing fibroblasts and capillaries in response to chronic inflammation.

Growth factors. Chemical substances that induce cells to initiate DNA synthesis.

Gubernacular cord. Fibrous cord connecting two structures; a connective tissue band uniting the tooth sac with the alveolar mucosa.

Hageman factor. The clotting factor XII that becomes activated following injury, and in turn activates the clotting complement kinin and plasmin systems.

Hard palate. Anterior part of the palate, consisting of the bony palate covered above by the respiratory mucosa of the floor of the nose and below by the keratinized stratified squamous oral mucosa of the roof of the mouth. The hard palate contains palatine vessels and nerves, adipose tissue, and mucous glands.

Haversian bone. Compact bone containing tubular channels with blood vessels, nerves, and bone cells with concentrically located lacunae that are termed the Haversian system or osteon.

Hemidesmosomes. Similar to a desmosome but representing only half of it. Located on the surface of some epithelial cells and forming the site of attachment between the epithelial cell and the basal lamina. Consist of single attachment plaque, the adjacent plasma membrane, and a related extracellular structure that attaches the epithelium to the connective tissue.

Hemostasis. The process that leads to stoppage of bleeding.

Heparan sulfate. A glycosaminoglycan consisting of N-acetyl-glucosamine alternating with D-glucuronic acid or D-iduronic acid. When covalently linked to protein, heparan sulfate proteoglycan is formed.

Heterotypic contacts. During development these represent the close approximation of epithelium and mesenchyme without an intervening basal lamina.

Histamine. A vasoactive amine that induces vasoldilation and increases vascular permeability.

Hormone. Chemical substance formed in one organ or part of the body and carried by the blood to another part where it stimulates or depresses functional activity.

Howship lacunae. Tiny depressions, pits, or irregular grooves on the surfaces of bones, the result of resorption by osteoclasts.

Hunter-Schreger bands. Alternating dark and light bands in enamel that result from absorption and reflection of light caused by differences in orientation of adjacent groups of enamel rods originating at the dentinoenamel junction and extending to near the outer enamel surface.

Hyalinization. A result of compression of the periodontal ligament in which all vascularity and most cells are lost from the zone of compression, creating a glasslike appearance. As a result, tooth movement will cease.

Hyaluronidase. Enzyme that catalyzes the hydrolysis of hyaluronic acid which forms the backbone of proteoglycan molecules in connective tissue.

Hydrodynamic. Branch of physics that deals with factors determining the flow of liquids. In dentistry, it refers to a theory of pain conduction through dentin.

Hypertrophic zone. Endochondral cartilage zone characterized by enlargement of existing cells.

Hydroxyapatite. The inorganic matrix of bone, enamel, cementum, dentin, and cartilage having the chemical formula $Ca_{10}(PO_4)_6(OH)_2$.

Hypomere. Portion of the myotome that extends ventrolaterally to form body-wall muscle and is innervated by the primary ventral ramus of a spinal nerve.

Hypoxia. Refers to low oxygen content of tissues.

Iatrogenic. An adverse condition resulting from the activities of a health professional.

IgA (secretory immunoglobulins). One of the classes of immunoglogulins; the principal immunoglobulin found in exocrine secretions—milk, intestinal and respiratory mucin, saliva, and tears. Antigens entering the oral cavity stimulate IgA synthesis and secretion in the salivary glands to protect the oral mucosa from pathogenic microbes.

Immunoglobulins. Serum proteins that function as antibodies and are responsible for humoral immunity. There are five classes of immunoglobulins: IgG, IgA, IgM, IgD, and IgE.

Impaction. Position of a tooth in the alveolus so that it is incapable of eruption into the oral cavity. Impaction may be due to crowding of teeth that results in a lack of available space for eruption. Teeth being driven into the alveolar process or surrounding tissues as a result of trauma.

Increment. The amount by which a given quantity is increased. A measurable amount.

Incremental deposition. Deposition of material in discrete amounts, rather than constant deposition. Rhythmic recurrent deposition of enamel, bone, dentin, or cementum.

Induction, embryonic. The act or process of causing the occurrence of a specific morphogenic effect in the developing embryo through the influence of organizers.

Innervation. Presence and distribution of nerves in a part or the supply of nerve stimulation of a part.

Instructive interaction. An embryonic interaction between two tissues in which the responding tissue differentiates by receiving specific signals (instructions) from the inducing tissue. The fate of the responding tissue is determined by the tissue with which it interacts.

Intercalated duct. Intralobular-type salivary gland duct draining the acinus. Intercalated duct cells are cuboidal and contain secretory granules and rough endoplasmic reticulum. They are the smallest ducts within the salivary gland.

Interdental septa. Bony partitions that project into the alveoli between the teeth; interalveolar.

Interglobular dentin. A zone of a globular- rather than linear-formed dentin in the crowns of teeth, underlying enamel specifically in the zone separating he mantle and circumpulpal dentin. Characterized by interglobular spaces that are unmineralized or hypomineralized dentin between normal calcified dentin layers.

Interlobular ducts. Ducts of the salivary glands that traverse in connective tissue septa between lobules; also termed excretory ducts.

Intertubular dentin. That dentin between zones of peritubular dentin that immediately surrounds the tubules.

Intralobular duct. Ducts within the lobules of the salivary glands of two types: intercalated, lined by low cuboidal epithelium, and striated, lined by tall cuboidal to columnar epithelium.

Intramembranous bone. Bone formation within or between connective tissue membranes. It does not replace cartilage, as does endochondral bone.

Intratubular dentin. The hypermineralized layer of dentin that lies between the sheath of Neuman and the dentinal tubule.

Junctional complex. Specialized region of contact between adjacent cells; it consists of three regions (moving in order from the apical region of the cell): zonula occludens, zonula adherens, and desmosome.

Junctional epithelium. Epithelial attachment. That epithelium adhering to the tooth or implant surface at the base of the gingival crevice and consisting of one or several layers of nonkeratinizing cells.

Keratinized. Having developed a horny layer of flattened cells containing keratin.

Keratinized mucosa. Stratified surface cornified epithelial cells that lack a nucleus and whose cytoplasm is replaced by large amounts of keratohyalin protein. Keratinized oral epithelium has four cell layers: basal, spinous, granular, and cornified.

Keratinocyte. Epithelial cells of the mucosa and skin whose main activity is the production of keratin.

Lamella. Thin leaf or plate as of bone.

Lamella enamel. Imperfectly calcified thin, leaf-shaped areas of enamel that extend from the outer surface toward the dentin.

Lamina dura. Radiographic term describing the hard compact bone layer lining the dental alveoli.

Lamina propria. Layer of connective tissue underlying the epithelium of skin or a mucous membrane.

Laminin. A glycoprotein found in the basal lamina. Laminin binds to type IV collagen; cells, particularly epithelial cells; and neurons through a laminin receptor (integrin) on the cell membrane, and glycosaminogly-cans. It is believed to provide a role in extracellular matrix regulation of cell migration and differentiation.

Langerhans cells. Clear or dendritic cells found in both superficial and deep layers of the epidermis and oral epithelium. Contain no desmosomes or tonofilaments. Probably arise from bone marrow and may have immunologic function in recognizing antigenic material.

Lateral lamina. Band of cells believed to be functionally and structurally similar to the parent dental lamina. Lateral lamina connects the developing tooth germs to the dental lamina.

Leukoplakia. Dysfunction of the keratinization process of stratified squamous epithelium resulting in a white appearance of the surface cells.

Lingual tonsil. Collection of lymphoid follicles on the base, posterior, or pharyngeal portion of the dorsum of the tongue.

Lining mucosa. Nonkeratinized oral mucosa that covers the cheeks, lips, soft palate, floor of the mouth, and ventral surface of the tongue.

Lobe. Subdivision of an organ bounded by structural demarcations such as connective tissue septa or fissures.

Lobules. Small lobes or subdivisions of a lobe that are separated by thin partitions of connective tissue.

Lymphokines. Cytokines produced by lymphocytes.

Macroglossia. Enlargement of the tongue, usually due to local lymphangiectasia or to muscular hypertrophy; megaloglossia.

Macrophage. Term generally used as a designation for the large mononuclear phagocytes that are found in various tissues and organs of the body, where they are called histiocytes, "wandering cells," or other terms. They are found in conspicuous numbers in the sinusoids of the spleen, lymph nodes, liver, lungs, and bone marrow. In the brain and spinal cord, they are designated microglia.

Major salivary glands. The paired parotid, submandibular (submaxillary), and sublingual salivary glands that are responsible for the production of enzyme amylase, mucins, secretory immunoglobulin A (IgA), and other constitutents of saliva.

Malassez' epithelial rests. Epithelial remnants of Hertwig's sheath in the periodontal ligament. These groups of epithelial cells appear near the surface of the cementum; occasionally they develop into dental cysts.

Mandible. Horseshoe-shaped bone forming the lower jaw and articulating, by its upturned extremities, the condyles, with the temporal bone on either side. The mandible is composed of the body and the ramus which is located posteriorly. The body includes the alveolar process which contains the teeth.

Mannose-6-phosphate (M6P). A marker on lysosomal hydrolases added only to the N-linked oligosaccharides in the cis-Golgi. M6P binds to M6P receptors that form on the clathrin-coated vesicles and provides the intracellular target signal to direct these enzymes into the lysosomal pathway.

Mantle dentin. The initially deposited portions of the dentin formed immediately beneath enamel.

Marginal leakage. Seepage of microorganisms, fluids, and debris along the interface between a dental restoration and the walls of a cavity preparation.

Mastication. Process of chewing food in preparation for swallowing and digestion.

Masticatory mucosa. The mucosa that functions in mastication. It tends to be bound to bone and is therefore immovable. It bears forces generated when food is chewed. The mucosa of the hard palate and gingiva.

Matrix vesicles. Membrane-bounded vesicles that arise by budding and lie free in the extracellular matrix. These vesicles may represent the initial sites of calcification in dentin, bone, and cartilage.

Maturation zone. Zone of cartilage characterized by chondrocyte enlargement.

Maxilla. Upper jaw bone; an irregularly shaped bone articulating with the nasal, lacrimal, zygomatic, palatine, ethmoid, sphenoid, and frontal bones of the face and containing teeth.

Maxillary sinus. Paired sinus cavities occupying the space beneath the floor of the orbit and above the roots of the posterior maxillary teeth.

Meatus. An opening, passageway, or channel.

Meckel's cartilage. The initial skeletal component of the first branchial arch. It is the supporting cartilage of the mandibular arch in the embryo.

Melanocyte. A cell that forms melanin pigment found in the skin and mucous membranes.

Membrane performativum. Basement membrane separating the enamel organ and the dental papilla preceding dentin formation.

Merocrine. Type of glandular secretion in which the secreting cells remain intact during the formation and release of the secretory product(s).

Mesenchyme. Loose undifferentiated embryonic type of connective tissue that usually is of mesodermal origin but that is a mixture of mesodermal and neural crest derivatives in the head and neck region. See *Ectomesenchyme*.

Mesial drift. Gradual movement of a tooth or teeth anteriorly toward the midline.

Mesoderm. Mesoblast; the third primary germ layer of the embryo to differentiate. It is positioned between the ectogerm and endoderm.

Microglossia. Smallness of the tongue.

Mineralization front. The junction between mineralized and unmineralized tissue—eg, between predentin and dentin, osteoid and bone, or cementoid and cementum.

Minor salivary glands. The numerous glands located throughout the oral cavity in the lips (labial), cheeks (buccal), hard and soft palate (palatine), tongue (lingual; eg, von Ebner's glands), and glossopalatine.

Mixed dentition. State of possessing primary and secondary teeth simultaneously.

Modulation. A reversible change in form and function.

Monokines. Cytokines produced by monocytes.

Morphodifferentiation. The process which occurs during tooth formation that is responsible for determining the shape of the tooth's crown.

Morphogenesis. The development process that creates the shape and form of an organ. The branching process that occurs during salivary gland development is an example of morphogenesis.

Morula. Mass of blastomeres resulting from the early cleavage divisions of the zygote.

Mucoceles. Retention cysts of the minor salivary gland ducts, which contain mucous secretion. Usually the result of rupture of the excretory duct of a minor salivary gland, causing pooling of saliva in the tissues. The resulting versicular elevation is a mucocele.

Mucoperiostem. A periosteum with a mucous surface. Close combination of mucous membrane (epithelium and lamina propria) with the periosteum of bone to form an apparent single layer.

Mucous acinus. Minute, saclike secretory portion of a mucous gland. This is the functional unit of the gland.

Mucous glands. Glands that secrete viscous proteinaceous secretions, such as the sublingual gland; glands of the hard palate.

Mumps. Parotitis. Enlargement of the parotid gland, an acute contagious viral infection marked by bilateral or unilateral inflammation and swelling and manifested by chills, fever, and headache.

Myoepithelial cells. Spindle-shaped cells with a stellate body and processes containing darkly staining fibrils found in all the glands of the oral cavity. They are located in the epithelium of the terminal portion of the salivary gland acini and are believed to have contractile ability that facilitates movement of the glandular secretion into the ducts.

Myofibrils. Fine longitudinal fibrils (parallel with long axis) occurring in a muscle fiber. They are composed of myofilaments.

Naris. One of the orifices of the nasal cavity; nostril. May be the anterior internal or posterior naris.

Nasal region. Relating to the area of the nose, subdivided into internal naris, olfactory region, and nasopharynx.

Neonatal line. Accentuated incremental line or hesitation line seen in hard tissue such as bone, dentin, and deposited enamel. Probably due to metabolic changes occurring at or near the time of birth.

Neovascularize. To form new blood vessels after an injury.

Nerves. Whitish cords composed of fibers arranged in bundles (fascicles) and held together by a connective tissue sheath. Nerves transmit stimuli from the central nervous system to the periphery or from the periphery to the central nervous system.

Neural crest. Ganglionic crest; a band of ectodermal cells that appear along either side of the line of closure of the embryonic neural groove. With the closure of the neural groove to form the neural tube, these bands then lie between the developing spinal cord and the superficial ectoderm and later separate into cell groups that constitute the primordia of the ganglia of cranial and spinal nerves. Other derivatives migrate ventrally to induce formation of various other tissues.

Neurocranium. That part of the skull enclosing the brain, as distinguished from the bones of the face.

Nociception. The process of responding to pain.

Nonkeratinocytes. Cells not producing keratin. Clear or dendritic cells found in oral epithelium such as pigment cells (melanocytes), Langerhans cells, Merkel cells, and inflammatory cells such as lymphocytes.

Nonkeratinized mucosa. Lining mucosa in which the stratified squamous epithelial cells retain their nuclei and cytoplasm. They contain no keratohyalin protein. Lining mucosa is found on the lips, cheeks, soft palate, vestibular fornix, alveolar mucosa, floor of the mouth, and undersurface of the tongue.

Occlusion. Relation of the maxillary and mandibular teeth when in functional contact during activity of the mandible.

Odontoblast. Layer of columnar cells with processes in the dentinal tubules, lining the peripheral pulp of a tooth. These cells function to form dentin.

Odontoblast process. Slender protoplasmic process in dentinal tubule. It is a cytoplasmic extension of the cell bodies of the odontoblasts in the dental pulp. They extend from the cell possibly as far as the dentinoenamel junction and the cementoenamel junction.

Odontogenesis. The entire process of tooth formation, which includes amelogenesis, dentinogenesis, and cementogenesis.

Olfactory mucosa. Site of most of the receptors for the sense of smell. It occupies the superior aspect of the nasal cavity between the superior nasal conchae, roof of the nose, and upper part of the nasal septum and is composed of three cell types: receptor cells, supporting cells, and basal cells.

Organic matrix. Formative portion of a tooth, as opposed to mineralized hydroxyapatite.

Oropharyngeal membrane. The embryonic transient membrane portion separating the oral and pharyngeal cavities. It ruptures and disappears during the fourth prenatal week. This membrane is located central to the pharynx and extends from the level of the palate to the vestibule of the larynx.

Osmiophilic. Tissue components stained easily with osmium or osmic acid.

Osseointegration. A direct structural and functional connection at the light microscopic level between living bone and the surface of a load-carrying implant.

Osteoblasts. Bone-forming cells derived from mesenchyme. They form the osseous matrix in which they may become enclosed to become osteocytes.

Osteoclasts. Larger multinucleated cells derived from monocytes with abundant acidophilic cytoplasm, formed in bone marrow and functioning in the absorption and removal of osseous tissue.

Osteocytes. Cells of the bone located in lacunae, which function in maintenance and vitality of bone.

Osteodentin. A form of reparative dentin in which cells become trapped in the matrix, giving it a bonelike appearance.

Oxytalan fibers. Type of connective tissue fiber histochemically distinct from collagen or elastic fibers and found in the periodontal ligament and gingiva. May

function in support of blood vessels and principal fibers of the ligament.

Palatal rugae. Transverse ridges located in the mucous membrane of the anterior part of the hard palate. They extend laterally from the incisive papilla. They have a core of dense connective tissue.

Palate, primary. That part of the palate formed from the median nasal process. The first palate to form, which is anterior to the secondary palate.

Palate, secondary. The palate proper, formed by fusion of the lateral palatine processes of the maxilla.

Palatine tonsils. Faucial; a large oval mass of lymphoid tissue embedded in the lateral wall of the oral pharynx bilaterally located between the pillars of the fauces.

Parakeratinized. Superficial epithelial cells that have retained their pyknotic nuclei and show some signs of keratinization; the stratum granulosum generally is absent, however.

Parenchyma. Functional elements of glandular tissue rather than the supporting framework (stroma) of the gland.

Parotid. The parotid salivary gland located anterior to the ear. It is encapsulated and produces 26% of the secretions of the major salivary glands.

Pellicle. Thin skin or film as on the surface of the teeth.

Perforating fibers (Sharpey's fibers). Penetrating connective tissue fibers by which the tooth's surface is attached to the adjacent alveolar bone. These bundles of collagen fibers penetrate both the cementum and the alveolar bone.

Perikymata. Wavelike grooves, believed to be the manifestations of the striae of Retzius, on the surface of enamel. They appear transverse to the long axis of the tooth.

Periodontal ligament. Connective tissue structure that is a mode of attachment of the tooth to the alveolus and consists of collagenous fibers arranged in bundles, between which are loose connective tissue, blood vessels, and nerves.

Peritubular dentin. That zone of dentin that forms the wall of the dentinal tubules. This dentin has a 9% higher mineral content than does the remainder of intertubular dentin.

Perivascular. Located around a blood vessel.

Permissive interaction. An embryonic interaction between two tissues in which the responding tissue differentiates along a predetermined path. Only the presence of inducing tissue is necessary for differentiation.

Phagocytosis. The engulfing and digesting of cells, debris, and other substances by cells.

Pharyngeal tonsil. Third tonsil; Luschka's tonsil; a collection of more or less closely aggregated lymphoid cells located superficially in the posterior wall of the nasopharynx, the hypertrophy of which constitutes the condition called adenoids.

Phosphoinositide cycle. A signal transduction pathway in which binding to a cell surface receptor activates a G protein that subsequently activates phospholipase C. This enzyme forms two important intermediates from phos-

phatidyl-inositol-bisphosphate: inositol triphosphate (IP3) and diacylglycerol (DAG). IP3 releases Ca^{++} from intracellular compartments, while DAG activates protein kinase C leading to phosphorylation within the cell.

Phosphoproteins. A conjugated protein in which phosphoric acid is esterified with hydroxyamino acid, usually serine.

Phosphophoryn. A unique highly phosphorylated protein found in the dentin matrix.

Placode. A platelike thickening or layer of ectoderm appearing in the embryo.

Plaque, dental. Deposit of material on the surface of a tooth, which may also serve as a medium for growth of bacteria. May serve as a site for formation of dental calculus.

Plasma cells. Cells derived from B-lymphocytes, which actively synthesize and secrete antibody (Ig) from an extensive rough endoplasmic reticulum. Under appropriate conditions, antigen stimulation induces proliferation and morphologic alterations in B-lymphocytes to form plasma cells.

Predentin. Organic fibrillar matrix of the circumpulpal dentin matrix before its calcification into dentin.

Preeruptive phase. Developmental stage preparatory to eruption of teeth and characerized by movements of the growing teeth within the alveolar process.

Primary curvatures of the dentinal tubule. These are the two curvatures of the dentinal tubule in the crown of the tooth which give the tubule its S shape.

Primary intention healing. The healing that occurs when wound edges can be sutured together thereby minimizing scar formation.

Proliferative cell zone. Zone in endochondral bone formation characterized by the presence of dividing chondrocytes.

Proliferative period. Time during which cells grow and increase in number by cell division.

Proline. Naturally occurring nonessential, heterocylic amino acid.

Prostaglandins. A group of hormones or hormonelike substances found in semen or menstrual fluid.

Proteoglycan (PG). A glycoprotein with a very high content of carbohydrate. These proteins are produced by odontoblasts and fibroblasts, are usually found in younger pulps or during active dentinogenesis, and are found reduced in older pulps.

Protein kinase A. Cyclic AMP–dependent protein kinase that is the intracellular effector molecule activated by cyclic AMP.

Proximate tissue interactions. Another term for secondary induction, referring specifically to the requirement that the epithelium and mesenchyme be in close proximity to one another.

Pulp bifurcation. Zone of branching of the pulp organ, as found in multirooted teeth.

Pulp organ. Soft tissue within the tooth, consisting of connective tissue blood vessels, nerves, and lymphatics.

Pulpal blood vessels. Characteristic capillary thin-walled blood vessels of the dental pulp. Large vessels in central pulp with loops among odontoblasts.

Pulpal stones (denticles). Calcified mass of dentinlike substance located within the pulp or projected into it from its attachment in the dentin wall. (See *Attached*, *Embedded*, and *Free pulp stones*.)

Pulp chamber. The space surrounded by dentin and in which the pulp organ resides.

Pus. A wound fluid that is mainly composed of dead neutrophils and their products.

Pyknotic. A reduction in size, condensation. Usually refers to a cell or nucleus of a degenerating cell in which the chromatin condenses to a structureless mass.

Radiation. Transmission of rays: light rays, short radiowaves, ultra-violet rays, or x-rays. The latter are used for treatment or diagnosis.

Radicular. Concerning a root.

Ramus. General term to designate a smaller structure given off a larger one or into which a larger structure divides.

Ramus of mandible. Quadrilateral process projecting superiorly and posteriorly from the body of the mandible.

Rathke's pouch. Ratheke's diverticulum; the pituitary diverticulum. A saclike opening extending from the roof of the stomodeum toward the base of the brain.

Red blood cell (corpuscle, erythrocyte). A non-nucleated, biconcave cell bearing hemoglobin and responsible for transport of oxygen to tissues via the circulatory system.

Reduced enamel epithelium. The several layers of the epithelial enamel organ remaining on the surface of the enamel after enamel formation is complete.

Regulated secretion. Secretion in a direct response to the binding of a secretagogue to a cell surface receptor, leading to stimulation of a signal transduction pathway (eg, cyclic AMP-G protein or phosphoinositide cycle-calcium) causing secretion. Typically, the secretion product is stored in secretory vesicles and released in response to a secretagogue. There is no secretion in the absence of the secretagogue.

Remodeling. Altering of the structure by reconstruction. The continuous process of turnover of bone carried out by osteoblasts and osteoclasts.

Reparative dentin. The deposition of new dentin by newly differentiated odontoblasts at the site of pulpal trauma. A defensive reaction whereby hard tissue formation walls off the pulp from the site of injury.

Reserve cell zone. Site in endochondral bone characterized by the presence of resting cells termed prechondroblasts. This zone lies adjacent to the perichondrium.

Respiratory mucosa. Lining of the respiratory system consisting of pseudostratified columnar epithelium containing numerous goblet cells and bearing true cilia in the apical region of the cell.

Retzius' striae. Lines reflecting successive incremental deposition of mineralized tissue (enamel).

Reversal lines. Lines separating layers of bone or cementum deposited in a resorption site from the scalloped outline of Howship's lacunae. The latter is obliterated by action of osteoblasts or cementoblasts. Deposition of new hard tissue leaving a visible line where the reversal of resorption took place.

Root canal. The space which contains pulp tissue of the tooth's root.

Root resorption. Dissolution of the root of a tooth by action of osteoclasts. May occur anywhere along the surface of the tooth root in response to caries, trauma, or the loss of a primary tooth.

Root sheath cells (Hertwig's). Merged outer and inner epithelial layers of the enamel organ, extending beyond the region of the crown to invest the developing root. The cells induce dentinogenesis of the root and atrophy as the root is formed, but when the cells persist, they are called (Malassez') epithelial rests.

Root trunk. That part of the tooth immediately below the crown neck, covered by cementum and fixed in the alveolus.

Sagittal plane. Median plane in the anterior-posterior direction.

Saliva. Clear, slightly alkaline, somewhat viscid mixture of secretions of the salivary glands and gingival fluid exudate. It functions to moisten the mucous membranes and food, facilitating speech and mastication. Contains water and 0.58% solids.

Salivary calculi. Calcium phosphate concretions (salivary stones) found within a salivary gland or duct, most commonly in the main excretory duct of the submandibular gland (Wharton's duct); the pathological state known as sialolithiasis.

Salivary corpuscle. One of the leukocytes or lymphocytes found in saliva.

Salivary gland. Exocrine glands whose secretions flow into the oral cavity.

Sclerotic dentin. Dentin in which tubules are occluded with mineral. This dentin then is nontubular and is termed transparent. Occurs mostly in elderly people, especially in the roots of teeth.

Sealant, dental. Agent that protects this enamel surface against the access of saliva. A resin capable of bonding to the surface of a tooth and offering protection against outside chemical or physical agents.

Secondary curvatures of the dentinal tubule. These are microscopic undulations of the dentinal tubule formed during deposition and mineralization of the dentin matrix.

Secondary dentin deposition. Deposition of dentin circumpulpally formed after tooth eruption.

Secondary induction. Embryonic induction other than the primary neural induction, which involves the interaction of epithelium and mesenchyme that occurs in the teeth and salivary glands. In induction one cell population (A) responds to a second group of cells (B), which causes a change in phenotype of the first population (A) to form a new cell type (C). The newly differentiated cells (C) will only form if the inducer (B) is present. After differentiation these cells may serve as inducers when they are proximate to other cells.

Secondary intention healing. The healing that occurs when wound edges cannot be approximated, which causes healing with significant scar formation.

Secretagogue. Signal in extracellular environment that stimulates the release of secretory product within the regulated pathway. β-Adrenergic and muscarinic drugs are secretagogues for salivary gland acinar cells.

Secretory canaliculus (secretory capillary). Canaliculus found between acinar cells. Spaces provide communication between the serous acinar cells and the lumen. They rarely are found between mucous cells.

Secretory granules. A prominent feature of the secretory cell accumulating in its apical cytoplasm. Granules are about 1 μm in diameter and have a distinct, limiting membrane and a dense homogenous content.

Senescence. The state of growing old; beginning old age.

Serotonin. A vasoconstrictor found in serum and body tissues that has the ability to modify neuronal function.

Serous. Relating to, containing, or producing a serious substance that has a watery consistency.

Serous demilumes. Half-moon or crescent-shaped serous cells associated with the terminal external surface of mucous alveoli.

Serous glands of tongue (von Ebner). Serous glands opening in the bottom of the trough surrounding the circumvallate papillae and functioning in cleansing action.

Sheath of Neuman. Boundary between the intratubular and peritubular dentin. It represents the initial boundary of the dentinal tubule prior to intratubular dentin deposition.

Sialography. Diagnostic x-ray technique visualizing salivary gland ducts by injection of a radiopaque substance into the main excretory duct.

Short-range matrix-mediated interaction. An embryonic interaction that is mediated by inductive molecules within the extracellular matrix, the matrix itself, or paracrine factors liberated in the immediate area.

Sinusoid. Resembles a sinus, a cavity. A form of terminal blood channel.

Sjögren's syndrome. Disease often associated with rheumatoid arthritis and believed to be an autoimmune disorder. Lymphoid infiltration of the parotid, submandibular, labial, and palatal glands leads to atrophy of gland parenchyma, which results in exocrine gland dysfunction.

Smear or smear layer. Debris formed by instrumentation of the tooth. The debris or smear particles form a layer that occludes dentinal tubules.

Soft palate. The posterior muscular portion of the palate, forming an incomplete septum between the nasopharynx and the oral cavity.

Somatic growth. The growth pattern of the body in general.

Specialized mucosa. Mucosa found on the dorsum of the tongue that consists of four types of papillae: filiform, fungiform, circumvallate, and foliate.

Squamosal. Relating to the flat squama, as of the temporal bone.

Squamous epithelium. Composed of a single layer of flat scalelike cells, as in the lining of the pulmonary alveoli; oral epithelium.

Stapedial artery. Artery that supplies the region of the middle ear (stapes). Important in prenatal facial development.

Stellate reticulum. A network of star-shaped cells in the center of the enamel organ between the outer and the inner enamel epithelium.

Stomodeum. The future oral cavity of the embryo; an invagination lined by ectoderm.

Stratified epithelium. A type of epithelium composed of a series of layers. The cells of each may vary in size and shape, as seen in skin and some mucous membranes.

Stratum germinativum. The inner layers of the epidermis resting on the corium; consists of several layers of polygonal cells (stratum spinosum) and a basal layer.

Stratum intermedium. That epithelial cell layer of the enamel organ which lies external and adjacent to the inner enamel epithelium and is attached to it by desmosomes. Stratum intermedium also refers to the intermediate layer of nonkeratinizing epithelia.

Striated duct. An intralobular salivary gland duct involved in ionic transport, located between the intercalated and interlobular ducts, and named for the basal striations produced by infoldings of the basal membrane that produce compartments containing numerous mitochondria.

Stroma. Supporting framework of a gland, such as the capsule and trabeculae, rather than the functional parenchyma.

Sublingual. Area beneath the tongue, subglossal.

Sublingual gland. The smallest of the three pairs of major salivary glands. A pure mucous gland located in the anterior floor of the mouth.

Submandibular. Area beneath the lower jaw.

Submandibular gland. Largest of the three paired major salivary glands contributing 65% of saliva. These two bilateral glands are a mixed seromucous type.

Submucosa. Layer of tissues that lies beneath the lamina propria underlying the mucous membrane of the lip, cheek, palate, and floor of the mouth.

Successional lamina. That portion of the dental lamina which is lingual to the developing deciduous teeth. It gives rise to the enamel organs that differentiate into permanent teeth.

Supporting bone. Bone tissue functionally related to the roots of the teeth. It surrounds, protects, and supports the tooth roots through the alveolar bone proper.

Sympathomimetics. Imitating the effects of postganglionic adrenergic nerves.

Synarthrosis. A suture between two bones, with the uniting medium being a fibrous membrane continuous with the periosteum.

Synchondrosis. A type of cartilaginous joint that usually is temporary. The intervening hyaline cartilage ordinarily converts to bone before the person reaches adult life.

Syndesmosis. A type of fibrous joint in which opposing surfaces are united by fibrous connective tissue, as in the union between most of the facial bones.

Synovial cells. Cells that secrete synovial fluid. These are of two types: A and B. Type A is thought to secrete hyaluronic acid, while type B produces a protein-rich secretion.

Synovial membranes. Membranes that line joint cavities and function to secrete a small amount of clear transparent alkaline fluid in the articular spaces. Synovial fluid acts as a lubricant and nutrient for the avascular tissue covering (ie, the condyle and articular tubercle of the temporomandibular joint). Also called synovial fluid.

Taste bud. Receptor of taste in the oropharynx. One of a number of goblet-shaped cells oriented at right angles to the surface by the epithelium. They consist of supporting cells and gustatory cells.

Tremporomandibular joint. Joint formed between the condyle of the mandible and the mandibular fossa (concavity of the temporal bone).

Temporomandibular ligaments. Four ligaments: on the medial surface, the sphenomandibular; on the posterior surface, the stylomandibular; on the lateral surface, the temporomandibular and capsular.

Tenascin. An extracellular matrix molecule, transiently expressed during development, that slightly resembles fibronectin. It interacts with fibronectin in the extracellular matrix to regulate cell adhesiveness, an important environmental factor in cell migration and tissue remodeling during development.

Teratogen. Agent or factor that causes the production of physical defects in the developing embryo.

Terminal bar apparatus. That part of the ameloblast that separates Tomes' process from the cell proper; localized condensations of cytoplasmic substance associated with the cell membrane.

Tic douloureux. Trigeminal neuralgia, repeated contraction, spasm, or twitching of the masticatory muscles usually resulting in extreme pain.

Tight junction. Fusions of the outer portions of adjacent cell membranes believed to provide a seal and communication between cells.

Tomes' granular layer. A granular-appearing layer in the dentin of the root adjacent to the cementum.

Tomes' process. Specialized apical zone of the ameloblasts. The apical Tomes' process is conical and interdigitates with the forming enamel rods.

Tonofibrils. Systems of fibers found in the cytoplasm of epithelial cells, which function with the desmosomal plaque to hold adjacent cells together.

Tooth crypt. Space filled by the dental follicle and developing tooth in the alveolar process.

Traction bands of the palate. Bundles of collagen that firmly attach the oral mucosa to the underlying bone of the hard palate.

Transduction. Conversion of physical force into biologic response. Theory proposing that odontoblasts are sensory receptors for pain stimuli transmitted through the dentin.

Transport vesicles. Vehicles for the transport of materials from the intracellular compartment to another compartment (eg, from the rough endoplasmic reticulum to the Golgi apparatus).

Trimer. A molecule composed of three identical, simpler molecules.

Tufts. Clump or cluster of organic filled spaces in enamel that extends from the dentinoenamel junction for one third of the thickness of enamel. Results in a defect in mineralization.

Turnover. Quantity of a material metabolized or processed in the body or a tissue within a given length of time.

Types I and III collagen. Two of the fibrillar collagens that form collagen fibrils after secretion into the extracellular milieu. Type I collagen is the most prominent form, accounting for about 90% of the collagen in the body. It is found in bone, tendon, and skin. Type III collagen is found in loose connective tissue, blood vessels, and in hematopoietic and lymphoid tissues, and is associated with the connective tissue side of the basement membrane.

Type IV collagen. The type of collagen associated with the basement membrane.

Vasculature. Reference to the blood vessels and circulating blood system.

Vermilion zone of the lip. Transitional zone between the skin of the lip and the mucous membrane of the lip known as the red zone. Color due to thin epithelium, the presence of eleiden in the cells, and superficial blood vessels apparent in humans.

Vestibular lamina. Lip furrow band labial and buccal to the dental lamina; forms the oral vestibule between the alveolar portions of the jaws and the lips and cheeks.

Vicerocranial. Those parts of the facial cranial skeleton that are of branchial arch origin.

Vomer. Flat unpaired bone located in the midline of the face, shaped like a trapezoid, and forming the inferior and posterior portion of the nasal septum. It articulates with the sphenoid, ethmoid, two maxillary, and two palatine bones.

Waldeyer's ring. Group or ring of tonsilar tissue at the oral-pharyngeal-nasal junction.

Zona pellucida. Translucent zone, noncellular secreted layer, surrounding an ovum. It has a striated appearance due to the numerous fine canals with which it is pierced.

Zonula adherens (intermediate junction). Part of the junctional complex of columnar epithelial cells located deep to the zonula occludens where the plasma membranes of two adjacent cells divert to form a 15-nm- to 20-nm-wide space.

Zonula occludens (tight junction). Part of the junctional complex immediately beneath the free surface and continuing all around the perimeter of the cell. There is no intercellular space, and the zonula occludens provides a permeability barrier to lumenal material.

Zymogen. An inactive precursor that is activated to an enzyme by the action of an acid and an enzyme. Granules in serous cells of enzyme-secreting glands, such as the salivary glands and the pancreas.

Index

Secular trend, 60
Serous cells, 366–369
Serous glands, 343
Serum proteins, 258
Sheath of Neuman, 246
Sialadenosis, 373
Sialography, 377
Simple coiled corpuscles, 339
Sinuses, 396–399
Sjögren's syndrome, 377, 378
Skeletal development, 11–12
Skeletal muscle, 8
Skull, 43–44
Smear layer, 259
Smoking, 17
Smooth muscle, 9
Soft palate, 307
Sphenoid sinus, 399
Stomodeum, 354
Stones, salivary duct, 379
Stratum basale, 299
Stratum corneum, 301
Stratum germinativum, 300
Stratum granulosum, 300–301, 303
Stratum spinosum, 300
Stratum synovial, 217–218
Striated ducts, 364–365
Sublingual gland, 361, 363, 376
Submandibular gland, 361, 362, 376
Submerged primary teeth, 127
Submucosa, 305
Successional teeth, 283
Supporting bone, 106, 145, 147–148
Supraosseous stage, 112
Suture, 46–48, 50, 59, 63
Synchondrosis, 47
Syndesmoses, 47
Synovial membrane/folds, 217–218, 224

Taste–bearing papillae, 342–343
Taste bud structure, 344–346
Taste receptors, 342, 400
    function, 348–349
    nerve supply, 347–348
Teeth
    abnormal behavior of primary, 127
    comparison of primary and permanent,
        282–295
        accessory root canals, 289
        arch shape and tooth position, 289–290
        development, 285
        enamel defects, 293
        number and size, 283
        pulp size and shape, 288
        root resorption and pulp degeneration,
            291–292

sequela to injuries, 292
    shape, 283–284
    structure, 286–287
dental tissue, 70–73, 113–117
development of, 70–92, 285
    agents affecting, 130–140
    amelogenesis, 83–89
    bud, cap, and bell, 74–76
    crown and tooth crypt, 89–91
    dentinogenesis, 77, 79–83
    epithelium and mesenchyme, 77–79
    pulp organ, 76–77
    root and supporting structures, 94–108
endosseous implants, 164–178
eruption,
    chronology of, 121–123
    movements leading to, 110–119
    theories of, 119–120
movement,
    fundamentals of, 181–188
    histologic changes during, 180–190
    rotation and bodily, 186–188
    stability and relapse, 189
    tipping and bodily, 184–185
resorption, 124–126, 176, 177, 183,
    291–292
shedding of primary, 123–124
structure of, 228–240, 286–287
wound healing, 205–209
    See also Dental pulp; Dentin; Enamel
Temporalis muscle fibers, 222
Temporomandibular fossa (glenoid fossa), 217
Temporomandibular joint, 214–225
    age changes in, 224
    ankylosis, 64, 223
    arthritis, 224
    developmental disturbances, 223
    dislocation, 223
    functional/clinical considerations, 222–224
    histological structure, 215–218
    injury to, 64, 223
    mastication muscles, 221–222
    neural supply, 219–220
    prenatal, 49, 51–53
    vascular supply, 218–219
Tertiary dentin, 247, 248, 249
Tetracycline, 17, 134, 135–138, 140
Thalidomide, 17
Thymus gland, 23
Thyroglossal cysts/fistulas, 36
Thyroid gland, 23
Tipping, 184
Tissue–tooth interphase, 205–206
T–lymphocytes, 199, 268
TMJ. See Temporomandibular joint
Tomes' fiber, 79

Tomes' granular layer, 250
Tomes' process, 83–87, 228, 230, 231, 233
Tongue, 27–28, 308, 310–312, 342
Tonsils, 315–319
Tooth crypt, 90–91
Touch receptors, 341
Traction bands, 309, 310
Transduction, 182
Transduction theory, 276
Transforming growth factor, 198, 258
Translucent dentin, 247
Transmucosal seal, 170
Transparent dentin, 247
Trauma, 277, 292
Treacher Collins' syndrome. See
    Mandibulofacial dysostosis
Trigeminal neuralgia, 345
Trophoblast, 4, 5
Type 1 dark cells, 345, 347
Type 2 cells, 346, 347
Type 3 cells, 346, 348

Undermineralized dentin, 245
Undermining resorption, 183

Vascular events, and connective tissue,
    202–203
Vascular triangle, 215
Vasculature
    of dental pulp, 270–271
    of face, 30–31
    of gingiva, 330
Vermilion border, 307
Viral infections, 16
Viscerocranium, 43
Vitamin A, 130–132, 139
Vitamin C, 132, 139
Vitamin D, 132–133, 139
Vomer, 46
von Willebrand factor, 193

Wharton's duct, 379
White spots, 238, 292, 293
Wound healing, 192–211
    associated with teeth, 205–209
    cellular events and establishment of acute
        inflammation, 196–200
    early events leading to clotting and
        inflammation, 193–196
    events leading to repair, 200–205
    maturation of wound, 204–205

Zygomatic arch, 45, 47
Zygote, 3